Breast Cancer

Nursing Care and Management

Edited by

VICTORIA HARMER

RN Diploma (Breast Care) BSc(Hons) AKC

Clinical Nurse Specialist
Breast Care Unit
St Mary's Hospital NHS Trust
London

W

WHURR PUBLISHERS
LONDON AND PHILADELPHIA

© 2003 Whurr Publishers

First published 2003 by
Whurr Publishers Ltd
19b Compton Terrace, London N1 2UN, England and
325 Chestnut Street, Philadelphia PA 19106, USA

Reprinted 2004

British Library Cataloguing in Publication Data

A catalogue record for this book is available from the British
Library.

ISBN 1 86156 353 1

Contents

Chapter 15   312

Psychological Issues for the Patient with Breast Cancer
Mary Turner

Chapter 16   334

The Differing Roles of Specialist Nurses
Emma Pennery

Index   353

ST. JAMES'S PALACE

It is of immense concern to us all that nearly 40,000 women are diagnosed with breast cancer every year. While the statistics speak volumes, there is nothing like first-hand experience to bring home the truly devastating effects of this disease; at some stage in our lives most of us will meet or know someone who has been diagnosed with cancer.

As Patron of Breakthrough Breast Cancer and through witnessing the work of the many Hospices with which I am closely involved, I have seen the terrible toll that breast cancer has taken.

Expert nursing care at this time is fundamental to treatment and recovery. Only with a thorough understanding of the disease and the treatments available, including complementary and alternative therapies, can nurses ensure that each patient receives the best, individualised care at this distressing and difficult time.

I am delighted that Victoria Harmer and her team of contributors have produced a book that will help nurses thoroughly to understand not only the physical aspects of the disease and its treatment, but also the emotional stresses faced by people with breast cancer, and so be able to offer relief, practical help and comfort. I am sure this inspiring book could become a handbook for every breast cancer nurse in the UK.

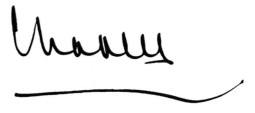

Contributors

Audrey Ardern-Jones RGN Dip(N) MSc
Senior Clinical Nurse Specialist in Cancer Genetics
The Royal Marsden Hospital NHS Trust
Sutton, Surrey

Karen Burnet RGN MSc BSc
Lead Breast Care Nurse
Cambridge Breast Unit
Addenbrooke's Hospital NHS Trust
Cambridge

Deborah Fenlon RGN MSc BSc(Hons)
Cancer Research UK Nursing Research Fellow
University of Southampton
Southampton

Helen Froyd RGN Dip(Onc) BSc(Hons)
Nurse Practitioner - Breast Care
St Mary's Hospital NHS Trust
London

Elisabeth Grimsey RN MSc
Macmillan Nurse Consultant – Breast Care
East Sussex Hospitals NHS Trust

Victoria Harmer RN Dip(Br Ca) BSc(Hons) AKC
Clinical Nurse Specialist – Breast Care
St Mary's Hospital NHS Trust
London

Rachael King RN BSc(Hons)
Clinical Nurse Specialist – Tissue Viability
Milton Keynes General Hospital
Milton Keynes

Pauline Koelling MCSP SRP
Senior Physiotherapist
The Royal Marsden Hospital NHS Trust
Sutton, Surrey

Linda Lee DCR MEd
Radiographic Services Manager
Breast Directorate
Nottingham City Hospital NHS Trust

Elizabeth Lomas RN Dip(N) BA(Hons)
Clinical Nurse Specialist in Palliative Care
St John's Hospice
London

Rosemary Lucey RGN RMN
Head of Drop-in Centre Services
Lynda Jackson Macmillan Centre
Mount Vernon Hospital
West Herts NHS Trust, Middlesex

Helen Macleod MCSP SRP
Senior Physiotherapist
The Royal Marsden Hospital NHS Trust
Sutton, Surrey

Joan McCoy RGN BSc(Hons)
Nurse Consultant Cancer Care/Lead Cancer Nurse
St Mary's Hospital NHS Trust
London

Emma Pennery RGN MSc
Formerly Senior Clinical Nurse Specialist (Breast Unit)/Honorary Clinical
    Research Fellow
The Royal Marsden Hospital NHS Trust
London

Mary Turner RGN PhD(Hons) BA
Macmillan Breast Care Specialist Nurse
Furness General Hospital NHS Trust
Cumbria

Nicola West RGN MA BN
Senior Clinical Nurse Specialist
Cardiff Breast Unit
Cardiff

Mary Woods RGN MSc BSc(Hons)
Clinical Nurse Specialist – Head of Lymphoedema Services
The Royal Marsden Hospital NHS Trust
Sutton, Surrey

Words of Encouragement

If it wasn't for your commitment to helping the needy, the world would certainly be a far crueller place. Your role in the fight against breast cancer starts from day one. You have the power to save a person from giving into the disease. It is your encouragement, patience and support which is invaluable ... thank you.

Warm regards
Stella
Stella McCartney

Preface

Although there is much literature available for people with breast cancer, there are very few books for nurses and other healthcare professionals.

Breast cancer is increasing in prevalence as the population ages. One in six women has a first-degree relative with breast cancer. This book aims to provide a well-balanced approach to all aspects of management of this malignancy. Generalities are not enough. Expert nurses in these topics deal with the specific details of special care. However, the importance of writing from a complete nursing perspective is underlined so that the essence of support and bedside care is not missed.

This book teaches us about breast cancer treatments, and how to manage, nurse and empower patients through each modality, as well as give sound, evidence-based information on possible side effects and how to combat them.

Nurses need to have the necessary information to enable seamless, individualized treatment for the patient. This book is applicable to any stage of the cancer journey, from the biological aspects of care to the psychological issues for people facing this potentially life-threatening disease.

This comprehensive book can act as a resource for any nurse or healthcare professional caring for a person with breast cancer.

Victoria Harmer
June 2003

Acknowledgements

I would first like to thank all the contributors for getting their chapters, alterations and illustrations to me so speedily.

It is then impossible to thank everyone who has helped me with this book, either practically or intellectually! You know who you are — thank you!

I am also grateful for the support of His Royal Highness The Prince of Wales, Stella McCartney and Sylvia Denton.

A special mention should go to Mr D. Hadjiminas, Director of St Mary's Hospital Breast Care Unit, London.

Particular thanks must also go to my family — my parents, Michael and Kasha.

CHAPTER 1

An Overview of Breast Cancer

ELISABETH GRIMSEY

Breast cancer is the most common cancer in women in the UK and accounts for one in four of all female cancers (CRC, 1997a). It is therefore very likely that most nurses will find themselves caring for women with breast cancer at some point in their career. To nurse these women with care and understanding it is vital to have a good theoretical and practical working knowledge regarding the breast and breast cancer.

This chapter will look at the anatomy and physiology of the normal breast, the incidence and aetiology of breast cancer, the risk factors of developing breast cancer and the different types of breast cancer.

Anatomy and Physiology of the Breast

Breast Development

The breasts, also known as mammary glands, exist in both males and females but are usually only enlarged in the woman. The breasts begin to develop in the fetus at around the seventh week of gestation and progress to the budding stage at the twelfth week. They are formed from the ectodermal mammary ridge that runs from the axilla to the groin, often referred to as the nipple line. Between weeks 13 and 20 the epithelial bud branches and canalizes to form the 16–20 major ducts found in the adult breast.

Occasionally at birth a baby may produce a small amount of milk. This is due to high levels of luteal and placental hormones crossing the placenta and entering the fetal circulation during the late stage of pregnancy, thus stimulating the fetal breast. At birth the fetal and maternal circulation are separated, resulting in the rapid fall of sex steroids in the baby's blood, whereas the baby's pituitary gland continues to secrete prolactin. The baby's prolactin level then declines and the secretions dry up. This is classed as a normal physiological event. Accessory nipples may also be found along the

1

ectodermal ridge, most commonly below the normal breast. These are harmless and only need to be removed if they cause distress to the individual.

Changes at Puberty

The female breast starts to change at the time of puberty. The pituitary gland begins to produce the gonadotropins, follicle stimulating hormone (FSH) and luteinizing hormone (LH). As the level of these hormones rises the egg follicles within the ovary start to produce oestrogen, which is responsible for the first stages of breast development. At around the age of 10 the mammary tissue behind the nipple enlarges producing the characteristic swelling referred to as a breast bud that may often be asymmetrical. Oestrogen also induces connective tissue and vascular growth that is required to support the ductal system. The connective tissue in turn stimulates fat deposition. Once the ovulating cycles begin, the increased output of progesterone balances the oestrogen output and results in the maturation of the glandular tissue (Hughes et al., 2000).

Anatomy of the Adult Breast

Gross structure

The breasts are situated on either side of the sternum between the second and sixth rib overlying the pectoralis major muscle. The shape of the breast is hemispherical with a tail of tissue extending into the axilla, known as the tail of Spence. The breasts are stabilized by a suspensory ligament know as Cooper's ligament, named after Sir Astley Cooper. The size of the breast will vary with the stage of development and age and will also vary between individuals. It is common to have one breast slightly larger than the other.

Centrally on each breast lies the nipple–areola complex. The areola is the pigmented circular area, measuring approximately 2.5 cm in diameter. The colour varies from pale pink in fair-skinned women to dark brown in dark-skinned women and will darken during pregnancy. On the surface of the areola are a number of small protuberances known as Montgomery's tubercles. These are modified sebaceous glands whose purpose is to lubricate the nipple during lactation. The nipple lies in the centre of the areola and is approximately 6 mm in length. The surface of the nipple is perforated by the openings of the lactiferous ducts. The nipple–areola complex is rich in smooth-muscle fibres that are responsible for nipple erection.

Microscopic structure

The breast is composed of fibrous, glandular and fatty tissue and is covered by skin.

Fibrous bands divide the glandular tissue into approximately 16–20 lobes. Clinical findings, however, show the number to be more in the region of 7–8 lobes (Hughes et al., 2000). Within each lobe is the milk-producing system. The lobe contains up to 40 lobules that contain 10–100 alveoli (or acini), which are the milk-secreting cells. The alveoli are connected to lactiferous tubules that in turn connect to the lactiferous duct, which is lined with epithelial cells. The lactiferous duct runs up towards the nipple and when approaching the nipple widens to form the ampulla, which acts as a reservoir for the milk to be stored. The lactiferous duct than continues on from the ampulla to open out onto the surface of the nipple (Figure 1.1).

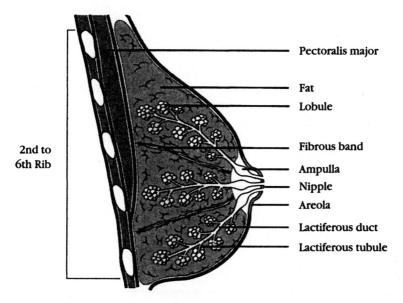

Figure 1.1: Microscopic structure of the breast.

The glandular tissue of the breast is surrounded by fat. If weight is lost or gained the breast will vary in size.

Blood supply

The blood supply is from the axillary artery and the internal mammary artery. The venous drainage is through the corresponding vessels into the internal mammary and axillary veins.

Nerve supply

The nerve supply to the breast is mainly from the somatic sensory nerves and the autonomic nerves accompanying the blood vessels. The most sensitive part of the breast is the nipple–areola complex that is supplied by the somatic sensory nerves. The rest of the breast is supplied by the autonomic supply.

The somatic sensory supply is served via the supraclavicular nerves (C3, C4) superiorly and laterally from the lateral branches of the thoracic intercostal nerve (3rd and 4th). The medial aspects of the breast receive supply from the anterior branches of the thoracic intercostal nerves that penetrate the pectoralis major to reach the skin. The nerve supply to the upper outer quadrant of the breast is provided by the intercostobrachial nerve (C8, T1) (Hughes et al., 2000).

Lymphatic system

The lymph fluid from the outer quadrants of each breast flows into the ipsilateral axillary lymph nodes along a chain which begins at the anterior axillary nodes and continues into the central and apical node groups. Lymph fluid from the medial quadrants drains towards the sternum via the inframammary nodes.

The major lymphatic drainage of the breast is to the axilla and the axillary nodes are the first place a breast cancer will spread to. The axillary nodes are divided into three levels (Figure 1.2):

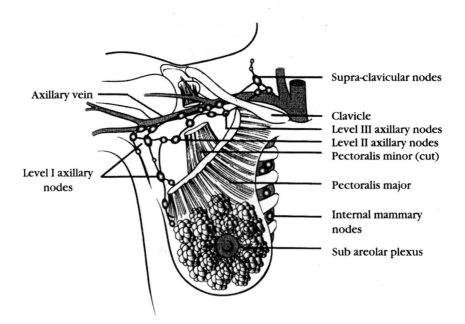

Figure 1.2: Lymphatic drainage of the breast illustrating levels of axillary nodes.

- Level [E1]I – the nodes lie lateral to the lateral border of the pectoralis minor muscle;
- Level II – the nodes lie behind the pectoralis minor muscle;
- Level III– the nodes are located medial to the medial border of the pectoralis minor muscle.

Cyclical Changes

During the menstrual cycle the breasts undergo cyclical changes due to the changing levels of the hormone prolactin which controls the secretion of the ovarian hormones, oestrogen and progesterone. These hormones cause the breast tissue and ducts to enlarge. The breast may change in size and consistency and become tender and nodular, usually 10–14 days prior to menstruation. These symptoms tend to resolve once menstruation occurs.

Changes during Pregnancy

Changes in the breast are often the first symptoms of pregnancy. The woman may complain of fullness, tenderness and an increase in size. Veins become more prominent as the blood supply is increased and the areola and nipple darken.

These changes are due first to oestrogen and progesterone and then to hormones produced by the placenta. Oestrogen stimulates the nipple and areolar complex causing it to darken and progesterone causes proliferation of the alveoli in preparation for milk production. As the placenta enlarges it secretes human placental lactogen that works alongside oestrogen and progesterone to stimulate the hypothalamus to secrete prolactin-releasing hormone (PRH). This hormone stimulates the anterior pituitary gland to secrete more prolactin that is responsible for milk production. After 12 weeks a clear watery fluid known as colostrum is secreted by the breasts and expressed from the nipple. Its main function is to clear the lactiferous ducts and tubules of dead epithelial cells to make way for the free flow of milk.

After birth and the expulsion of the placenta an alteration in the levels of the hormone oestrogen and progesterone occurs resulting in the release of prolactin from the anterior pituitary gland. Oestrogen suppresses the action of prolactin so it is not until about three days post-birth that the milk 'comes in'. In the meantime the baby feeds off the colostrum, which is low in fat and contains vitamin A, protein and minerals.

Post-menopausal Changes

When ovarian activity ceases at the menopause, causing the fall of oestrogen and progesterone, the glandular tissue in the breast starts to involute and atrophy. The glandular tissue is replaced by fat. The breasts tend to feel softer and become more pendulous. If hormone replacement therapy (HRT) is prescribed the breasts may become fuller and can be tender.

Incidence and Aetiology of Breast Cancer

Cancer is a common disease with a lifetime risk of more than one in three. Of all the cancers diagnosed in the UK breast cancer is the most common female cancer, accounting for 30 per cent of all new cases. Approximately 38,000 cases were diagnosed in the UK in 1997. The estimated lifetime risk is now quoted to be one in nine (CRC, 1997a). Breast cancer in men is rare. There are approximately 250 new cases annually (CRC, 1997a).

Although the incidence of breast cancer is seen to be rising, the mortality rate is fortunately on the decrease. In the UK in 2000 approximately 12,770 died from breast cancer. This reduction is thought to be due to earlier detection and improvement in treatment (Cancer Research UK, 2002). The five-year relative survival rate for women with breast cancer is now estimated to be over 70 per cent (CRC, 1997a).

Risk Factors

The cause of breast cancer is not yet fully understood; however, some risk factors have been identified. The risk factors can be divided into two: definite risks and potential risks.

Definite Risks

These are the known risks which research has shown to increase the risk of developing breast cancer.

- *Sex*: being female increases the risk of breast cancer. As stated earlier, males do get breast cancer but it is rare.
- *Age*: As we get older our chance of getting breast cancer increases. Breast cancer is rare in women under the age of 35 but after that age the incidence stars to rise. It is most common in women aged between 45 and 75 (CRC, 1996).
- *Strong family history*: having a strong family history of breast cancer increases the risk of developing breast cancer. Much research is being undertaken to identify faulty genes that are associated with the increased risk. Two such genes have been identified so far: *BRCA1* and *BRCA2*. This will be discussed in depth in Chapter 3.

Not everyone who has a family history of breast cancer will be at a higher risk of developing breast cancer than the average population. Those in the high-risk category will have a strong family history of:

- a first-degree relative (parent, sibling or children under 40 years old);
- two second-degree relatives (aunts, uncles, nieces or nephews) on the same side of the family diagnosed under the age of 60 with breast or ovarian cancer;
- three or more first- or second-degree relatives on the same side of the family with breast or ovarian cancer;
- a first-degree relative with bilateral breast cancer
- a first-degree male relative with breast cancer. (CRC, 1997b)

Those deemed to be in the high-risk category can be offered a referral to a Family History Clinic where they can have regular screening.

- *Exposure to hormones*: the number of menstrual cycles a woman undergoes is a powerful determinant of breast cancer risk. A woman who has an early menarche and late menopause has an increased risk of developing breast cancer. It has been shown that women who undergo a bilateral oophorectomy under the age of 50 have a 50 per cent reduction in breast cancer for up to nine years post-surgery (Fentiman, 2001). A woman who has her first baby after the age of 35 or is nulliparous also carries a higher risk of developing breast cancer.

These findings lead to the understanding that the unopposed circulating oestrogen increases the breast tissue's susceptibility to other risk factors for breast cancer (MacPherson et al., 1995).

- *Benign breast disease*: There have been several studies looking at the correlation between breast cancer and benign breast disease (Fentiman, 2001). A consensus paper published by the American College of Pathologists (Winchester, 1985) based on the work of Dupont and Page (1985), uses three classifications: no risk, slight risk and moderate risk. Those in the slight risk group (1.5–2 times) include: moderate or florid hyperplasia with no atypia; intraduct papillomas. Those in the moderate risk group (5 times) include: atypical lobular or ductal hyperplasia.
- *Ionizing radiation*: Exposure to ionizing radiation is known to increase the risk of breast cancer. This has been found in studies in the use of radiation to treat benign conditions such as ringworm and enlarged thymus (Hildreth et al., 1989, Modan et al., 1989).

It must be stressed that the amount of radiation delivered by a screening mammogram is very small and the potential benefits obtained outweigh the small risk.

Potential Risks

These are risks that have not been proved but have led scientists to research further.

Oral contraceptive pill

The Collaborative Group on Hormonal Factors in Breast Cancer (CGHFBC, 1996) carried out a meta-analysis of results of 54 studies which included 53,297 breast cancer cases and 100,239 controls. It found that those who had used oral contraceptives (both combined or progesterone only) had a small but statistically significant risk that disappeared 10 years after cessation. It is important to remember that breast cancer is uncommon in young women (the age group more likely to use oral contraception) so this only leads to a few extra cases per year. The combined pill also reduces the risk of ovarian cancer.

Hormone replacement therapy

There is still much debate about the risk associated with the use of hormone replacement therapy (HRT). HRT is known to reduce menopausal symptoms and prevent coronary artery disease and osteoporosis. In general, the benefits outweigh the risks. It is of interest to note that a nationwide study is to be undertaken looking at the use of HRT on those who have had breast cancer.

The CGHFBC (1997) performed a meta-analysis of 51 studies comprising 52,705 breast cancer patients and 108,411 controls. It was found that taking HRT for more than 10 years increased the risk of developing breast cancer by 34 per cent. The relative risk returned to unity within two years of stopping HRT.

Diet

As yet there is no scientific evidence to link breast cancer with diet (McPherson et al., 1995). The intake of fat in the diet has been studied, showing no significant risk. Hunter et al. (1996) pooled the results from eight major cohort studies and showed no effect of fat intake on the risk of breast cancer. It showed that women whose intake of fat comprised less than 20 per cent of their calorie intake did not have any reduction in risk. Therefore, if western women reduce their fat intake, it is unlikely to lead to any significant reduction in breast cancer risk reduction.

Obesity

Most studies have shown that obesity is a protective factor in pre-menopausal women but increases the risk in the post-menopausal. This is because in postmenopausal women the major source of oestrogen comes from peripheral aromatization of adrenal adrogens in fat. Therefore obesity increases the risk of breast cancer (Sellers et al., 1992; Ziegler et al., 1996).

Height

There has been inconsistency in the research findings regarding the influence of height on breast cancer risk. In studies where height was self-recorded there was no increased risk identified but in studies where the participants were formally measured there was found to be a positive association between height and breast cancer risk (Fentiman, 2001).

Alcohol intake

In a pooled analysis of cohort studies looking at the effect of alcohol consumption on the risk of breast cancer, Smith-Warner et al. (1998) found that it is associated with an increased risk. The type of alcohol consumed did not strongly influence risk estimates.

Types of Breast Cancer

Breast cancer is not a single disease. There are different types with different prognostic features. Breast cancers arise in the terminal duct lobular unit. They are classified according to the type of tissue from which they arise and their appearance under the microscope. When making treatment decisions the type of breast cancer may affect the choice. This chapter will look at the common breast cancers only, as rare breast cancers will be discussed in Chapter 2.

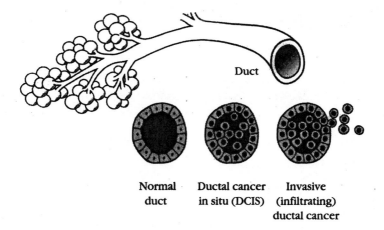

Duct

| Normal duct | Ductal cancer in situ (DCIS) | Invasive (infiltrating) ductal cancer |

Figure 1.3: Types of Breast Cancer.

In situ Disease

Carcinoma cells confined within the terminal duct lobular unit and adjacent ducts, but which have not yet invaded the basement membrane, are known as carcinoma in situ. Two types have been identified: ductal carcinoma in situ (DCIS) and lobular carcinoma in situ (LCIS). DCIS arises from the ducts and is more common than LCIS that arises from the lobules.

Both DCIS and LCIS are 'non-invasive' but it is not possible to predict when they will become invasive, therefore surgical excision is advised.

DCIS

This is commonly diagnosed via the National Breast Screening Programme, as it tends to present as microcalcifications that are identified on mammography. It can be classified into five different types: papillary, micropapillary, cribriform, solid and comedo (Silverstein, 1999). Commonly these classifications are divided into two groups: non-comedo (papillary, micropapillary, cribriform and solid) and comedo.

There are several classification systems used to describe DCIS. In the UK the United Kingdom Coordinating Group for Breast Screening Pathology classified DCIS according to nuclear grade into: high, intermediate and low grade (NHSBSP, 1995).

High-grade (comedo) DCIS

This is the most common type of DCIS accounting for 85 per cent of all high-grade lesions. It presents as linear, branching microcalcification on the mammogram or as an ill-defined mass or Paget's disease of the nipple (Chinyama and Wells, 1998). It tends to have a high proliferation rate, HER-2 gene amplification or protein over-expression and is clinically more aggressive (Silverstein, 1999).

Low-grade (non-comedo) DCIS

This is often an incidental finding on biopsy for a benign lesion. It rarely presents as a palpable lesion and mammographically appears more granular (Chinyama and Wells, 1998). According to Silverstein (1999) non-comedo DCIS is less aggressive.

Intermediate grade DCIS

This is a group of DCIS that does not fall easily into the above two categories. Its features lie midway between the two.

LCIS

This is often an incidental finding as it tends to have no specific mammographic or clinical features. Seventy per cent of women with LCIS are pre-menopausal and the condition is present in 1 per cent of screen-detected lesions (Page et al., 1995). LCIS tends to be multifocal, bilateral and predisposes to invasive carcinoma (Chinyama and Wells, 1998). Page et al. (1995) calculate the relative risk for developing invasive cancer to be 10-11 times that of the general population.

Invasive Ductal Carcinoma

This is the most common type of invasive breast cancer accounting for approximately 85 per cent of all breast cancers (Dixon and Sainsbury, 1998). It usually presents as a palpable lump or an irregular spiculated soft tissue density on mammography. An invasive ductal carcinoma arises from the ductal epithelium and breaks out of the ducts into the surrounding breast tissue. There it meets with the blood and lymphatic systems and it has the potential to invade these vessels (vascular and lymphatic invasion) and metastasize to a secondary location (King, 1996).

Invasive Lobular Carcinoma

This cancer is less common than invasive ductal carcinoma, accounting for approximately 15 per cent (Letcher, 1998). It originates from the lobules of the breast and behaves in the same way as invasive ductal carcinoma although it has the tendency to be bilateral and multifocal.

Staging Breast Cancer

The pathologist is responsible for reporting the histological findings. The results should be discussed at a multidisciplinary audit meeting. The core members of this team should include a Consultant Pathologist, Consultant Radiologist, Consultant Surgeon, Consultant Medical Oncologist, Consultant Clinical Oncologist and Breast Care Nurse. The histological factors will help to determine the appropriate treatment for the patient.

The pathologist will report different characteristics of the tumour including:

- *Size*: the size of the tumour is one of the most significant prognostic indicators. The smaller the cancer the better the prognosis.

- *Grade*: the tumour is graded according to the cellular differentiation, i.e. the degree to which the cancer cells resemble their tissue of origin (King, 1996). A commonly used grading system is the modified Bloom and Richardson system (Elston and Ellis, 1998). It uses three grades: grade I, grade II and grade III. Grade I is a well-differentiated tumour with the cells closely resembling their tissue of origin. Grade II is a moderately differentiated tumour where the cells are less like their tissue of origin and Grade III is a poorly differentiated tumour where the cells look very unlike their tissue of origin.

Grade alone is an important prognostic indicator. It is known that 85 per cent of patients with a grade I tumour are alive and well at five years as opposed to 45 per cent of those with a grade III tumour (Ellis et al., 1992).

- *Vascular and lymphatic invasion*: if the tumour has invaded the blood or lymphatic vessels this is a poor prognostic feature.
- *Lymph node status*: the number of lymph nodes involved with cancer cells determines the chance of survival for that individual and is one of the most important prognostic indicators. If positive nodes are identified it will impact on the type of treatment offered.
- *Receptor status*: the tumour is analysed to test for the presence of the steroid hormone receptors, oestrogen (ER) and progesterone (PR). The presence of such receptors will determine the effectiveness of endocrine therapy such as tamoxifen. It has been shown that those with an oestrogen-receptor-positive tumour have a better outcome.

The Early Breast Cancer Trialists' Collaborative Group (1998) presented an overview of the randomized trials of adjuvant tamoxifen among women with early breast cancer over a period of five years or more. This overview showed that if tamoxifen was taken for five years in women who had ER-positive tumours, the recurrence rate was reduced by 50 per cent as compared with 10 per cent in those whose tumour was ER negative. A benefit was also demonstrated by a reduction in mortality of 28 per cent in women with ER-positive tumours as compared with 10 per cent in those whose tumour was ER negative.

- *Oncogenes*: changes to the genes in a normal cell can result in cell proliferation and malignant proliferation. Proto-oncogenes are involved in stimulating the cell through the normal cell cycle resulting in proliferation, while tumour suppressor genes inhibit excessive cell proliferation. However, either mutation or amplification of proto-oncogenes and inactivation or loss of tumour suppressor genes can result in uncontrolled cell proliferation and cancer formation (Cooke et al., 1999).

Many proto-oncogenes encode for growth factors or growth receptors. One of these growth factors is the human epidermal growth factor receptor - 2 (HER-2). This is sometimes referred to as c-erbB2. It is located on chromosome 17. HER-2 has been shown to be over-expressed in 25–30 per cent of all human breast cancers; women whose tumour over-expresses HER-2 have a shorter disease-free survival and overall survival (Slamon et al., 1987; Slamon et al., 1989).

Classification of Stage

Staging refers to the grouping of patients according to the extent of their disease. The purpose of this is to:

- aid the clinician in the planning of treatment;
- give some indication of prognosis;
- assist in evaluation of the results of treatment;
- facilitate the exchange of information between treatment centres;
- contribute to the continuing investigation of human cancer. (Sobin and Wittekind, 1997)

There are several classification systems in use, most commonly the TNM system, UICC system and the Nottingham prognostic indicator.

TNM system

This system was developed in France between 1943 and 1952. It is used for all tumour types, not solely breast.

The TNM system is based on three main components:

- T – the extent of the primary tumour;
- N – the absence or presence and extent of regional lymph node metastasis;
- M – the absence or presence of distant metastasis.

The TNM system is summarized in Table 1.1.

To put this into practice any woman who presents with a 3 cm tumour with a moveable node in her ipsilateral (same side) axilla but has no evidence of metastatic disease is said to have a T2 N1 M0 invasive breast cancer.

The Union International Contre Centre Cancer staging system (UICC)

This classification system has five stages:

- stage 0
- stage I

- stage II
- stage III
- stage IV

Table 1.1: TNM classification

Stage	Characteristics
T – Primary Tumour	
TX	Primary tumour cannot be assessed
T0	No evidence of primary tumour
Tis	Carcinoma in situ, intraductal carcinoma, lobular carcinoma in situ or Paget's disease of the nipple with no associated tumour mass
T1	Tumour 2.0 cm or less in greatest dimension
	T1mic: Microinvasion 0.1c m or less in greatest dimension
	T1a: More than 0.1 cm but not more than 0.5 cm in greatest dimension
	T1b: More than 0.5 cm but not more than 1 cm in greatest dimension
	T1c: More than 1 cm but not more than 2 cm in greatest dimension
T2	Tumour more than 2 cm but not more than 5 cm in greatest dimension
T3	Tumour more than 5 cm in greatest dimension
T4	Tumour of any size with direct extension to chest wall or skin
	T4a: Extension to chest wall
	T4b: Oedema (including peau d'orange), or ulceration of the skin of the breast, or satellite skin nodules confined to the same breast
	T4c: Both 4a and 4b, above
	T4d: Inflammatory cancer
N – nodal status	
NX	Regional lymph nodes cannot be assessed (e.g. previously removed)
N0	No regional lymph node metastasis
N1	Metastasis to moveable ipsilateral axillary node(s)
N2	Metastasis to ipsilateral axillary node(s) fixed to one another or to other structures
N3	Metastasis to ipsilateral internal mammary lymph node(s)
M – distant metastasis	
MX	Presence of distant metastasis cannot be assessed
M0	No distant metastasis
M1	Distant metastasis present (including metastasis to ipsilateral supraclavicular lymph nodes)

It combines these stages with the TNM system as summarized in Table 1.2.

Table 1.2: UICC staging system combined with the TNM classification

UICC Stage	TNM classification
0	Tis, N0, M0
I	T1, N0, M0
IIA	T0, N1, M0
	T1, N1, M0
	T2, N0, MO
IIB	T2, N1,M0
	T3, N0, M0
IIIA	T0, N2, M0
	T1, N2, M0
	T2, N2, M0
	T3, N1, M0
	T3, N2, M0
IIIB	T4, any N, MO
	T, N3, M0
IV	Any T, any N, M1

Source: Dixon and Morrow (1999).

Nottingham prognostic indicator (NPI)

This is an integrated prognostic index that combines tumour size, lymph node status and grade. The index is calculated by 0.2 x the tumour size (cm) + grade (1-3) + lymph node status (1 = no nodes, 2 = 1-3 nodes, 3 = 3 or more nodes are involved). This separates patients into three prognostic groups: good, moderate and poor (see Table 1.3).

Table 1.3: Nottingham prognostic indicator

Prognosis	NPI score	Survival (15 years)
		(%)
Good	<3.4	80
Moderate	3.4-5.4	40
Poor	>5.4	15

Source: Dixon and Morrow (1999).

Conclusion

This chapter has given an overview of breast cancer including anatomy and physiology. It will hopefully provide a good knowledge base for healthcare professionals caring for women with breast cancer.

References

Cancer Research Campaign (1996) Breast Cancer UK Fact Sheet 6.1–6.5. London: Cancer Research Campaign.

Cancer Research Campaign (1997a) Breast Cancer UK, Fact Sheet 6.1–6.5. London: Cancer Research Campaign.

Cancer Research Campaign (1997b) Cancer Genetic Fact Sheet. London: Cancer Research Campaign.

Cancer Research UK (2002) Statistics: Mortality. London: Cancer Research UK.

Chinyama CN, Wells CA (1998) Pre-malignant, borderline lesions, ductal and lobular carcinoma in situ. In Morgan MWE, Warren R, Querci della Rovere (Eds) Early Breast Cancer: From Screening to Multidisciplinary Management. Amsterdam: Harwood Academic Publishers.

Collaborative Group on Hormonal Factors in Breast Cancer (1996) Breast cancer and oral contraceptives. Lancet 347: 1713–27.

Collaborative Group on Hormonal Factors in Breast Cancer (1997) Breast cancer and hormone replacement therapy. Lancet 350: 1047–59.

Cooke T, Rovelon P, Slamon D, Bohme C (1999) I am HER2-positive – what does this mean? Providing answers to patient concerns. Program and abstracts of European Cancer Conference, EONS Symposium, 12–16 September, Vienna, Austria.

Dixon JM, Morrow M (1999) Breast Disease - A Problem-based Approach. London: WB Saunders.

Dixon JM, Sainsbury R (1998) Diseases of the Breast, 2nd edn. London: Churchill Livingstone.

Dupont WD, Page DL (1985) Risk factors for breast cancer in women with proliferative breast disease. New England Journal of Medicine 312: 146–51.

Early Breast Cancer Trialists' Collaborative Group (1998) Tamoxifen for early breast cancer: an overview of randomised trials. Lancet 351: 1451–67.

Ellis IO, Galea M, Broughton N, Locker A, Blamey RW, Elston CW (1992) pathological prognostic factors in breast cancer – relationship with survival in a large study with long-term follow-up. Histopathology 27: 479–89.

Elston CW, Ellis IO (1998) The Breast. Edinburgh: Churchill Livingstone.

Fentiman IS (2001) Fixed and modified risk factors for breast cancer. International Journal of Clinical Practice 55(8): 527–30.

Hildreth NG, Shore RE, Dvoretsky P (1989) The risk of breasts cancer after radiation for the thymus in infancy. New England Journal of Medicine 321: 1281–4.

Hughes LE, Mansel RE, Webster DJT (2000) Benign Disorders and Disease of the Breast: Concepts and Clinical Management. London: WB Saunders.

Hunter DJ, Spiegelman D, Adami H-O, Beeson L, van deb Brandt PA, Flostom AR, Fraser GE, Goldbohm RA, Graham S, Howe GR (1996) Cohort studies of fat intake and the risk of breast cancer – a pooled analysis. New England Journal of Medicine 334(6): 334–61.

King RJB (1996) Cancer Biology. Harlow: Longman.

Letcher M (1998) Invasive carcinoma of the breast. In Morgan MWE, Warren R, Querci della Rovere. Early Beast Cancer: From Screening to Multidisciplinary Management. Amsterdam, Harwood Academic Publishers.

MacPherson K, Steel CM, Dixon JM (1995) Breast Cancer: Epidemiology, Risk Factors and Genetics. In Dixon JM (Ed) ABC of Breast Diseases. London: BMJ Publishing.

Modan B, Chetrit A, Alfanary E (1989) Increased risk of breast cancer after low-dose radiation. Lancet ii: 629–31.

NHS Breast Screening Programme (1995) Pathology reporting in breast cancer screening: national co-ordinating group for breast screening pathology. NHSBSP Publication No 3, 2nd edn. Sheffield: NHS BSP Publications.

Page DL, Steel CM, Dixon JM (1995) Carcinoma in situ and patients at high risk of breast cancer. British Medical Journal 310: 39–42.

Sellers TA, Kushi LH, Potter JD, Kaye SA, Nelson CL, McGovern PG, Folsom AR (1992) Effect of family history, body fat distribution and reproductive factors on the risk of post-menopausal breast cancer. New England Journal of Medicine 326: 1323–9.

Silverstein MJ (1999) Ductal carcinoma in situ of the breast – can we tailor treatment to pathological findings? In Fentiman IS (ed) Breast Cancer. Oxford: Blackwell Science.

Slamon DJ, Clark GM, Wong SG, Lewin WJ, Ullrich A, McGuire Wl (1987) Human breast cancer: correlation of relapse and survival with amplification of the Her-2 /neu oncogene. Science 235: 177–82.

Slamon DJ, Godolphin W, Jones LA, Holt JA, Wong SG, Keith DE, Levin WJ, Stuart SG, Udove J, Ullrich A (1989) Studies of the HER-2/neu oncogene in human breast cancer and ovarian cancer. Science 244: 707–12.

Smith-Warner SA, Spiegelman D, Yaun SS, van den Brandt Folsom AR, Goldbohm RA, Graham S, Holmberg L, Howe GR, Marshall JR, Miller AB, Potter JD, Speizer FE, Willett WC, Wolk A, Hunter DJ (1998) Alcohol and breast cancer in women – a pooled analysis of cohort studies. Journal of the American Medical Association 279(7): 535–40.

Sobin LH, Wittekind CH (1997) TNM – Classification of Malignant Tumours, 5th edn. New York: Wiley-Liss.

Winchester DP (1985) ACP consensus statement: the relationship of fibrocystic disease to breast cancer. In Hughes LE, Mansel RE, Webster DJT (2000) Benign Disorders and Disease of the Breast: Concepts and Clinical Management. London: WB Saunders.

Ziegler RG, Hoover RN, Nomura AM, West DW, Wu AH, Pike MC, Lake AJ, Horn-Ross PL, Kolonel LN, Siiteri PK, Fraumeni JF Jr (1996) Relative weight, weight change, height, and breast cancer risk in Asian-American women. Journal of the National Cancer Institute 88: 650–60.

CHAPTER 2

Rare Breast Cancers

HELEN E. FROYD

Introduction

Breast cancer is often curable, particularly if it is diagnosed at an early stage. This requires early detection of the disease and a knowledge and awareness of all types of the disease, including the rarer forms of breast cancer, by healthcare professionals. This chapter is devoted to understanding this group of breast cancers that are by definition rare or 'unusual'. They are recognized as rare based on their architecture, growth pattern or cytological characteristics (layout of the nucleus, cytoplasm and cell membrane). Some rare breast cancers behave differently. The specific incidence, pathological features, diagnosis and treatment will also be described, as will possible issues that may lead to psychological and social problems.

Pathology of the Breast

The breast develops as a modified sweat gland with functional units called breast lobules that secrete during periods of breast-feeding. There are 15–20 breast ducts that conduct the secretion to the nipple.

The two main groups of breast cancer are ductal carcinoma and lobular carcinoma. The connective tissue within the breast consists mainly of fat, fibrous tissue, lymphatics and blood vessels (stroma), which can also give rise to malignant tumours. These stromal tumours are called sarcomas. The breast may also be the site of metastatic deposits from other tumours such as the ovary, lung, kidney, or skin (melanoma).

Table 2.1: Incidence of special types of breast cancer

Classification	Incidence	Reference
Inflammatory cancer	1%	Harris et al. 1999
Pregnancy-associated breast cancer	1%	National Cancer Institute 2001
Papillary	0.4–1%	Ellis et al. 1992
Intracystic	0.5%	Fletcher 1995
Phylloides	0.5%	Roses 1999
Paget's disease	2%	Haagensen 1986
Mucinous	1–4%	Page and Anderson 1987
Young women under 30	0.0005%	Xiong et al. 2001
Male breast cancer	1%	Office for National Statistics 1994

Source: Reprinted from Waller A, Caroline NL (2000) Handbook of Palliative Care in Cancer, 2nd edn, with permission from Elsevier Science.

Table 2.2: Age and incidence of breast cancer

Age	Incidence
Up to age 25	1 in 15,000
Up to age 30	1 in 9,000
Up to age 40	1 in 200
Up to age 85	1 in 10

Source: Office for National Statistics (2002) [www.cancerscreening.nhs.uk/breastscreen]

Inflammatory Carcinoma

These are a sub-type of ductal cancers that occur in approximately 1% of breast cancers (Harris et al., 1999).

Biological Features

An inflammatory breast cancer has specific features which include oedema of the skin and an 'orange peel' appearance. Other characteristics include a warm, red colour to the breast, and lymphatic involvement in the skin, the latter being present in at least 80% of women (Page and Anderson, 1987). These cancers are associated with a clinical picture of inflammation and are most likely to be high grade (poorly differentiated cancers). They are biologically very aggressive, so present frequently as locally advanced disease.

Treatment

Inflammatory cancers usually involve a large area of the breast including the skin. Breast conservation surgery is usually not appropriate where the cancer involves the skin. There is evidence that in locally advanced disease, primary medical treatment (chemotherapy prior to surgery) is recommended to induce shrinkage of the cancer (Israel et al., 1986) as it has been shown in women to significantly improve survival rates with a poor-prognosis breast cancer (Buzdar et al., 1982).

Following a course of chemotherapy, mastectomy with an axillary clearance is considered the safest option. Radiotherapy is also given to reduce local recurrence rates.

Breast Cancer Associated with Pregnancy

Breast cancer associated with pregnancy occurs with an incidence of 1% of all breast cancers (National Cancer Institute, 2001). According to Petrek et al. (1991) the standard definition of pregnancy-associated breast cancer is defined as a diagnosis of breast cancer during pregnancy or within a year after delivery.

Biological Features

The hormone-receptor status includes the oestrogen (ER) and progesterone (PR) receptor expression. This determines whether a cancer could respond to hormonal therapy. A low incidence of less than 25% ER positive cancers has been reported in breast cancer during pregnancy.

The breast undergoes enormous changes in pregnancy, including an increase in volume, dilation of ducts, and increasing hormonal levels of oestrogen, progesterone, prolactin, lobular growth and cell proliferation. Blood flow increases by up to 180% by the time the baby is at full term (Hughes et al., 1989). These changes present a challenge to the clinician as the breasts are often dense, and may double in size (hypertrophy) so masking the clinical features of an underlying breast cancer.

Diagnosis

Mammography is of limited value in pregnancy due to the high water content of the breasts, which can lead to difficulties in differentiating benign from malignant masses. Exposure of the fetus must be avoided during the first eight weeks due to the risks of radiation.

Ultrasound is by far the safest radiological tool during pregnancy. Together with ultrasound all palpable breast masses should be biopsied. To achieve an accurate diagnosis fine-needle aspiration cytology (FNAC) is required. Fine-needle aspiration cytology is technically more difficult to perform when the breast is engorged with milk. Gupta (1997) showed that FNAC in pregnant and lactating women could be very accurate. In one cancer centre in the USA, Keleher et al. (2001) preferred the use of image-guided core biopsy. These biopsies are important to obtain information on the histology including the ER and PR status of the cancer.

Treatment

The treatment sequence for each patient is individualized. It is important that treatment is not postponed because of pregnancy. The management of the breast cancer and the different treatment options follow the same principles as in a non-pregnant woman. However, the risks to the fetus and its protection are important considerations in planning treatment. Close monitoring of fetal development by an obstetrician is important throughout the pregnancy.

Although termination of the pregnancy is not recommended, it may be considered an option under specific circumstances. The following factors must be considered: whether the patient/partner/family is able to cope with a new baby, whether the patient has a poor prognosis, or whether the effects of treatment on the fetus could lead to patient or infant death (Carol et al., 1995).

Breast surgery can be performed at any time during pregnancy, with little risk to the fetus (Gianopoulos, 1995). The delivery date is usually brought forward to 30–32 weeks, and labour induced to be able to commence treatment as soon as possible. Usually immediate breast reconstruction is avoided during pregnancy.

Breast conservation therapy, which includes wide local excision with axillary surgery followed by a course of radiotherapy, is acceptable in a selection of patients (Kuerer et al., 2002). If the diagnosis is in the third trimester radiotherapy can commence after delivery. Although radiotherapy in pregnancy has been reported, it is not widely accepted (Antypas et al., 1998) since there is a risk of congenital abnormalities from radiation and risk of premature delivery (Willemse et al., 1990). If therefore the normal radiotherapy schedule would fall within the pregnancy, then a mastectomy should be performed.

At present little is known about the effects of pregnancy on lymphatic spread. Dixon et al. (2000) reported that 65% of all breast cancers in pregnancy involved axillary lymph glands. It is likely that surgeons perform axillary clearance of the glands as the role of sentinel node biopsy is not recommended. The main reason is that the safety of the radioactive isotope and blue dye in pregnancy has yet to be determined. However, pregnant women should not be excluded from clinical trials (Moirta et al., 2000).

Chemotherapy is not given during the first trimester of pregnancy, to prevent damage to the development of the fetus. Chemotherapy should be avoided during the three weeks before delivery to avoid myelosuppression in the baby, increased risk of infection and death (Giacalone et al., 1999).

If the cancer is over 3.5 cm, the treatment usually considered is primary chemotherapy. Breast cancers in pregnancy are frequently oestrogen-receptor negative, and therefore insensitive to hormonal therapy. No studies of tamoxifen in pregnant women are likely since the drug can cause vaginal bleeding, spontaneous abortions, birth defects and fetal death. Therefore hormonal therapy is never commenced until after delivery.

Breast-feeding Issues

Radiotherapy to the breast can cause fibrosis of the ducts, consequently reducing the amount of milk produced. Women should be advised that future breast-feeding is rare. Although future milk production may be compromised, breast-feeding is possible on the affected side, depending on the volume of breast tissue treated.

Papillary Carcinoma

These cancers are uncommon in a pure form and may present as a cystic mass in 0.5% of all breast cancers (Ellis et al., 1992).

Biological Features

Papillary carcinoma is characterized by the architectural arrangement of the malignant cells forming finger-like projections.

Diagnosis

Papillary carcinoma is picked up on mammography as a mass with irregular margins. The presence of bloodstained cystic fluid on fine-needle aspiration provides a clue to the true nature of the lesion, and an ultrasound examination may reveal irregular margins with solid areas inside the cyst cavity (McCulloch et al., 1997).

Treatment

There is no consensus in the management of this condition (Harris et al., 1999). Retrospective analysis of 23 patients over 18 years recommended that local excision is adequate. These lesions have the potential to spread to the lymph nodes and lead to metastatic disease.

Intracystic Papillary Carcinoma

Intracystic papillary cancers occurs in less than 1% of all breast cancers, although more frequently in the elderly (Ellis et al., 1992; Fletcher, 1995).

Biological Features

Invasive papillary carcinoma should be clearly distinguished from in situ or DCIS papillary carcinoma. Intracystic papillary cancer is an invasive tumour within a thick cyst cavity. Usually these cancers are small, between 1 and 3cm in size. Mucin secretion is a pathological feature.

Diagnosis

It is important to obtain a core biopsy for histological confirmation of invasive disease.

Secretory Carcinoma

These cancers were first seen in children (McDivett and Stewart, 1966) but are known in all age groups. They usually presenting as a lump measuring less than 2 cm. In children, secretory carcinoma carries an excellent prognosis, but there is limited evidence available to suggest the outlook in adults is as favourable (Tavassoli and Norris, 1980).

Phylloides Tumours

Phylloides are stromal tumours, which resemble benign fibroadenomas, accounting for approximately 0.5% of all breast cancers (Roses, 1999).

Biological Features

The behaviour of these tumours varies according to the size and certain microscopic features appearing as leaf-like structures. There are three subtypes of phylloides: benign, borderline and frankly malignant. They are derived from stromal tissue, and the malignant form is known as cystosarcoma. They can vary in size from 2 to 10 cm but are normally over 5 cm and may grow rapidly. They mainly occur in middle-aged or elderly women and occur in a population of people who are 10–15 years older than those who develop fibroadenomas.

Diagnosis

It is often difficult to distinguish between a fibroadenoma, a common benign breast tumour, and benign phylloides. On mammography phylloides present as benign masses and may contain large calcifications. Cytology is usually suspicious if there are increased numbers of cellular stromal elements or isolated abnormal cells are present. A core biopsy usually provides a definitive diagnosis.

Treatment

As these lesions pose a threat of recurrence, it is important that there are clear surgical margins, thus a wide local excision with negative margins is the principal approach to the management of these tumours (Schnabel, 1993).

As with other stromal cancers such as sarcomas, the preferred pathway of spread is through the blood vessels to the lungs, liver or bones (Kessinger et al., 1972). These cancers rarely affect the lymphatics, which means there is no indication for axillary node surgery.

Sarcoma of the Breast

Sarcomas are extremely rare in the breast; the most common types are angiosarcoma, fibrosarcoma, liposarcoma and malignant fibrous histiocytoma.

Biological Features

These cancers arise from the stroma or connective tissue of the breast and blood vessels, thus they are vascular and grow quickly.

Diagnosis

These cancers frequently present with a large lump which has rapidly increased in size. Mammography is usually non-specific.

Treatment

The surgical approach to sarcomas depends on the size of the tumour. If large it may require mastectomy; otherwise, wide local excision is appropriate. There is some suggestion that radiotherapy may be beneficial in local control (Johnstone et al., 1993). They are usually locally aggressive and spread via the blood with a poor response to chemotherapy.

Angiosarcomas

Angiosarcomas are the commonest stromal tumours of the breast. The overall five-year survival is poor, 33% (Chen et al., 1988).

Diagnosis

Such a tumour often presents as a painless lump, varying in size from 1 cm to 11 cm, although sometimes there is diffuse breast enlargement without a mass. It may involve both breasts. The most common sites of spread are liver, lung, skin and to the contralateral breast.

Lymphangiosarcoma (Stewart-Treves lesion)

Lymphangiosarcomas are associated with post-treatment lymphoedema.

This is a rare complication of radical mastectomy developing usually 10 years after surgery, frequently involving only the arm. It has a very aggressive quality, with rapid spread to an area of lymphoedema and then wide spread throughout the body. The five-year survival rate is poor (Stewart and Treves, 1948; Martin et al., 1984).

Paget's Disease of the Breast

Paget's disease of the nipple occurs in approximately 2% of all breast cancers (Haagensen, 1986). It is now believed that Paget's disease is a variant type of comedo DCIS (ductal carcinoma in situ) supported by the fact that DCIS is usually found in at least one nipple duct (Ellis and Elston, 1995). From the patients who present with a lump, 90–94% will have an invasive cancer. For patients where no palpable lump can be clinically felt, far fewer are found to have invasive carcinoma but all have DCIS. For these patients, the prognosis is more favourable.

Diagnosis

The most common features of Paget's disease are changes to the nipple, associated with a rash, eczema, scaling, bleeding, itching or ulceration. If a patient presents with any eczematous lesion of the nipple, mammography should be performed to determine whether there is a lesion that cannot be felt, and its degree of involvement with the rest of the breast. However, in many patients mammography is entirely normal. Some 40–50% of patients are diagnosed with Paget's disease without a clinical lump (Maier et al., 1969; Ashikari et al., 1970). The most reliable method of obtaining a histological diagnosis is by nipple-skin biopsy.

Treatment

Historically, the standard treatment has been a mastectomy, because of the goal of ensuring that the surgical excision margins of the cancer are clear. However, there are increasing reports of successful use of breast conservation techniques involving removal of the nipple and areola. Radiotherapy alone or partial central excision of the breast and nipple have also been used (Fourquet et al., 1987; Stockdale et al., 1989; Bulens et al., 1990; Pierce et al., 1997). Dixon et al. (2000) suggested that in both male and female Paget's disease that presents without a lump, wide local excision followed by radio-therapy produces good results. If the nipple is removed, the breast care nurse can arrange for a prosthetic nipple to improve the cosmetic result. Possibilities for later stage nipple reconstruction, such as grafting or tattooing, can be discussed.

Mucinous Carcinoma

Mucinous carcinoma is also referred to as mucoid or colloid cancer, because these tumours contain mucin, representing 1–4% of breast cancers, and occur mainly in older women (Page and Anderson, 1987).

Biological Features

Mucinous cancers arise from the ductal epithelium. Compared with other breast cancers, pure mucinous carcinomas have a good prognosis, with survival of 70–90% at 10 years.

Breast Cancer in Young Women (under 30)

Breast cancers that occur in women under 40 are rare. Women under age of 40 are usually described as 'younger women' although some authors suggest this age group includes women under 30 years old (Xiong et al., 2001). The incidence of breast cancer in younger women is shown in Table 2.2 (see page 19).

Biological Features

The literature on breast cancer in young women focuses on the disease being more aggressive compared with older women, with repeated reports that young age is a poor prognostic factor (Xiong et al., 2001). Breast cancer in young women is more likely to be high grade, hormone insensitive (ER/PR negative), to have HER2/neu over-expression, and the presence of vascular invasion compared with older women (Colleoni et al., 2002; Dubsky et al., 2002; Kothari and Fentiman, 2002). However, young age is not an independent prognostic determinant. Providing tumours are of similar grade, size and nodal status, prognosis is independent of the patient's age.The sensitivity to hormones is different in young women as 33% of cancers in young women are oestrogen receptor negative (ER-ve) whereas over 70% of cancers in post-menopausal women are oestrogen sensitive (ER+ve).

One of the most important features of these cancers is the increased likelihood that a genetic mutation is causing the disease (see Chapter 3). Approximately 30% of all breast cancers in women under 35 years old are caused by a genetic mutation. The option of referral to a regional cancer genetics service, which provides genetic counselling and genetic testing, should be offered. Genetic counselling should be made available for the women's siblings and female relatives, who may carry an increased risk or susceptibility to developing breast cancer.

Treatment

Chemotherapy is increasingly being considered appropriate for all women under the age of 35 years but poses the difficult problem of infertility.

Most young women are pre-menopausal. If their cancer is oestrogen receptor positive, there are two methods of ovarian ablation (Clive and Dixon 2002). The permanent method involves either surgical removal with oophorectomy or radiotherapy.

If the woman wishes to conserve her fertility, the most common method is to use a LHRH analogue (luteinizing hormone-releasing hormone) such as goserelin or leuprorelin. These are injections given monthly for two years, either by the general practitioner, the practice nurse or a member of the breast care team.

Male Breast Cancer

Male breast cancer occurs in approximately 1% of all breast cancers, affecting 189 men in 1994 in England and Wales (Office for National Statistics, 1994) and 70 deaths in 2000 (Office for National Statistics, 2000). The average age for male breast cancer is approximately between 60 and 70 years old, 10 years older than in women.

Biological Features

The pathology is similar to that of female breast cancer, with infiltrating ductal carcinoma the most common type, and intraductal carcinoma (DCIS) is well described. Inflammatory carcinoma and Paget's disease have also been seen in men. Breast cancer can develop following radiotherapy for previous cancers such as lymphoma. In 75% of men the tumour presents as a mass under the nipple. As men have less breast tissue than women, skin infiltration is more likely (Donegan, 1991). Overall survival has been reported as similar to that of women (Borgen et al., 1992; Cutuli et al., 1995).

The causes of male breast cancer remain largely undetermined; however, it is known that men with a family history of the disease are at a higher risk that men who have no such history. Two breast cancer genes (*BRCA1* and *BRCA2*) have been mapped and may be responsible for as much as 20% of all male breast cancers (Vetto et al., 1999) (see Chapter 3).

Diagnosis

Mammography is performed on men together with an ultrasound. A core biopsy is necessary to obtain an accurate histological diagnosis.

Treatment

Current treatments for male breast cancer are the same as those for women with the disease (Fenlon, 1996). The main treatment for men with breast cancer is surgery, most commonly modified mastectomy (Borgen et al., 1992; Jaiyesimi et al., 1992; Ravandi-Kashani and Hayes, 1998). In a recent study comparing treatments between men and women with breast cancer it was found that men were more likely to have mastectomy combined with radiotherapy than women (Scott-Corner et al., 1999).

A higher percentage of male than female breast cancers are hormone-dependent (Rosen et al., 1976), which means they are responsive to adjuvant hormonal therapy such as tamoxifen. Anelli et al. (1994) reported that the side effects of tamoxifen in 24 men with breast cancer were decreased libido, weight gain, hot flushes, mood alteration and depression.

Research on systemic therapy with chemotherapy in male breast cancer has not been well established over the last decade and is based largely on anecdotal or retrospective reports (Bunkely et al., 2000).

Psychological Issues

Psychological problems can occur following any cancer diagnosis. It is therefore important to consider the specific concerns and difficulty patients with rare breast cancer may face in adjusting to their diagnosis.

A delay in diagnosis can occur where the clinician may not recognize the symptoms of a rare breast cancer, and therefore not refer the patient urgently to the hospital as a suspicious case. This group includes patients with inflammatory cancer, women under 30, women who are pregnant, men with breast cancer and those with sarcomas. Paget's disease may be mistaken clinically as eczema or treated as a chronic form of dermatitis with topical steroids. Inflammatory carcinomas may be diagnosed as a breast infection and be treated with antibiotics. Often these patients wait longer to be seen by specialist breast teams, which could potentially influence their long-term prognosis, and this often causes anxieties about the disease spreading.

Breast Cancer in Pregnancy

A diagnosis of breast cancer associated with pregnancy raises a number of difficulties and psychological issues. A delayed diagnosis is not uncommon and may contribute to some women presenting with more advanced disease (Byrd et al., 1962).

The focus of attention is not only on the woman but on securing the future of her unborn child. In one study, Bandyk and Gilmore (1995) found the major concerns of pregnant women treated with chemotherapy were: 'living to see my child grow up', the cancer treatments and their effects on the baby, and 'the risk of not being there for other children if the pregnancy continues'. The unpredictability of cancer with all of its uncertainties, plus the additional stress of treatment effects on the unborn child, can make the situation very difficult. Prior to and during chemotherapy, there may be fears of potential congenital abnormalities in the unborn child.

Another poignant issue raised is the possible loss of future offspring where treatments are likely to cause infertility. Treatments for preservation of oocytes or eggs are currently limited and largely experimental, such as cryopreservation of ovarian tissue.

A possible effect of chemotherapy is a premature menopause, as the ovaries are temporarily, or in some cases permanently, affected. Menopausal symptoms may be experienced and include weight gain, hot flushes, vaginal dryness, reduction in bone density and low libido. There may be fears over whether ovarian function will resume, and the possible loss of fertility altogether. As healthcare professionals we need to seek ways to help women cope with menopausal symptoms (see Chapter 10).

The nurse should always carry out a full social assessment to ascertain the psychological concerns and social needs of the patient and her/his family. Important issues relevant for these women are childcare if the woman needs to return to work, and financial concerns. Some women may require further therapy following delivery of their child, which may require time off work and consequently a drop in income. If a job carries no maternity rights or sickness pay, financial difficulties may be on the horizon. A social worker may be required to help the woman access child benefit and income support.

Many of the issues relating to pregnant women may be pertinent to those young women who are diagnosed in their twenties and thirties. If unmarried, a young woman may be concerned about the possible threat to future relationships, or revealing scars and the diagnosis to a new or old partner, coupled with concerns over future sexual function and fertility.

The breast care nurse specialist and multidisciplinary team need to be involved in women's psychological adjustment to their diagnosis and reaction to illness, and may be key players in exploring further concerns or difficulties. Support is available through cancer charities such as Breast Cancer Care.

Male Breast Cancer

There is an assumption that the impact and male response to a breast cancer diagnosis and its treatment is the same as for women (Peate, 2001). Breast cancer mainly affects women, so the majority of psychosocial literature has considered breast cancer within this group (Smyth et al., 1995). Thus our understanding of the supportive care needs for men with breast cancer are limited. Whilst male breast cancer may be rare, the emotional impact has remained largely ignored.

The breast, like many organs in the body, is present in both sexes and yet it is symbolically represented as belonging only to woman. Within western society the breast is not embodied as a part of the male body but is perceived as the 'chest'. For men 'breasts' are part of the female anatomy, related to childbearing, lactation and female sexuality.

Men's knowledge of breast awareness is constrained by the inadequate information available for men on the disease and its symptoms. Froyd (2002) studied men's narratives of their breast cancer and found symptoms of cancer were not taken seriously, as they did not recognize the condition as a 'normal' man's illness. Therefore symptoms including nipple changes or lumps were not taken seriously, and were dismissed as fat, an infection, damage, or a blocked duct. By dismissing symptoms of illnesses, Charmaz (1995) found that men with chronic illnesses often work hard to hide their diagnosis in an effort to preserve their masculinity. The rarity of the disease caused even more ambiguity owing to poor understanding and lack of information on the disease.

For men with breast cancer, adjustment to the diagnosis may be difficult for a number of reasons. Despite occurring in both men and women, breast cancer is represented as a woman's disease. Men may feel their diagnosis a threat to their masculinity. Froyd (2002) found men did not talk about their illness or want to meet other men with the same condition because they felt like an 'oddity'. Other fears included ridicule by others, believing 'he must be a woman' or that something is 'physically wrong', led men to feel embarrassment.

It is important for the multidisciplinary team to recognize that the needs and concerns of those with male breast cancer are different from women's. In addition, with any rare disease, disbelief and feelings of being the only person with the condition can cause difficulties with psychological adjustment.

If mortality from breast cancer is to be reduced, greater knowledge and improved awareness by all healthcare professionals is fundamental in reducing the number of delayed diagnoses, and ensuring that these cancers are treated appropriately by specialist cancer teams. A difference in the quality of care and availability of specialist cancer care should not exist for any woman or man with a common or rare breast cancer.

Providing effective interventions aimed at minimizing the impact of side effects of treatment, assisting the patient in adjustment to changes resulting from the disease and its treatment, and giving emotional support are important roles for all nurses.

Conclusion

Those facing a diagnosis of a rare breast cancer have specific physical and psychological difficulties and needs. Most of the studies of special types of breast cancer focus on the pathology and prognosis rather than how nurses can offer appropriate care and support. More research is required to recognize the supportive care needs of these patients. There is a paucity of research and information on the psychological and social impact of rare breast cancers. Subsequently there may be a lack of awareness amongst healthcare professionals concerning the possible psychological consequences. So what is the solution?

An Agenda for Change

Most healthcare professionals believe they do recognize the person behind the treatment but all too often the person is obscured from view. It is easy to assume what you see is a true reflection of how the patient really feels. Patients may hide their distress or think their symptoms are an inevitable consequence of treatment or symptoms of a previous condition, so they do not seek help, yet they should not have to ask for help. Saillent (1990) illustrates this through recounting a story of a young woman with advanced breast cancer with bone pain in her hips that she believed was caused by a previous stillbirth, rather than cancer in the bone. She did not disclose her pain to her carers as she believed her explanation would not be acceptable, so her pain went unrecognized.

The following items should be on an agenda for change:

1. We must start thinking about examining ways in which we can be available to talk, to volunteer information and to help the carers who might also be affected. There are too many unknowns: verbal information is poorly absorbed and inadequately reinforced. As a result, patients experience uncertainty, powerlessness, isolation and loss of control. Patients need knowledge, even if it does not banish fear.
2. As nurses, we need to be aware of the sensitive nature of the impact of diagnosis for these patients and provide appropriate assessment and treatment. The breast care nurse's involvement is vital.
3. We should recognize the complexity of these special cancers and their impact and 'recovery' from treatment. It is important to acknowledge that patients may have treatments that continue to affect them as they try to rebuild their lives. Young women may fear loss of their fertility for years after their treatment is completed.
4. Breast care services are designed for women. This may have significant implications for affected men, who may feel uncomfortable being in a

clinic full of women. Male breast cancer patients could be seen at the beginning or end of breast clinics to reduce the embarrassment and isolation of being the only man in the clinic. We must not assume or ignore the possibility that following breast surgery a man may not have the same difficulties that a woman might experience.

Breast cancer is not simply one disease but many. To improve a patient's cancer journey with a rare type of breast cancer, we need to improve our understanding of the impact of these cancers, deliver accurate and timely information, and recognize how our practice can make a difference.

Appendix 1: Patient Information

Breast Cancer Care (2000) Breast Cancer and Childcare. Factsheet 25. London: BCC.
Breast Cancer Care (2000) Breast Cancer in Pregnancy. Factsheet 13. London: BCC.
Breast Cancer Care (2000) Inflammatory Breast Cancer. Factsheet 11. London: BCC.
Breast Cancer Care (2000) Paget's Disease. Factsheet 26. London: BCC. London: BCC.
Breast Cancer Care (2001) Breast Cancer Treatment and Fertility. Factsheet 16.
Breast Cancer Care (2001) Information and Support for Younger Women. London: BCC.
Breast Cancer Care (2001) Male Breast Cancer. Factsheet 2. London: BCC.
Cancer BACUP (2002) Genetics in Bowel, Breast and Ovarian Cancer. London: BACUP.
Cancer BACUP (2002) Male Breast Cancer. London: BACUP.
Cancer BACUP (2002) Paget's Disease. London: BACUP.

Support Organizations and Websites

Breast Cancer Care:
Younger women's volunteer network, volunteers with male breast cancer.
Website: www.breastcancercare.org.uk

Cancer During Pregnancy:
Telephone support for women diagnosed with cancer during pregnancy.
Tel: 0208 9428759

National Breast Screening Program:
Website: www.cancerscreening.nhs.uk/breastscreen

References

Anelli TF, Anelli A, Tran KN, Lebwohl D E, Borgen P (1994) Tamoxifen administration is associated with a high rate of treatment-limiting symptoms in male breast cancer patients. Cancer 74(1): 74-7.
Antypas C, Sandilos P, Kouvaris J, Balafouta E, Karinou E, Kollaros N, Vlahos L. (1998) Fetal dose evaluation during breast cancer radiotherapy. Internal Journal of Radiation Oncology, Biology, Physics 40: 995-9.

Ashikari R, Park K, Huvos AG, Urban JA (1970) Paget's disease of the breast. Cancer 26: 680-5.

Bandyk EA, Gilmore MA (1995) Perceived concerns of pregnant women with breast cancer treated with chemotherapy. Oncology Nursing Forum 22: 975-7.

Borgen PI, Wong GY, Vlamis V, Potter C, Hoffman B, Kinne DW, Osbourne MP, McKinnon WM (1992) Current management of male breast cancer: a review of 104 cases. Annuals of Surgery 215(5): 451-7.

Bulens P, Vanuytsel L, Rjinders A, van der Schueren E (1990) Breast conserving treatment of Paget's disease. Radiotherapy and Oncology 17: 305-9.

Bunkley DT, Robinson JD, Bennett NE, Gordon S (2000) Breast cancer in men: emasculation by association? Journal of Clinical Psychology in Medical Settings 7(2): 91-7.

Buzdar AU, Smith TL, Powell KC, Blumenschein GR, Gehan EA (1982) Effect of timing of initiation of adjuvant chemotherapy on disease-free survival in breast cancer. Breast Cancer Research and Treatment 2(2): 163-9.

Byrd BF, Bayer DS, Robertson JC, Stephens SE (1962) Treatment for breast tumors associated with pregnancy and lactation. Annuals of Surgery 155: 940-7.

Carol EH, Conner S, Schorr S (1995) The diagnosis and management of breast problems during pregnancy and lactation. American Journal of Surgery 170: 140-4.

Charmaz K (1995) Discovering chronic illness: using grounded theory. Social Science and Medicine 30(11): 1161-72.

Chen KT, Kirkegaard DD, Bocian JJ (1988) Angiosarcoma of the breast. Cancer 46: 368-71.

Clive S, Dixon JM (2002) The value of adjuvant treatment in young women with breast cancer. Drugs 62(1): 1-11.

Colleoni M, Rotmensz N, Robertson C, Orlando L, Viale G, Renne C, Luini A, Veronesi P, Intra M, Orecchia R, Catalano G, Galimberti V, Nole F, Martinelli G, Goldhirsh A (2002) Very young women (<35 years) with operable cancer features of disease at presentation. Annals of Oncology 13(2): 273-9.

Cutuli B, Lacroze M, Dilhuydy J M, Velten M, Lafontan B, Marchal C, Resbeut M, Graic Y, Campana F, Moncho-Bernier V (1995) Male breast cancer: results of the treatments and prognostic factors in 397 cases. European Journal of Cancer 31A(12): 1960-4.

Dixon AR, Sainsbury JRC, Rodger A (2000) Breast cancer: treatment of elderly patients and uncommon conditions. In Dixon AR (Ed) ABC of Breast Diseases. London: BMJ Publishing.

Donegan W (1991) Cancer of the breast in men. CA-A Cancer Journal for Clinicians 41(6): 339-54.

Dubsky PC, Gnant MF, Taucher S, Roka S, Kandioler D, Pichler-Gebhard B, Agster I, Seifert M, Sevelda P, Jakesz R (2002) Young age as an independent adverse prognostic factor in premenopausal patients with breast cancer. Clinics in Breast Cancer 3(1): 65-72.

Ellis IO, Galea M, Broughton N (1992) Pathological prognostic factors in breast cancer, II: Histological type. Relationship with survival in a large study with long-term follow-up. Histopathology 20: 479-89.

Ellis IO, Elston CW (1995) Tumors of the breast: In Fletcher CDM (Ed) Diagnostic Histopathology of Tumors, Vol. 1. New York: Churchill Livingstone.

Fenlon D (1996) Endocrine therapies for breast cancer. In Denton S (Ed) Breast Care Nursing. London: Chapman & Hall.

Fletcher CD (Ed) (1995) Diagnostic Histopathology of Tumors, Vol. 1. London: Churchill Livingstone.

Fourquet A, Campana F, Vielh P, Schlienger P, Jullien D, Vilcoq JR (1987) Paget's disease of the nipple without detectable breast tumor: conservative management with radiation therapy. International Journal of Radiation Oncology, Biology, Physics 13(10): 1463-5.

Froyd HE (2002) An exploratory study of men's experiences of breast cancer and prostate cancer. Unpublished MSc thesis, University of London.

Giacalone PL, Laffargue F, Benos P (1999) Chemotherapy for breast carcinoma during pregnancy. A French national survey. Cancer 86: 2266-72.

Gianopoulos JG (1995) Establishing the criteria for anaesthesia and other precautions for surgery during pregnancy. Surgical Clinics of North America 75: 33-43.

Gupta RK (1997) The diagnostic impact of aspiration cytodiagnosis of breast masses in association with pregnancy and lactation with the emphasis on clinical decision making. Breast 3: 131-4.

Haagensen CD (1986) Diseases of the Breast, 3rd edn. Philadelphia, PA: WB Saunders, pp. 824-32.

Harris KP, Faliakou E , Exon DJ, Nasiri N, Sacks NP, Gui GP (1999) Treatment and outcome of intracystic papillary carcinoma of the breast. British Journal of Surgery 86(10): 1274.

Hughes LE, Mansel RE, Webster DJT, Gravelle IH (1989) Benign Disorders and Diseases of the Breast. Philadephia, PA: Baillière Tindall.

Israel L, Breau JL, Morore JF (1986) Two years of high dose cyclophosphamide and 5-fluorouracil followed by surgery after 3 months for acute inflammatory breast carcinomas: a phase II study of 25 cases with a median follow-up on 35 months. Cancer 57(1): 24-8.

Jaiyesimi IA, Buzdar AU, Sahim AA, Ross MA (1992) Carcinoma of the male breast. Annals of Internal Medicine 117(9): 771-7.

Johnstone PA, Pierce L, Merino MJ, Yang JC, Epstein AH, DeLaney TF (1993) Primary soft tissue sarcomas of the breast: local-regional control with post-operative radiotherapy. International Journal of Radiation Oncology, Biology, Physics 27(3): 670-5.

Keleher AJ, Theriault RL, Gwyn KM, Hunt KK, Stelling CB, Singletary E, Ames FC, Buchholz TA, Sahin AA, Kuerer HM (2001) Multidisciplinary management of breast cancer concurrent with pregnancy. Journal of the American College of Surgeons 194(1): 54-64.

Kessinger A, Foley JF, Lemon HM, Miller DM (1972) Metastatic cystosarcoma phylloides: a case report and review of the literature. Journal of Surgical Oncology 4(2): 131-47.

Kothari AS, Fentiman IS (2002) Breast cancer in young women. International Journal of Clinical Practice 56(3): 184-7.

Kuerer HM, Cunningham JD, Bleiweiss IJ, Doucette JT, Divino CM, Brower ST, Tarter PI (1998) Conservative surgery for breast carcinoma associated with pregnancy. The Breast Journal 4(3): 171-6.

Kuerer HM, Gywn T, Ames FC, Theriault RL (2002) Conservative surgery and chemotherapy during pregnancy for breast carcinoma. Surgery 131(1): 108-10.

Maier WP, Rosemond GP, Harasym EL, Al- Saleem TI , Tasoni EM, Schor SS (1969) Paget's disease in the female breast. Surgery, Gynecology and Obstetrics 128: 1253-63.

Martin MB, Kon ND, Kawamonto EH (1984) Post mastectomy angiosarcoma. American Journal of Surgery 10: 541-5.

McCulloch GL, Evans AJ, Yeoman L, Wilson AR, Pinder SE, Ellis IO, Elston CW (1997) Radiological features of papillary carcinoma of the breast. Clinical Radiology 52(11): 865-8.

McDivett RW, Stewart FW (1966) breast carcinoma in children. Journal of the American Medical Association 195: 388-90.

Moirta ET, Chang J, Leong S (2000) Principles and controversies in lymphoscintigraphy with emphasis on breast cancer. Surgical Clinics of North America 80: 1721-37.

National Breast Screening Program (2002) Breast screening. Available at: http://www.cancerscreening.nhs.uk/breastscreen; www.cancerscreening.nhs.uk/breastscreen

National Cancer Institute (2001) Breast cancer in pregnancy Cancer-Net. Available at: http://cancernet.nci.nih.gov/ cgi-bin/srchcgi.exe

Office for National Statistics (1994) Cancer Statistics: Registrations 1994, Series MBI, No 27. London: HMSO.

Office for National Statistics (2000) Annual Reference Volume: Mortality Statistics, Cause: 2000, Series DH2, No. 27. London: HMSO.

Office for National Statistics (2002) Cancer Trends in England and Wales in 1950-1999. London: HMSO.

Page DL, Anderson J (1987) Diagnostic Histopathology of the Breast. London: Churchill Livingstone.

Peate I (2001) Caring for men with breast cancer: causes, symptoms and treatment. British Journal of Nursing 10(15): 975-81.

Petrek JA, Dukoff R, Rogatko A (1991) Prognosis of pregnancy associated breast cancer. Cancer 67(4): 699-702.

Pierce L, Haffty B, Solin L, McCormick, Vicini F, Wazer D, Recht A, Strawderman M, Lichter A (1997) The conservative management of Paget's disease of the breast with radiotherapy. Cancer 80(6): 1065-72.

Ravandi-Kashani F, Hayes TG (1998) Male breast cancer: a review of the literature. European Journal of Cancer 34(9): 1341-7.

Rosen PP, Menendez-Botet CJ, Nisselbaum JS, Schwartz MK, Urban JA (1976) Estrogen receptor protein in lesions of the male breast: a preliminary report . Cancer 37(4): 1866-8.

Roses DF (1999) Breast Cancer. New York: Churchill Livingstone.

Schnabel FR (1993) Cytosarcoma phylloides. Surgical Oncology Clinics of North America 2: 107-19.

Scott-Corner CEH, Jochimsen PR, Menck HR, Winchester DJ (1999) An analysis of male and female breast cancer treatment and survival among demographically identical pairs. Surgery 126(4): 775-81.

Smyth MM, McCaughan E, Harrison S (1995) Women's perceptions of their experiences with breast cancer: are their needs being addressed? European Journal of Cancer Care 4: 86-92.

Stewart FW, Treves N (1948) Lymphangiosarcoma in post mastectomy lyphoedema. A report of six cases in elephantiasis chirurgica. Cancer 1: 64-81.

Stockdale AD, Brierly JD, White WF, Folkes A, Rostom AY (1989) Radiotherapy for Paget's disease of the nipple: a conservative alternative. Lancet 2(8664): 664-6.

Tavassoli FA, Norris HJ (1980) Secretory carcinoma of the breast. Cancer 45: 2404-13.

Vetto J, Jun S-Y, Padduch D, Eppich H, Shih R (1999) Stages at presentation, prognostic factors and outcome of breast cancer in males. American Journal of Surgery 177(5): 379-83.

Waller A, Caroline NL (2000) Handbook of Palliative Care in Cancer, 2nd edn. Oxford: Butterworth-Heinemann.

Willemese PHS, vd Sijde R, Sleijfer Dt (1990) Combination chemotherapy and radiation for stage IV breast cancer during pregnancy. Gynecological Oncology 36: 281.

Xiong Q, Valero V, Kau V, Kau S, Taylor S, Smith TL, Buzdar AU, Hortobagyi GN, Theriault RL (2001) Female patients with breast carcinoma age 30 years and younger have a poor prognosis. Cancer 92(10): 2523-8.

CHAPTER 3

Breast Cancer Genetics

AUDREY ARDERN-JONES

Introduction

In the UK, one in three people develop cancer in their lifetime and there are 25 000 cases of breast cancer and just over 5000 cases of ovarian cancer diagnosed per year (ONS, 1998). The majority of cancer cases occur by chance alone. Therefore, clustering of cancer cases in a family is not uncommon. In a small proportion of cases this may be due to the familial inheritance of a piece of genetic damage (mutation) in a gene responsible for cellular growth control or DNA repair. Cancer is always genetic at the cellular level in that a cancer is the end result of a series of genetic changes.

Biological Explanation of Inherited Breast Cancer

Mutations or changes within a gene accumulate in every somatic cell during the course of an individual's lifetime. Somatic cells are the cells in the body that are not the sex cells. Not all mutations occur in somatic cells. Mutations also occur in the ova and spermatocytes. Some of these mutations can be inherited via the germ line to cause an inherited cancer predisposition.

There is a long process of cumulative genetic changes that take place in a single breast cell before it becomes malignant. The malignant cell divides many times before an outward physical change manifests as a lump in a breast.

All cells in the human body contain a chemical substance called deoxyribonucleic acid (DNA). Chromosomes are structures that contain DNA and are arranged in pairs. There are 23 pairs, or a total of 46 chromosomes. The 23rd pair of chromosomes is the sex chromosomes. Males have one X and one Y chromosome and females have two X chromosomes. The reason why chromosomes are arranged in pairs is due to the fact that one set of the 23 chromosomes comes from the mother in the egg and the other set comes from the father in the sperm. When a sperm and an egg unite, together they form a new cell with 46 chromosomes. The fertilized egg then divides, and all 46 chromosomes are copied and passed on to every cell, where DNA is arranged in sequences or units that are known as genes. Genes direct the growth, development and function of the human body: everything from the colour of our hair to our height and how often cells divide. Metaphorically speaking they are like a booklet of complex instructions. As we have inherited two copies of every chromosome, one from our mother and one from our father, we also have two copies of every gene - one copy from each parent.

Sometimes a gene is altered, so that it does not function as it should - it gives the cell the wrong set of instructions. This is known as a gene mutation or an altered gene, which does not function in the normal way.

Each gene has a specific function in the body. One of the main functions of the cell is to replicate itself and therefore some genes control cell division. When mutations occur in these genes, a cell may begin to divide without control. Such a cell, once altered and therefore not functioning in a normal manner, may then change into a cancer cell. Thus all cancer is the result of gene mutations. Mutations may be caused by ageing or by exposure to environmental factors such as radiation, chemicals, hormones or other factors such as smoking and alcohol. Over time, a number of mutations may occur in a particular cell, thus allowing the cell to divide and grow in a way that may turn into a cancer. This usually takes many years, and this therefore explains the fact that the older a person is, the higher the risk of developing cancer. Thus the population risk figure of 1 in 3 people developing cancer in our western society relates to an older population.

If an individual has inherited a gene fault it means that every single cell in his/her body has the mutation. This mutation may or may not pass down to the offspring (Figure 3.1). The diagram reflects the premise that there is always a 50/50 chance of the offspring inheriting or not inheriting the faulty copy of the gene. Each circle represents a person's two copies of a gene. The copy with the mutation is darkened and has a line through it.

It is understandable that if a person has inherited a faulty gene predisposing to cancer there is an increased risk over and above that of other people of developing the disease. Inherited gene mutations explain why, in some families, there are more cases of cancer throughout the different generations. In particular in inherited cancer one finds bilateral disease, younger onset of cancer and the same types of cancer throughout the generations, e.g. breast.

About 5-10% of breast cancer cases are thought to be due to heritable genetic influences. This means that most breast cancers are not hereditary.

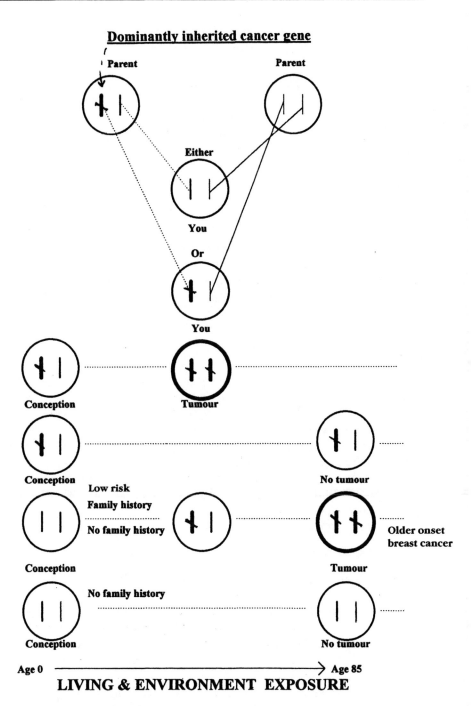

Figure 3.1: Mode of inheritance.

However, if a woman outlines her family history there is sometimes an explanation as to why breast cancer may have developed in her family. It is important to note that currently there is limited knowledge to explain the reasons why some families seem prone to developing breast cancer. The most likely cause relates to a combination of environmental exposures interacting with various genes that are yet to be identified. Indeed any woman who has a first-degree relative who has developed breast cancer under the age of 50 has an increased risk over and above other women who do not have this. Very often the increased risk is marginal, and extra screening is not recommended for these women other than the UK National Screening programme.

Many family members are under the illusion that if they look like their relative they will automatically develop cancer (Richards et al., 1995). Genetic counselling seeks to explain simply the basics of genetic inheritance to dispel these beliefs, and elucidate information about family members so that cancer cases can be independently confirmed. Cancer risk should be explained in a way that is comprehensible to everyone involved (Ardern-Jones and Mitchell, 1999).

Family Concerns

If a woman develops breast cancer she may well be concerned about the risk for her daughters. Studies have shown the profound effect of the impact of a mother's breast cancer diagnosis on a daughter. These fears need to be translated into the reality of relative risk for the daughter (Wellisch et al,, 1996). Family contacts and dynamics are an important part of the counselling process and sadly many families have experienced having young-onset cancer relatives who may have died. Time needs to be taken to understand these families and help them, as many have a distorted perception of their risk (Ardern-Jones, 1997).

Confirming a Cancer Family History

Talking about the past with an individual who is bereaved of loved ones is sometimes very upsetting for that person. It is imperative that the health professional collecting the family history is sensitive to the past experience of the client. For some families it is hard to know what sort of illness a relative may have had. It takes a considerable amount of work to search through hospital records and collect histological evidence of different cancer illnesses. There are methods of collecting information that are not too problematic if a person is dead. These include writing to Cancer Family Registers that exist all around the UK. However, not all registers are complete and in some areas were only started in the 1970s. Collecting a death certificate is possible if the family member is prepared to pay and submit accurate information on the relative concerning her/his birth and death. Not all cancers are recorded, particularly if a person developed cancer many years before he/she died. If a relative is alive, it is essential to receive written consent before searching for information.

Dominantly Inherited Breast Cancer Susceptibility Genes

The gene *BRCA1* (breast cancer 1 gene) for breast cancer is located on chromosome 17, and was the first breast cancer predisposition gene characterized after many years of research (Miki et al., 1994). *BRCA1* mutations are linked with more than 45% of inherited breast cancers and 90% of families with broth breast and ovarian cancer. Statistical evidence shows that up to 80% of women who carry *BRCA1* mutations develop breast cancer by the age of 80 and have an estimated 15–60% risk of ovarian cancer, the risk increasing from the early thirties for breast cancer and 40 for ovarian cancer. The important information for a family is to know that this risk is distributed over a lifetime. Thus the presence of a cancer-predisposition gene increases cancer risk but does not mean that cancer will definitely develop (Figure 3.2).

The *BRCA2* gene is located on chromosome 13 and is another breast cancer predisposition gene (Wooster et al., 1994). This gene also confers an

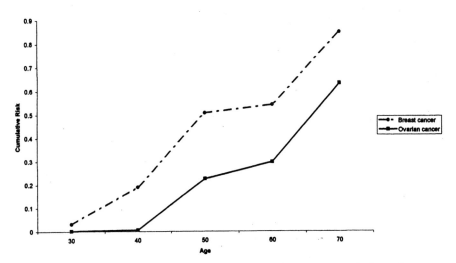

Figure 3.2: *BRCA1* Breast/Ovarian Cancer Risks. Source: Breast Cancer Linkage Consortium (1998).

increased risk of breast cancer and ovarian cancer. Both genes are dominantly inherited and can be passed down through the germ line either through the mother or the father (Figure 3.3).

Risk Assessment

Risk assessment may be divided into 'absolute risk' and 'relative risk'.

- Absolute risk: This risk refers to the frequency that a particular disease occurs in a particular group. For example, 1 in 10 women will develop breast cancer if they live to 85 in the UK.
- Relative risk: This risk compares the risk of the disease among the people who have a certain risk factor with the people that do not have this risk factor. For example a woman with a maternal history of breast cancer in several relatives is compared with a woman of the same age who has no family history of breast cancer.

The determination of which risks are meaningful and therefore contribute towards the disease depends on the latest research findings published in peer-reviewed journals. The question remains as to how many factors such as the use of the oral contraceptive in high-risk breast cancer younger women, ethnicity and age of onset of menarche alter the risk of breast cancer. True associations between risk factors and the disease being questioned are

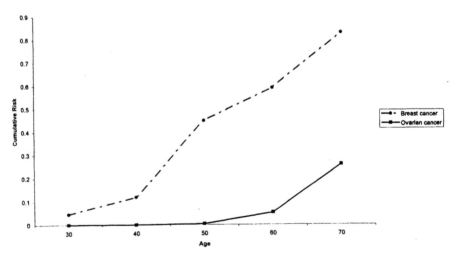

Figure 3.3: *BRCA2* Breast/Ovarian Cancer Risks. Source: Breast Cancer Linkage Consortium (1998).

usually answered by large case-control studies analysed for statistical significance (Claus et al., 1994).

The chance that breast cancer is inherited is determined by assessing the family history pattern. Both males and females can carry cancer predisposition genes and so multiple cases of breast and other cancers may occur either on the maternal or paternal sides of the family. Risk estimates for the presence of a cancer predisposition gene in a family depend on the number of cases plus the ages of diagnosis of cancer and the age of the person who is seeking advice for risk. For example, if a mother or sister develops breast cancer at the age of 35 there is a 30% chance that this is because of a genetic susceptibility. If both the mother and sister developed breast cancer at the age of 35 this then increases the chance that this was due to a gene to approximately 90% (Figure 3.4). This estimate does not identify the predisposition genes involved, and is based on epidemiological data and consulting the risk assessment tool developed by Claus (et al.) in 1994.

The breast cancer risk for a female in a high-risk family starts at the age of 30 and steadily rises until she reaches 75. In rare families this may start at an earlier age if there are younger cases. The older a family member is without developing cancer, the less likely it is that she has inherited the cancer predisposition gene. In other words, the person 'lives through their risk period' and does not develop breast cancer.

The other model used to measure breast cancer risk is the Gail model (Gail and Green, 2000). This model evaluates risk factors that include: current age, age at first live birth, number of primary relatives with breast cancer, number of breast biopsies, biopsy with hyperplasia and age at first menstruation. It does not take into account other cancers.

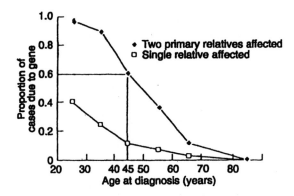

Figure 3.4: Probability curve for breast cancer (Claus et al., 1994).

Both the *BRCA1* and *BRCA2* genes are associated with an increased risk for individuals who are carriers of germ-line mutations. This estimate varies according to ethnic group and age of the individual. However, there is a significant risk of developing breast and/or ovarian cancer and family members need to be counselled accordingly.

Definitions of Hereditary, Familial and Sporadic Breast Cancers

- Hereditary breast cancer: There is evidence of high-incidence breast cancer in the first- and/or second-degree relatives. Typically early age at onset (under 45), bilateral disease. May be associated with cancer of the ovary. May sometimes be associated with other tumours.
- Familial breast cancer: Evidence of breast cancer involving one or more first- or second-degree relatives but does not fit the definition of hereditary breast cancer.
- Sporadic breast cancer: No family history of breast cancer through two generations including both sets of grandparents, parents, aunts and uncles and siblings and offspring, or limited scattering of breast cancer in older women in a family.

Classifications of hereditary breast cancers all involve pre-menopausal onset of the disease and increased risk of bilateral disease.

1. Site-specific hereditary breast cancer: Predominantly breast involvement. No other tumours present.
2. Breast/ovarian syndrome: Association of breast and ovarian cancer and BRCA genes.
3. Li-Fraumeni syndrome: Association of breast cancer with sarcoma, brain tumour, leukaemia and adrenocortical cancers. This may be associated with a mutation in the TP 53 gene.
4. Cowden's syndrome: Association of breast cancer with mouth and skin lesions and thyroid tumours. This is associated with mutations in the PTEN gene.
5. Breast/gastrointestinal syndrome association with cancers of the stomach, colon and pancreas. This could be associated in some families with a mutation in the genes responsible for Hereditary Non-Polyposis colorectal cancer or Peutz Jegher Syndrome (Goodwin, 2000).

Screening and Prevention Options for At-risk Women

There is uncertainty regarding the efficacy of screening women with a family history of breast cancer. These women may understandably have increased anxiety levels and false-positive screens may increase their fears. Reasonable screening for women in high-risk hereditary families includes the following:

(1) Breast self-examination (BSE): The evidence that this is an effective screening technique is weak in the general population. Several studies have failed to demonstrate that it impacts on mortality, stage or tumour size (Semiglazov et al., 1996; Thomas et al., 1997). There is limited evidence to suggest that in high-risk women it is an effective option (Gui et al., 2001). Women should be educated about BSE and choose whether they practise it. If done, it should be performed monthly, preferably 5–10 days after a period has finished. A trained breast care nurse should teach the procedure. Although scientific evidence is limited, there are arguments to suggest that this procedure empowers women (Lerner, 2000).

(2) Clinical breast examination: There is debatable evidence that this process is effective. However, it is generally considered a key component of screening and young women at risk should have this available from a trained health professional in a screening centre if they are at high risk. Indeed Gui et al. (2001) report in their study on younger women the effectiveness of both clinical breast examination and mammography screening.

(3) Mammography screening: Data regarding the efficacy of mammography screening comes from a series of randomized trials that were conducted in the general population. It is known that in women over the age of 50, regular mammography screening reduces breast cancer by about one-third. Mammography as a screening tool under the age of 50 years has a lower overall accuracy. The subject of screening and its value is controversial but Fieg (1996) suggests that the benefit of mammography screening far outweighs any recorded risk of radiation-induced cancer. Furthermore, there have been recent papers that suggest that screening younger women (40–50) has been found to be beneficial for those with a family history (Kollias et al., 1998; Lalloo et al., 1998). In the UK mammography screening in high-risk women does not usually start until a woman reaches the age of 35. However, in rare cases where there are very young onset cases screening may occur at an earlier age. It is recommended that mammography screening begin no earlier than the age of 30.

(4) Ultrasound and MRI: These are currently used for investigation of symptoms. Ultrasound plays a role when an abnormality is detected to differentiate between cystic and solid. There is not enough evidence to support the use of these tools as effective screening options. Currently both modalities are being evaluated in the research process for high-risk women and results will be known in a few years.

(5) Ovarian screening: This is recommended for those women with an increased ovarian cancer risk. This includes women in families where there is at least one case of breast and ovarian cancer in the family as well as those families with only ovarian cancer. This is normally performed annually and involves annual transvaginal ultrasound and an annual blood test to measure CA 125. Women who have developed breast cancer and who may be a BRCA carrier with no ovarian cancer in the family should have this arranged. Ovarian screening is currently being evaluated in a national UK study of efficacy in high-risk women.

(6) Chemoprevention: A recent overview of tamoxifen prevention trials has shown a 38% reduction in breast cancer incidence (Cuzick et al., 2003). However, this was only in oestrogen receptor positive cancers.

(7) Prophylactic surgery: The role of prophylactic surgery in high-risk breast cancer gene carriers is unproven. However, a recent study has reported that prophylactic bilateral total mastectomy reduces the incidence of breast cancer at three years' follow-up (Meijers-Heijboer et al., 2001). The Hartman et al. (1999) study suggested a risk reduction of breast cancer of at least 90% after prophylactic mastectomy.

(8) Prophylactic oophorectomy in high-risk women is thought to reduce the risk of ovarian cancer considerably from a range of 16–60% to approximately 2–3%. The risks are not reduced to exactly those of the general population because of the 2–3% risk of peritoneal adenocarcinomatosis (Rebbeck, 1999). The impact of this surgical procedure on reduction of breast cancer risk as well as ovarian cancer risk has been highlighted by Rebbeck et al. (2002) in a study of women with *BRCA1* and 2 mutations. This risk persisted beyond 10 years of follow-up and is encouraging. As this can be a keyhole surgical procedure, many women at high risk are opting after full counselling for this procedure as a preventive option.

Preventive measures rely on screening procedures to reduce death from breast cancer by picking up a tumour at its early stage of development and treating it accordingly. Familial breast cancer is usually associated with breast cancer occurring at a young age.

Anybody with a blood relative under the age of 40 with a diagnosis of breast cancer, or a family history of two relatives on the same side of the family diagnosed with breast cancer under the age of 60, is at some increased risk. Such women should be seen for early mammography screening and follow-up which can be arranged at the local screening unit through their general practitioner. Currently, the NHS provides mammography screening on a three-yearly basis between the ages of 50 and 65 years. It is not routinely offered to women under the age of 50.

Genetic Testing and Counselling

The most likely individuals to be carrying a breast cancer predisposition gene are those with a dramatic family history of breast and ovarian cancer. Those at highest risk are women with a family history of four or more cases of breast cancer at less than 60 years of age, or breast and ovarian cancer (Eeles, 1999). Others who are at high risk and may wish to be tested are families with two cases of breast cancer and one case of ovarian cancer, families with male and female breast cancer, or Ashkenazi Jewish women with breast cancer aged 40 years with or without a family history.

There are several options open to high-risk women. They may wish to consider genetic counselling and discuss in a private and confidential setting the pros and cons of genetic testing. If they choose this option an affected person with cancer in the family must be tested first, to search for the mutation that is specific to that particular family

Testing the Cancer Patient

In order to start the process of genetic testing it is the current practice to look for the alteration in the gene in the affected person. The reason for this is that in most situations only by looking in the DNA make-up of an individual who has already developed cancer is it possible to interpret the results of the genetic test for the whole family.

If an alteration in the gene is found in the affected member, unaffected family members may then be tested. The process of genetic counselling for the affected individual is essential to give the cancer patient the chance to consider all the implications of the test. It is sometimes thought that a patient who has already developed cancer may not need time to discuss all the issues. However, this is not the case and it is essential that the individual seeking counselling fully understands the risks. These risks include the development of other cancers, in particular ovarian cancer. Furthermore, there is the knowledge that if he/she is a gene carrier there is a 50/50 chance that each of the offspring may carry the same alteration. The test for the cancer patient may take anything up to six months to screen the gene in a National Health Laboratory. This current test is only 60% sensitive: many people have the test and no mutation is found, and this then becomes an uninformative result. In America genetic testing is more specific but very costly.

If a mutation is not picked up in the genetic test, this may be for several reasons:

- the wrong gene is being tested;
- the limited test (i.e. 60% specific) may have missed the mutation, as it is present in a region of the gene not tested;
- the person undergoing the genetic test developed cancer by chance alone and was unlucky rather than having an inherited gene fault, despite a strong family history. This may happen in high-risk families but of course is very rare.

The individual with cancer is given his/her genetic test result, and if nothing is found in the test he/she is informed that the test is inconclusive and the family must continue with the guidelines for appropriate screening as advised at the time of counselling. Some women find the information that no mutation has been found confusing (Hallowell, 2002) and need further time to reflect with a health professional on the limits of the test. If a mutation is identified the individual returns to meet the counsellor and is informed. The counsellor always follows up this session. Individuals vary as to how they handle the information and whom in the family they inform. This may be problematic in some families. Confidentiality is paramount within the genetic counselling programme and a professional is unable to inform the family other than through the index case. This may present problems for some families where communication has broken down.

Options Available for Families in which a Mutation is found

There is the possibility of prophylactic surgery for risk reduction. This option needs to be carefully considered with the specialists caring for the patients. The status of the cancer patient needs to be carefully considered and balanced with regard to any further surgery. It is essential that all carriers of genetic mutations should be followed up annually for the rest of their lives (Ardern-Jones and Eeles, 2002).

Predictive Genetic Testing

This test is usually carried out on someone in the family who wishes to know his or her genetic status and has not developed cancer. In this case the affected person has been tested and a mutation has been identified. It usually takes 6–8 weeks from the test date before results are given in the NHS Clinical Testing Programme. The individual has a session that includes outlining all the risks available and taking time to consider all the implications of undergoing such a test. This includes mentioning insurance issues. It is up to the patient to make all the necessary enquiries of his/her company before undergoing such a test. Time is taken to discuss the emotional implications of undergoing such a test and to check with whom the individual will have to share her/his concerns and how she/he will cope following the results. Follow-up support is always offered. Communication may well be a problem for some families as family members do not always feel comfortable informing other relatives about their gene test result (Foster et al., 2002).

This normally takes place over several sessions and time must be allowed for the person to consider all the issues of finding out her/his genetic status. The first session with the Cancer Genetics Consultant in the clinic informs the individual about all the risk estimates associated with the mutation in the family gene, and discusses the options that are available to that individual should she/he find out that she/he is a carrier of the gene. Currently the lifetime risk of developing breast cancer for an individual who carries either the *BRCA1* or *BRCA2* gene is up to 60–80%. The risk starts at the age of 30 but is very low at this age. The risk for ovarian cancers varies between 15% and 60% depending on the gene, ethnic group and previous medical history. For example, oral contraceptives taken for more than three years may reduce the risk of developing ovarian cancer (see Figures 3.2 and 3.3). These risks may be different for Ashkenazi Jewish women (Struewing et al., 1997).

It is important that the individual be aware of potential problems such as depression and anxiety, which may occur following disclosure of the genetic status. It may be that a further session is arranged before a blood sample is taken. The final session is when the results are given, and this will depend on the turnaround time for mutation analysis after the blood was taken. It is recommended that another person should attend the clinic with the patient for support. In rare cases, it is necessary to speed through this test as the results may alter clinical management (Mitchell et al., 2001).

If a predictive test is negative, the person having the test then is informed that her/his risk for cancer is that of the general population. It is not necessary for a woman who does not carry the family gene alteration to continue with early screening unless there is a history on the other side of the family. All women should practise breast awareness and arrange to take part in the National Screening Programme for those over the age of 50. If a woman or man does not carry the gene it means that she/he cannot pass it on to her/his children. In particular, some of the gene-negative persons under-going testing express disbelief or an emotion called 'survivor guilt'. These emotions need time to heal and such individuals should be followed up by the nurse (Ardern-Jones and Eeles, 1997).

Men do seek predictive testing as they have the same chance of inheriting the gene as women in the same family. It has been reported that their uptake is lower. This may be due to many factors including the fact that men do not attend health appointments so readily as women.

Ethical Issues

Ethical issues can be considered in three different categories:

1. individual rights;
2. obligations of health professionals;
3. likely conflicts between the individual's rights and others' rights.

Individual Rights

It is straightforward that an individual seeking genetic testing should have the nature of the tests and the implications of the results explained to her/him before she/he gives consent. The individual should be prepared well for the results, and for the impact that the results may have on his or her psychological well-being. Furthermore, the discussion of confidentiality and the consequences associated with the result should be made clear before testing.

Rights of Other Individuals

Should a woman or man be obliged to inform her/his family about her/his genetic status? Should she or he inform her/his partner and general practitioner about the test? There are major consequences for the family in terms of emotional burden and the implications of the risk for all first-degree relatives. The individual's right to the confidentiality of test results may conflict with the interests of employers and insurance companies. For these reasons, some people refuse the test. Currently, legislation to protect gene carriers from possible discrimination does not exist in the UK.

The Obligation of Healthcare Professionals

There are important ethical obligations for healthcare providers and policy makers with regard to the criteria for testing. They include identifying those who test positive and providing systems, personnel and training.

One of the principles of an appropriate screening test is that an effective preventive strategy is available for those testing positive for the condition. It could be argued that it is unethical to test unless one can do something about it. Currently, there are no proven preventive measures, but there are early detection options. Prophylactic surgery does not offer complete protection although it reduces risk very substantially.

When should genetic testing be undertaken? The age of adult consent in the UK is 18 years. This could be an appropriate time if a young person is interested in this option. However, there are no screening programmes available for young persons of this age. Neither ovary or mammography screening is offered before the age of 30 due to the low risk of cancer. It would be ethically essential for the young person to be counselled about not being eligible for screening at this age, and time should be taken to remind them of the normal levels of risk and the appropriate ages of screening.

Psychological assessment of the individual choosing testing is essential. The counsellor caring for high-risk women must be aware that mood disorders, anxiety and depression are common, and severe in women at risk of breast cancer.

Thus, if genetic testing is chosen, then genetic counselling must be provided. This is a multidisciplinary practice where the individual will meet the medical Consultant and have access to the Clinical Nurse Specialist in Cancer Genetics (or Genetic Counsellor) for ongoing follow-up.

Four Vignettes to Outline the Principles of Breast Cancer Genetic Counselling

(Note: All the family trees for the purpose of this chapter are fictional; see Figure 3.5.)

Family 1

The family tree comprises a woman aged 41 who has developed unilateral breast cancer, whose sister developed breast cancer aged 34. Her father is well and healthy at the age of 70. However, it transpires that his sisters developed bilateral breast cancer aged 44 and 51. There is another aunt who developed breast cancer aged 56. The paternal grandmother developed ovarian cancer at 49 and is now dead.

Q: Does the family history represent any known syndrome?
A: This family represents a family with a possible BRCA mutation.
Q: Are there any significant issues?
A: If this family has a significant risk of both breast and ovarian cancer, are all the histologies checked? For example, if the ovarian cancer was in fact uterine cancer and if the breast cancers in one of the younger cases were not cancers but benign disease this would lower the risk of there being a gene mutation present in the family.
Q: If the cancers in the family are confirmed by histology, what are the options?
A: All the females in the family should have both breast and ovarian screening on an annual basis for breast from the age of 30 and for ovary from the age of 35. Genetic testing may be arranged after full counselling on a person who has developed cancer. The person most likely to carry the mutation is the youngest person affected with cancer in the family. However, this depends on the person wishing to know her/his status. The individual with cancer having the

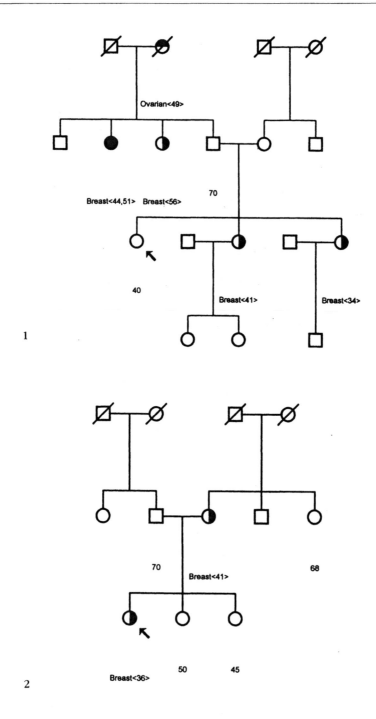

Figure 3.5: Principles of breast cancer genetic counselling.

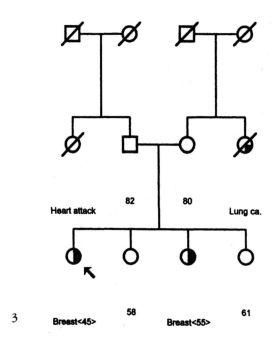

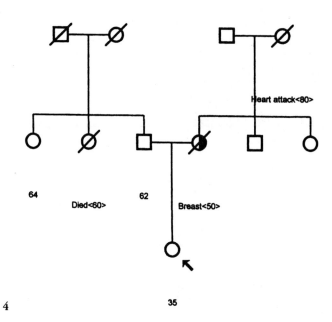

Figure 3.5: (contd)

test must appreciate that if she is a mutation carrier, she has a significant risk of another cancer developing in the other breast, and if she is BRCA carrier there is a significant risk of ovarian cancer developing. If after testing a mutation is identified unaffected members of the family may come forward for genetic testing and there is a 50/50 chance that they may or may not have inherited the gene mutation that exists in the family.

Q: What are the ethical and social implications related to this family?

A: First, it may well be that the person seeking advice with regard to genetic testing does not fully appreciate that other family members may need to be given screening advice. In some families where communication is difficult, revealing information about one's self becomes a difficult and unexpected role. The genetic nurse may have difficulty obtaining accurate information from live affected members of the family, as written consent may not be forthcoming because of barriers in the family communication system. Second, if one person has developed breast cancer and is very ill, the partner of that particular person may be very reluctant to involve the family member in genetic testing. It may then become a sensitive and very traumatic time for other members in the family who are desperate to find out more information. Third, men may not realize that their offspring are at risk of developing both breast and ovarian cancer. Fourth, there may be insurance implications, and worries and scares regarding employment issues. Fifth, the father of the daughter seeking counselling may not realize that he is a potential carrier of a gene mutation and be devastated if he finds that he is the carrier in the family who put his daughters at high risk of developing cancer. This may be problematic in a relationship. Sixth, there may be issues surrounding further surgery for the person who is only 41; i.e. if she is a gene carrier should she have prophylactic surgery on the other breast with possible reconstruction, and perhaps have her ovaries removed? All these are very serious issues and the thought of surgery versus current health status, situation and quality of life are complex and difficult decisions for someone in this situation. Finally, the worry that relates to children and their risk is always stressful for the person who has developed cancer. This is exacerbated if an experience with another family member has been traumatic and frightening. Despite being assured that young children are not at risk, family members sometimes find it hard to appreciate this knowledge in a factual light.

Family 2

In this case, the person seeking advice developed breast cancer at the age of 36 and her mother developed breast cancer at 41. There are no other recorded cancers in the family. This family has a high risk of there being a genetic factor that is causative for the development of breast cancer. This is calculated by factoring in the epidemiological data and conferring with the risk assessment tool developed by Elizabeth Claus et al. in 1994 (see Figure 3.2).

However, although there is a high genetic risk, the pattern of the cancers does not reflect a *BRCA1* or *2* gene mutation. It is highly likely that there is another gene not currently identified to explain the development of these two cancers. There could be a different explanation if the family has Jewish ancestors, as there is significant risk of BRCA mutations for younger onset cases who are of a Ashkenazi Jewish background (Struewing et al., 1997).

Q: If the gene has not yet been identified to represent this family, is it likely that the cases with breast cancer have an increased risk of developing further cancers?

A: It is unknown at this time. The thinking is that the risk for these families is related only to the onset of breast cancer; the risk of bilateral disease is unknown.

Q: As regards ethical and social issues, would you arrange genetic testing on this family?

A: Currently, such testing would not be arranged as there is not enough evidence to suggest that a mutation in the *BRCA1* or *2* genes is present and therefore it would be a waste of resources. This would alter if the patient has an Ashkenazi Jewish background.

Q: What would you recommend?

A: It would be possible to store a sample from an affected person as in the future this may become informative for the family if further genes are identified.

Q: What issues would be of concern for the unaffected members in the family?

A: The main issues relate to the appropriateness of preventive surgery and screening. As there is a 90% chance of there being a gene in the family, other family members would be informed that there is a high risk of developing the disease. If a person is very worried and seeks surgery, a test would then be arranged to check the low likelihood that there is a *BRCA1* or *2* mutation present – if the affected person consents.

Family 3

There are two sisters in a family who have developed unilateral breast cancer at the ages of 45 and 52. Two other sisters have not developed breast cancer, nor has the mother. This represents a moderate risk family. There is a 50% chance that the two women in this family developed breast cancer due to an inherited genetic predisposition. This predisposition may be polygenic. Thus there may well be several genes involved in the chance that there is an inherited predisposition. Therefore there is a 50% chance that both these women developed cancer by chance alone, and are not linked with an inherited genetic predisposition (see Figure 3.4).

One would not arrange genetic testing for unaffected members in the family as there is an extremely low likelihood of there being a *BRCA1* or *BRCA2* mutation in the family. There may well be worried people in this family who need to have the situation explained, and appropriate screening should be arranged for other women in these families. This would be reconsidered for Jewish families.

Q: My daughter is convinced that she will develop breast cancer and she wishes to have her breasts removed as a prevention option. Should she do so?

A: With the moderate level of risk for your daughter of the development of breast cancer, this would need very careful discussion with the breast surgeon and consultant geneticist. Evidence of the cancer diagnosis would need to be proved in the family and time taken to explain the genetic risk and the possibility of the chance occurrence of the cancers in the family. The long-term effects of surgery are unknown and the psychological factors underlying the fear of developing breast cancer need to be addressed. However, annual breast screening from the age of 35 is recommended. Appropriate psychological counselling may be needed to help the worried person cope with her cancer fear.

Q: Are there any other reasons why my mother and her sister both developed cancer at the age of 50?

A: If both these women were exposed to high levels of radiation for reasons of treatment, the chances may be increased that environmental reasons contributed to the development of breast cancer (Shore et al., 1986). If there are other familial influences, i.e. obesity, diet high in fat and early menarche, the risk may be increased. There are many factors that may not relate to a high-risk gene that cause two members in one family to develop breast cancer.

Family 4

This is a family with only one relative who has developed breast cancer. The young woman's mother developed unilateral breast cancer at the age of 50 and sadly died two years later. She has two sisters who are well and no other members of the family have developed cancer except an uncle who was a smoker and developed lung cancer at the age of 63.

This daughter aged 35 is very worried about her risk of breast cancer and underwent a very traumatic experience looking after her mother for many years. As the only girl in the family, she feels very vulnerable. In this case breast screening would not be recommended above what is offered to the general population because she is not at substantial increased risk. Careful explanation with regard to risk and psychological support is needed to help a woman in this situation. The nurse would need to take time to understand and help this person through a very difficult time.

In Conclusion

Risk interpretation may well be subjective, and the nurse caring for a worried family relative may need to spend time with that person exploring the many contextual reasons as to why the individual is very worried about his/her risk. It is essential not to focus on statistics but to consider the social and cultural implications in order to help women make decisions. In today's climate of rapidly developing new technology, families with a high genetic risk should have the opportunity to receive in-depth genetic counselling from experts. Thus referrals should be made to the local genetics service. Furthermore, gene carriers should be followed up annually for support and advice in a suitable clinic with both oncological and genetic expertise (Ardern-Jones & Eeles, 2002). This is a changing area of knowledge and nurses should be able to confidently reassure some women regarding their risk and refer others on either to screening services or to the local Regional Genetics Service for advice.

References

Ardern-Jones A (1997) The experience of hereditary cancer in the family. Unpublished MSc thesis, London University.

Ardern-Jones A, Eeles R (1997) Predictive gene testing for breast cancer. Trends in Urology, Gynaecology and Sexual Health January/February.

Ardern-Jones A, Eeles R (2002) Forum for applied cancer education and training – cancer genes. Management of carriers of breast cancer genes who have already developed cancer: the Carrier Clinic Model. European Journal of Cancer Care 11: 63-8.

Ardern-Jones A, Mitchell G (1999) Family inheritance. Journal of Women's Health 4, (2): 7-9.

Breast Cancer Linkage Consortium, Ford D et al. (1998) Genetic heterogenity and penetrance analysis of the BRCA1 and BRACA2 genes in breast cancer families. American Journal of Human Genetics 62: 676-89.

Claus EB, Risch N, Thompson WD (1994) Autosomal dominant inheritance of early onset breast cancer. Implications for risk prediction. Cancer 73: 643-51.

Cuzick J, Powles T, Veronesi U, Forbes J, Edwards R, Ashley S, Boyle P (2003) Overview of the main outcomes in breast-cancer prevention trials. The Lancet Vol 361 (9354): 296-300.

Eeles R (1999) Screening for hereditary cancer and genetic testing epitomised by breast cancer. European Journal of Cancer 35(14): 1954-62.

Fieg SA (1996) Assessment of radiation risk from screening mammography. Cancer 77(5): 818-22.

Foster C, Watson M , Moynihan C, Ardern-Jones A, Eeles R (2002) Genetic testing for breast and ovarian cancer predisposition: cancer burden and responsibility. Journal of Health Psychology 7(4): 469-84.

Gail MH, Green MH (2000) Gail model and breast cancer. Lancet 1999 27(354): 1846-50.

Goodwin P (2000) Management of familial cancer risk. Breast Cancer Research and Treatment 62: 19-33.

Gui G, Hogben R, Walsh G. A'Hern R, Eeles R (2001)The incidence of breast cancer from screening women according to predicted family history risk: does annual clinical examination add to mammography? European Journal of Cancer 37: 1668-73.

Hallowell N, Foster C, Ardern-Jones A, Eeles R, Murday V, Watson M (2002) Genetic testing for women previously diagnosed with breast/ovarian cancer: examining the impact of BRCA1 and BRCA2 mutation searching. Genet Test Summer 6(2): 79-87.

Hartmann LC, Schaid DJ, Woods JE, Crotty TP, Mpyers JL, Arnold PG, Petty PM, Sellers TA, Johnson JL, McDonnell SK, Frost MH, Jenkins RB (1999) Efficacy of bilateral prophylactic mastectomy in women with a family history of breast cancer. New England Journal of Medicine 340(2): 77-84.

Kollias J, Sibbering Dm, Blamey RW, Holland PA, Obuszko Z, Wilson AR, Evans AJ, Elis I, Elston CW (1998) Screening women aged less than 50 years with a family history of breast cancer. European Journal of Cancer 34(6): 937-40.

Lalloo F, Boggis CRM, Evans DG Shenton A, Threlfall AG Howell A (1998) Screening by mammography, women with a family history of breast cancer. European Journal of Cancer 34: 937-40.

Lerner BH (2002) When statistics provide unstatisfying answers: revisiting the breast self-examination controversy. CMAJ Jan 22; 166(2): 199–201.

Meijers-Heijboer H, van Geel B, van Putten WL, Henzen-Logmans SC, Seynaeve C, Menke-Pluymers MB, Bartels CC, Verhoog LC, van den Ouweland Am, Niermeijer MF, Brekelmans CT, Klijn JG (2001) Breast cancer after prophylactic bilateral mastectomy in women with a *BRCA1* or *BRCA2* mutation. New England Journal of Medicine 345(3): 159.

Miki Y, Senesen J, Shattuck-Eidens D, Futreal PA, Harshman K, Tavtigian S, Liu Q, Cohran C, Bennett LM, Ding W (1994) A strong candidate for the breast and ovarian cancer susceptibility gene, BRCA1. Science 226: 66–71.

Mitchell G, Kissen M, Ardern-Jones A Tayor R, Eeles RA (2001) Urgent genetic testing - a paradox. Familial Cancer 1: 25–9.

Office for National Statistics (1998) Mortality Statistics by Cause – England and Wales 1996, Series DH2 NO23. London: HMSO.

Rebbeck T, Lynch H, Neuhausen S, Narod S, van't Veer L, Garber J, Evans G, Isaacs C, Daly M, Matloff E, Olufunmilay I, Olapade M, Weber B (2002) Prophylactic oophorectomy in carriers of BRCA1 or BRCA2 mutations. New England Journal of Medicine 346(21): 1616–22.

Rebbeck TR, Levin AM, Eisen A, Snyder C, Watson P, Cannon-Albright L, Isaacs C, Olopade O, Garber J, Godwin A, Daly M, Narod S, Neuhausen S, Lynch H, Weber B (1999) Breast cancer risk of bilateral prophylactic oophorectomy in BRCA1 mutation carriers. Journal of the National Cancer Institute 91: 1475–9.

Richards MPM, Hallowell N, Green JM, Murton F, Statham H (1995) Counselling families with hereditary breast and ovarian cancer: a psychosocial perspective. Journal of Genetic Counselling 4(3): 219–33.

Semiglazov VF, Sagaidak VN, Moiseenko VM, Protsenko SA (1996) Preliminary results of the Russia (St Petersberg/WHO) program for the evaluation of the effectiveness of breast self-examination. Voprosy Onkologii 42: 49–55.

Shore RE, Hildreth N, Woodard E, Dvoretsky P, Hempelmann L, Pasternack B (1986) Breast cancer among women given X-Ray therapy for acute postpartum mastitis. Journal of the National Cancer Institute 77(3): 689–96.

Struewing JP, Hartge P, Wacholder S, Baker SM, Berlin M, McAdams M, Timmerman MM, Brody CC, Tucker M (1997) The risk of cancer associated with specific mutations of BRCA1 and BRCA2 among Ashkenazi Jews. New England Journal of Medicine 336: 1401–8 .

Thomas DB, Gao DL, Self DG, Allison CJ, Tayuo Y, Maholoch J, Ray R, Qin Q, Presley P, Pister P (1997) Randomized trial of breast self-examination. Cancer in Shanghai: methodology and preliminary results. Journal of the National Cancer Institute 89: 355–65.

Wellisch DK, Schain W, Gritz ER, Wang H-J (1996) Psychological functioning of daughters of breast cancer patients, Part 111: Experiences and perceptions of daughters related to mother's breast cancer. Psycho-Oncology 5: 271–81.

Wooster R, Neuhausen Sl, Mangion J, Quirk Y, Ford D, Collins N, Nguyen K, Seal S, Tran T, Averill D, Stratton M (1994) Localisation of breast cancer susceptibility gene to BRCA2 to chromosome 13Q 12-13. Science 265: 2088–90.

Bibliography

Schneider K (2002) Counseling about Cancer, 2nd edn. New York: Wiley.

Tingle J, Cribb A (eds) (1995) Nursing Law and Ethics. Oxford, UK: Blackwell Science Ltd.

CHAPTER 4

Breast Screening

LINDA LEE

Wilson and Junger (1968) first devised the principles of screening for the World Health Organisation. Any proposed national screening programme should be considered against these criteria before it is implemented. In order to consider the role of a breast-screening programme for the England, Scotland, Wales and Northern Ireland a report was commissioned by the Health Ministers of the time, which was chaired by Sir Patrick Forrest. Two previous studies were particularly to influence the outcome of the enquiry (Shapiro et al., 1982; Tabar et al., 1985). At the time of the Forrest enquiry, the evidence supporting the implementation of the programme against the criteria was as follows (Forrest, 1986):

1. *The condition being screened for should pose an important health problem.* Some 24 000 new case of breast cancer were diagnosed every year. There were 15 000 deaths annually from breast cancer.
2. *The natural history of the disease should be well understood.* Breast cancer was known to be a progressive disease with early cancer development confined to the ductal system. This is followed by an early invasive stage when the cancer cells break through the basement membrane of the ducts and there is the potential to spread to other parts of the body and produce metastases.
3. *There should be a recognizable early stage.* At the time of the Forrest report it was well established that 20% of cancers were too small to be identified by clinical examination by either the woman or a clinician but these cancers were evident on mammography.
4. *Treatment of the disease at an early stage should be of more benefit than treatment started at a later stage.* Previous studies had indicated that there was a reduction in mortality when comparing women who had attended a screening programme with those who had not been invited.

5. *A suitable screening test should exist.* The aim of a screening test is to identify those who are normal and those who may have mammographic signs of possible breast cancer. The test should be able to maximize the number of true positives (high sensitivity) and minimize the false positives (high specificity). Evidence indicated a range of 80–90% sensitivity and 95% specificity for mammography.

6. *The test should be acceptable to the population.* A test is deemed acceptable if attendance is high, particularly on repeat visits. Attendance of 60% had been achieved in previous studies but these had covered a greater age range than that intended for the UK programme. It was in women over 65 that attendance had been limited.

7. *There should be adequate facilities for the diagnosis and treatment of abnormalities detected.* Staff and facilities to provide a screening and assessment service varied across the UK. It was noted that these would need to be developed to address the needs of the programme on a national basis.

8. *For diseases of insidious onset, screening should be repeated at intervals determined by the natural history of the disease.* Evidence at the time varied and previous screening studies and trials had different intervals from 12 to 33 months.

9. *The chance of physical or psychological harm should be less than the chance of benefit.* Although the test involved ionizing radiation, the dose delivered for mammography was felt to be small enough not to pose any significant threat to the women. Concern was also expressed that women who did not have breast cancer might require an excision biopsy to establish their normality. Women might also receive treatment for a cancer that would not have become invasive and therefore life threatening in their lifetime. Finally there was a risk of psychiatric morbidity. There was little evidence to suggest that women who were returned to normal screening suffered any long-term psychological sequelae.

10. *The cost of the screening programme should be balanced against the benefits it provides.* Many factors were considered. Financial cost was considered in terms of the cost of life years gained and the Quality Adjusted Life Year (QALY) gain. Compared with other costs within the health service, breast cancer screening equated to the QALY of kidney transplantation, although being more costly than hip replacement and less costly than heart transplantations. Other factors considered were the psychological costs to the women invited and the cost of time and travel.

As a result of their deliberations, the Forrest committee, in their report of 1986, recommended the following proposal for a national programme:

- Women should be invited for screening once every three years.
- Women attending should have one view taken of each breast.
- The age range of the women invited should be from 50 to 64 years of age.

The Forrest report recognized that further work needed to be undertaken to develop and refine the national programme. They therefore recommended continued research into five specific areas:

1. number of views;
2. screening age group;
3. screening frequency;
4. natural history and treatment;
5. risk factors.

UK wide, the number of women expected to be invited within the three-year programme was 4 857 000. The recommendations of the report were accepted and in 1988 the National Health Service Breast Screening Programme was implemented. Similar programmes were agreed and implemented in both Wales and Scotland. Throughout the history of national breast screening, Wales and Scotland have acted independently of the NHS but in the main they mirror the service in the NHS.

The aim of the programme was to reduce mortality from breast cancer in the screening age group. In 1992 the Department of Health made this target more specific by stating that the programme should reduce mortality by 25% by 2000 (Department of Health, 1992). It was against this background that later discussions about the success or otherwise of the programme would occur.

Introducing the National Health Service Breast Screening Programme

The first screening mammogram was performed in England in the last months of 1988. The first centres to take part were those that had already been offering a mammography service for women with breast symptoms and had both equipment and skilled personnel in place. As was noted in the Forrest report (1986), the implications for training and educating the workforce were considerable, and supply of good quality equipment would take some time. Many programmes were therefore unable to commence until staff were trained and equipment in place. It was not until 1993 that every programme had commenced screening, and it was 1995 before every woman in the programme had received an invitation. This was later to have an impact on how the effectiveness of screening would be demonstrated in breast cancer mortality data.

Screening in Action

Identifying Eligible Women

Screening procedures differ from the normal route to investigation when a patient reports a symptom to the General Practitioner. With the breast-screening process, women invited are 'well women' and normally asymptomatic. Lists of women within the relevant age group are obtained by the screening service. The list is then sent to the general practice so that they can identify those who no longer live in the area, those who may have recently died or those who are believed not to be suitable for breast screening at this particular time. The introduction of information technology for patient records at the surgery has meant that in recent years the lists provided are more easily kept up to date and accurate.

It is important to note that women can only be removed from the lists temporarily. Women who are unable to attend at the time of invitation because of ill health can request an appointment for breast screening as soon as they are well enough to attend. They should automatically receive an invitation at the next round of screening in three years' time. In some cases women who are on follow-up for breast cancer are removed from the screening list as they are on mammographic follow-up with the surgical/oncological team.

Invitations and Written Information

All women receive a letter of invitation for screening. Women are invited for an appointed time approximately three weeks ahead. They are able to request a change of time and date, and an alternative site if they work near one unit but live near another. The design of the letter will vary to some degree between units but each should contain essential information about the invitation clearly presented (Austoker and Ong, 1994). Additional information about the process is provided by the inclusion of a leaflet, 'Breast Screening, the Facts 2001' (NHSBSP 2001a). The current format of this nationally agreed leaflet is based on research into several factors affecting women's anxiety associated with an invitation to be screened and the issue of informed consent (Austoker, 1999).

Liaison with General Practitioners

Throughout the screening process, general practices are kept informed of the key information. Whenever women are recalled for further tests, the practice is informed and advised of the likelihood of malignancy. It is then able to respond if women enquire at the surgery as to the reasons for recall.

The practice is also informed when a woman is being referred for treatment. Usually the woman is referred to the local specialist breast surgical team but if the woman or General Practitioner feels another referral pathway is more appropriate she or the practice have the right to seek a change of referral. Since the development of highly specialized breast care teams within the locality, changes of referral pattern are now rare. At the end of a screening round, practices are advised of those women who have not responded to their invitation and a note is attached to the practice notes. This alerts health professionals within the practice team, and the issue can be raised when the woman next attends the surgery.

The Screening Unit

Each breast screening unit delivers the mammography service in different ways according to the geographical area and population density. To achieve the target attendance of 75% the service needs to be easily accessed by the women invited. Most centres now combine a static unit based within a local Acute Trust with a mobile service that can be taken to rural or socially deprived areas. Mobile units are only used for the basic screening mammogram. Women with potential abnormalities will all need to attend the static screening unit for assessment (Figure 4.1).

The Basic Screening Method: Mammography

Mammography is the name given to X-ray imaging of the breast. At the present time mammography is based on the use of X-ray film and cassettes (film container). The cassette contains a fluorescent screen which when hit by X-rays converts this into light. X-ray film is very similar to photo film and although it does respond to X-rays to produce a latent image, the film responds more effectively to light. The use of an intensifying screen can reduce the dose received by patients considerably. The use of cassettes and screens in combination with film is standard practice for all basic radiography imaging.

The use of digital imaging is becoming widespread in radiology departments but as yet the quality of the image required for mammography cannot be fully reproduced with a digital system, although considerable progress has been made in the last five years. It is likely that this technique will continue to improve to a point where it is as good as plain-film mammography. However, there are now digital systems designed to be used for screening assessment. This will be referred to later in this chapter.

Mammography films/screen systems and the X-ray equipment used to produce the image are very specialized. In mammography the system needs to enhance areas of minimal contrast, i.e. the difference between fat and the

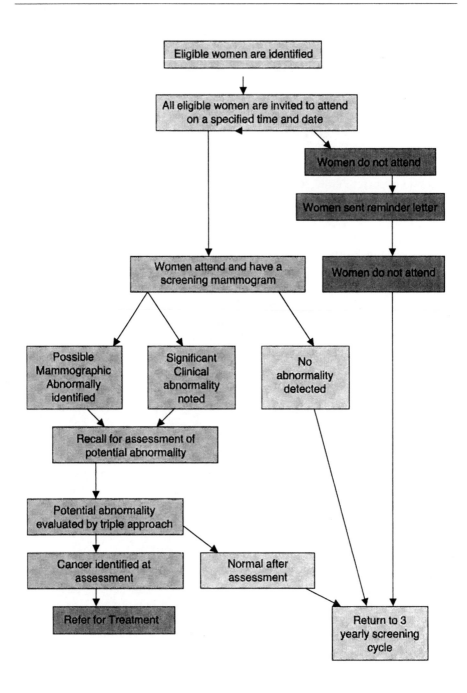

Figure 4.1: Screening process.

breast parenchyma. The inherent contrast differences between these areas are minimal when compared with differentiating between bone and soft tissue as in the majority of plain-film imaging.

The mammography equipment is also designed for ease of use for both the women attending and the radiographer. The machine is designed to rotate through 360 degrees and is able to be raised and lowered by counter-balanced and electronic drives to raise and lower the machine to suit the individual stature of the women (Figure 4.2).

Screening mammography clinics are very labour intensive. The norm is for approximately 70 appointment slots to be made available each day. One woman is invited every five to six minutes. These screening sessions take place on one machine with two radiographers performing the examination in turn. In a static unit the radiographer who is not performing the examination will put the films through the film processor and check the resultant images for quality and accurate patient identification marking. While on a mobile screening service the non-examining radiographer will perform reception duties and the films will be processed at the end of the day back at the base unit. Where more than one machine and sufficient radiography staff are available additional screening sessions can scheduled each day.

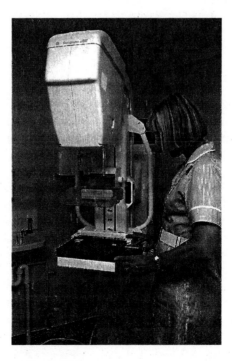

Figure 4.2: Mammography machine.

The radiographer needs to produce a high-quality examination and also make sure the women feels welcome, unembarrassed and able to make an informed choice about proceeding with the examination (Lee et al., 1995). The radiographer must also make sure that the compression to the breast is sufficient to produce a good examination on which a diagnosis can accurately be made but also that the compression is not painful for the women. If women experience extreme discomfort or pain they are less likely to return for the subsequent examination.

Compression

All mammographic examinations of the breast require that the breast be compressed during the procedure. The benefits of compression cannot be underestimated (Lee et al., 1995). Application of compression to the breast:

- reduces movement and therefore the risk of motion blur;
- brings the breast tissue nearer to the film, which increases the detail of breast tissue demonstrated;
- reduces the dose;
- ensures even X-ray penetration of the breast by equalizing the depth of the majority of tissue;
- spreads and separates the tissue to improve visualization of potential abnormities.

Positioning

As a general rule women are placed in the erect position, which helps with patient mobility and speed of examination (which is of significance in an NHS-funded programme of this type). This does not preclude, however, the possibility of imaging women who are seated. Mammography positioning requires that the whole body of the woman is placed in the appropriate position to facilitate the accurate positioning of the breast on the machine. With patients who are seated this flexibility of position can occasionally be compromised with the result that films may not be of optimal quality.

The two views now used for the Breast Screening programme and for any first attendance at a symptomatic service are the cranio-caudal projection and the lateral oblique projection. The cranio-caudal projection means that the X-ray beam is sent from the superior surface of the breast through to the inferior surface of the breast on to the film below. This position can demonstrate the majority of the breast tissue but with a very small amount excluded from both the lateral and medial borders (Figures 4.3 and 4.4).

The medio-lateral oblique projection has the X-ray beam coming from an angle of 45 degrees from the medial (upper inner quadrant of the breast) through to the lateral side (lower outer quadrant). This view is the one most

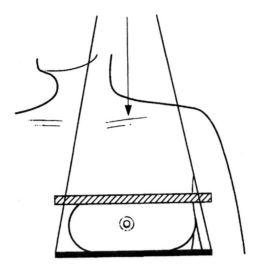

Figure 4.3: Positioning for the cranio-caudal projection. (Reprinted from Fundamentals of Mammography, 2nd edition. Lee, Stickland, Evans and Wilson (2003) by permission of W.B. Saunders.)

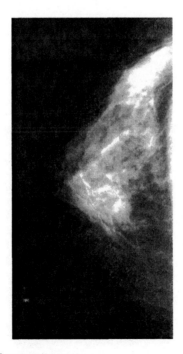

Figure 4.4: Cranio-caudal mammogram.

likely to demonstrate the whole breast tissue, and in particular the upper outer quadrant of the breast which is excluded from the cranio-caudal projection and is also the most common site for cancers to be found (Figures 4.5 and 4.6).

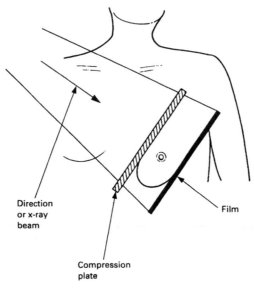

Direction or x-ray beam

Film

Compression plate

Figure 4.5: Positioning for the 45-degree medio-lateral oblique projection. (Reprinted from Fundamentals of Mammography, 2nd edition. Lee, Stickland, Evans and Wilson (2003) by permission of W.B. Saunders.)

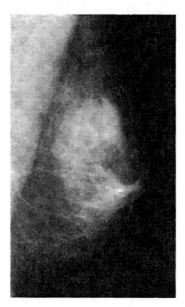

Figure 4.6: Oblique mammogram.

Film Reading

When the mammogram has been completed and checked for diagnostic quality it will need to be examined for potential abnormalities. The mammography films are loaded on to a multi-viewer. This has the capacity to hold between 70 and 150 mammographic examinations depending on the manufacturer. A film reader reviews all mammograms. The film reading process is designed to identify the women who are normal and those who have a possible abnormality. This is not a definitive report but will enable women to be:

- returned to routine screening invitation;
- recalled for further assessment.

Each examination is identified as within the one of five categories:

1. benign;
2. probably benign;
3. indeterminate;
4. probably malignant;
5. malignant.

Women in category 1 will not require recall; > 90% of women attending for screening should be in this category. Women who are in categories 2 to 5 will be recalled for screening assessment. The categorization will also help in identifying the pathway of care on reaching the screening assessment clinic.

Screening Assessment

There should be only two outcomes from screening assessment:

- return to routine screening invitation;
- refer for treatment.

In the early days of the screening programme the use of early recall (between six and 12 months) was comparatively common. Research indicated that the psychiatric morbidity associated with early recall was detrimental to the well-being of women attending and all screening centres are encouraged to eliminate this as an outcome (Ong and Austoker, 1997; Ong, Austoker and Brett, 1997). There will inevitably be one or two cases where this will occur but these should be less than 1% of women screened.

When the Forrest (1986) and Pritchard (1988) reports were published, the role of the multidisciplinary team and the use of the triple approach were recommended. The triple approach refers to the use of the three modalities used to differentiate accurately between benign and malignant. These are (1) imaging (mammography and ultrasound), (2) clinical examination and (3) cyto/histopathology.

When a woman is recalled for screening assessment the imaging characteristics of the abnormality will define which investigative techniques will be employed to determine the nature of the abnormality. Various procedures can be performed and these are outlined below.

Additional Mammography

Within the assessment clinic one of the options available for patient work-up is additional mammography. This can comprise additional views, paddle views and magnification views. A paddle or localization view will require the replacement of the normal full field compression plate with one of approximately three inches in diameter. The potential abnormality is measured from the film and the compression applied to the appropriate area of the breast. If an abnormality is real, it will be demonstrated on the resultant film. If it appeared coincidentally, it will disappear on compression (Figures 4.7 and 4.8).

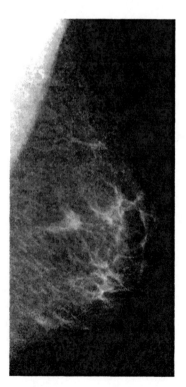

Figure 4.7: Potential solid mass.

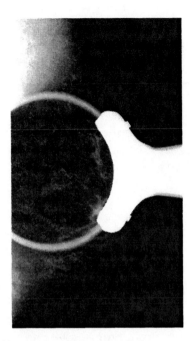

Figure 4.8: Mass spread by compression – normal tissue.

Magnification views are mainly used to examine areas or specks of micro-calcification more closely. These can signify early malignant disease or ductal carcinoma in situ, or can be produced by normal breast processes. The differentiation between these two is obviously critical. Magnification can also be combined with the use of the three-inch compression device. This will clarify the situation where there is a potential parenchymal deformity with associated micro-calcification.

Ultrasound

Ultrasound is a non-invasive procedure that is painless and does not use ionizing radiation. It is an invaluable tool for work-up of a potential abnormality in breast screening and in the symptomatic service. A mass can be examined to see whether it is solid, fluid filled or mixed. Appearances on ultrasound are not definitive and any mass confirmed as solid will require cytology or histopathology. Ultrasound is particularly useful for estimating the size of a lesion as accurate measurements can be taken.

As the quality and sensitivity of ultrasound equipment have improved the procedure is very useful in identifying invasive disease including both masses and parenchymal deformities. High-frequency ultrasound can also demonstrate calcification but this is a coincidental finding and ultrasound has not yet been demonstrated to be sufficiently sensitive to be able to detect ductal carcinoma in situ. Ultrasound cannot be used as a screening tool as examining both breasts thoroughly is time consuming and lacks specificity.

Clinical Examination

Not all women receive a full clinical examination. Women who have a potential abnormality on mammography that proves to have been superimposition shadowing on paddle compression will be discharged after imaging. The role of clinical examination in the screening situation is twofold:

1. to examine all women who are about to undergo needle biopsy. Examination of women post-needle biopsy is compromised by haematoma;
2. to examine women who have reported a significant clinical sign to the radiographer or when the radiographer has noticed a significant clinical sign while performing the original screening mammogram.

Approximately 5% of cancers are occult and are not demonstrated on a mammogram. The noting of symptoms is therefore a small but significant factor within the programme.

Fine-needle Aspiration Cytology and Core Biopsy

These are two techniques that are regularly used in screening assessment to establish the nature of a confirmed abnormality. Fine-needle aspiration cytology was widely used in the first years of the programme. More recently automated core biopsy devices have been developed. This has resulted in the increasing use of core-cut biopsy over the last five years, and the use of fine-needle aspiration has declined. The degree of use of these two tests will vary according to local practice. However, the main benefits of core biopsy are that it can indicate invasive disease, which helps in deciding on the treatment required and in cases of micro-calcification will demonstrate inclusion of the calcification, which confirms the accuracy of the test. In a screening situation these tests are generally performed under X-ray or ultrasound guidance.

Methods of core biopsy and fine-needle aspiration biopsy

Even in the case of women who have been recalled for a reported clinical abnormality the lesion will be sampled by imaging whenever possible. This ensures accuracy as the site of the needle can be identified. Ultrasound is the more desirable technique, as women are supine throughout the procedure reducing the risk of syncope. The abnormality and the needle can be seen in real time providing greater accuracy of sampling. Ultrasound is therefore used for palpable abnormalities, parenchymal deformities and masses detected in mammography.

In the case of micro-calcification stereotactic (X-ray guided) localization will be used. This requires a special add-on attachment to be placed on the mammography machine. This attachment enables images to be taken while the woman is seated at the machine and check images can be taken while the sampling is taking place. In the past this equipment was film based, requiring additional time while images were processed. In the last few years digital imaging systems have been developed for this procedure, reducing the time women spend seated at the machine. The images are produced on a monitor within the mammography room almost instantaneously. This allows adjustment of the needle position and increased accuracy of sampling. The samples taken from the breast are also imaged to ensure that calcification has been included in the specimen.

A few units within the UK have a prone table biopsy system. This is beneficial for the patient because if she is prone throughout she cannot see the procedure as it is being performed and therefore is less likely to suffer from syncope. However, these units are extremely expensive and a large amount of space is taken up by a machine that cannot be used for anything except invasive procedures. The upright add-on system more commonly used means that the equipment can be used for both screening and assessment. Bearing these factors in mind it is unlikely that prone tables will be adopted throughout the service.

Diagnostic Excision Biopsy

The screening process can proceed up to the point of diagnosis; this means that if a preoperative diagnosis is not achievable by needle biopsy technique, it will be necessary for the woman to undergo a diagnostic excision biopsy. Owing to the recent aggressive sampling of identified lesions with core biopsy techniques, the potential to accurately identify a malignant lesion is greatly improved, and the need to resort to operative procedures has been reduced. The target for benign biopsy is less than four per thousand women screened. In the Breast Screening Programme Annual Review (NHSBSP, 2001b) for the years 1999–2000 the achieved rate was 0.7 per 1000 women screened.

Quality Assurance

Subsequent to the Forrest report (1986), another document was produced called the Pritchard Report (1988). This outlined the need for extensive training and education for the radiographers and radiologists and supported that the programme should be based on several quality assurance principles. The quality assurance (QA) mechanism is one of the great strengths of the programme and in the Calman Hine report (Calman and Hine, 1995), QA in the NHSBSP was raised as an exemplar of practice that should be applied in a wider health service arena. There are now numerous NHSBSP publications to underpin the quality of the service. These relate to the technical aspects of the programme, the call and recall system, guidance for quality assurance visits and guidance for each professional group involved in the programme. All these publications should be available within each breast-screening unit, at the local Quality Assurance Reference Centre and from the National Coordinating Office in Sheffield (www.cancerscreening. nhs.uk).

The programme is subject to rigorous and regular monitoring of a variety of factors. The full details of the standards and targets for the programme are available in the majority of NHSBSP publications. Each standard relates to one of the domains defined in 'The New NHS: Modern and Dependable' (DoH, 1998):

- fair access;
- effective delivery of appropriate healthcare;
- efficiency;
- patient/user experience;
- health outcomes of NHS care. (NHSBSP, 2001b)

Updating the Breast Screening Programme

Screening Age Group

Over 65

The age group selected by the Forrest report (1986) after due consideration of the evidence was 50 to 64. In the previous studies women of 65 and above had not attended when invited for breast screening. In the NHSBSP women over 65 were not excluded from breast screening but were not sent a specific invitation to be screened. Women over 65 were able to refer themselves to the screening unit for an appointment via their GP.

Women are now living longer, many to 85 years and above. With this increase in life expectancy, women between 65 and 70 would benefit from regular mammography screening. The women in this age group have already participated in the screening programme while they were between the ages of 50 and 64. A demonstration study was commenced in 1996 within three centres in England: Nottingham Breast Screening Service; East Sussex, Brighton and Hove Breast Screening Service; and Leeds and Wakefield Breast Screening Service. The results of the study were reported in 2001 (Moss et al., 2001). The study established that attendance rate for women in this age group was 71% and that overall a programme offered to women in this age group was as beneficial as the existing programme for women of 50 to 64. As a result the NHS and Cancer Plans (DoH, 2000a and 2000b) stated the intention to extend invitations for routine screening to women up to 70 years of age. This change to the programme will be implemented across England by 2004.

Number of Views

The Forrest report (1986) suggested a one-view screening technique. This had been based on the results of the previous studies. The NHS Breast Screening Programme was therefore funded on this basis. Some centres, however, adopted two views at the first visit, the prevalent screen, whereas others opted to perform two views at both prevalent and incident screens. The units that took this path had to identify the additional funding locally.

In 1995 research (Wald et al., 1995) indicated that the number of cancers detected at the prevalent round was increased in units that used two views at each visit. As a result of this research the NHSBSP was adjusted so that all women had two views at the prevalent screen. Further research ensued (Blanks et al., 1997; Blanks et al., 1998) and in the NHS and Cancer Plans a two-view policy was announced for all women at all visits. This change will be implemented across the country by 2003.

Contentious Issues

Over the years several aspects of the breast-screening programme have been subject to adverse comment.

Authors (Baum et al., 1995; Baum 1996) have suggested that the cost of the programme far outweighs any benefits and that the money would be better spent on improving treatment. The process of detection would then rely solely on reported symptoms via the GP. Treatment has improved considerably and is improving life expectancy for women, but the recent paper by Blanks (2000) clearly demonstrates that screening is beginning to have a direct impact on mortality rates. As some programmes did not complete their first screening round until 1995 the full effect of breast screening on mortality is unlikely to be demonstrated until 2005.

Over-treatment

Within the screening programme a large number of cases of ductal carcinoma in situ are detected. The detection of DCIS in the screening programme can lead to a mastectomy in patients where those who are demonstrated to have small invasive tumours may have a wide local excision. DCIS may or may not ultimately lead to invasive disease depending on its grade and the sojourn time. Women who are treated with a mastectomy for low-grade DCIS may never develop invasive disease but will live with the knowledge that they have cancer for their lifetime. The nature and progression of ductal carcinoma in situ into invasive disease is not clear and continues to be the subject of considerable research.

Interval Cancers

These are cancers that are detected between the three-yearly screening invitations. There are three main categories of interval cancers:

- the true interval which, despite a review of previous mammography examinations, shows no evidence at the previous visit;
- the false negatives which, on review of the previous examinations, showed some evidence of a malignant process that was not detected at the previous visits;
- the occult cancer, which is detected after referral from the GP and confirmed on clinical examination alone and which is not evident on the current or previous mammographic examinations.

The majority of interval cancers occur in the third year after screening. A research study, referred to as the Frequency Trial, examined the issue of the screening interval. The results of this trial have not yet been published. Many of the amendments to the programme implemented in recent years should have an impact on the number of interval cancers. Research continues into the false-negative mammogram and will inform clinical practice (McCann et al., 2001).

Ages 40 to 49 years

The incidence of breast cancer within this age group is lower than that of women of 50 and above (Figure 4.9). The breast is more likely to be dense mammographically and identifying a small cancer more difficult. Several studies have been reviewed and further studies undertaken, regarding a screening programme in this age group. To date there is insufficient evidence to suggest that a national programme would bring similar benefits to those offered by the current programme for women between 50 and 70. Research continues in this area.

Anxiety Associated with the Screening Process

A large number of papers have examined the issue of anxiety raised by the invitation to screening attendance (Ellman et al., 1989; Fallowfield et al., 1990; Sutton et al., 1995; Steggles et al., 1998; Aro et al., 1999), and anxiety

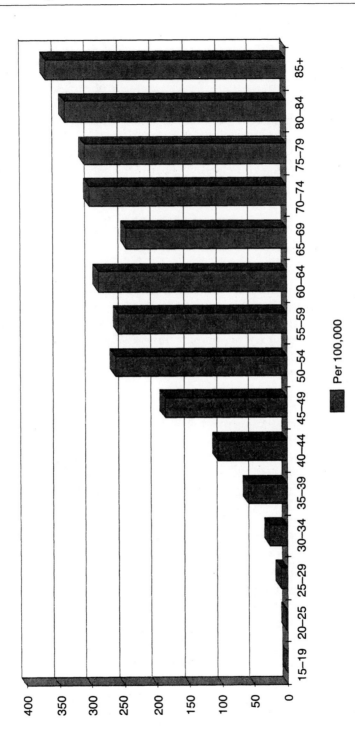

Figure 4.6: Breast cancer incidence according to age.

relating to recall for assessment (Sutton et al., 1995; Ong and Austoker, 1997; Rimer and Bluman 1997; Scaf-Klomp et al., 1997; Brett et al., 1998; Pisano et al., 1998; Steggles et al., 1998; Aro et al., 2000). It is clear that anxiety does exist and it is the responsibility of every member of staff within the service and those in general practice to try to alleviate some of the symptoms of anxiety. All staff within a breast-screening unit should have excellent communication skills, in particular those of effective listening and empathy. Each member of the clinical team needs to have an awareness of the potential impact of the screening and assessment process on the women attending.

Nurse's Role

Breast Care Nurses

Since the beginning of the programme the need for good quality psychological support has been recognized. In the early days of the programme specialist breast care nurses were not available for the majority of services. In recent years it has become essential practice to provide good emotional support for women attending for screening assessment (Ong and Austoker, 1997). The role of the breast care nurse has developed over this time and all units have the benefit of a breast care nurse to a greater or lesser extent (NHSBSP, 1998).

In the assessment clinics, breast care nurses are those who have been trained to have a greater understanding of the psychological impact of recall, and in particular are well versed in the impact of a malignant diagnosis and options available to women in terms of treatment and psychological support. In many assessment clinics, nurses come into contact with the women when they first attend the clinic. They are therefore a familiar face when women receive the final results of their diagnosis, and can not only provide emotional support and guidance at that time but also continue to be available for women on an ongoing basis throughout their treatment. Many women are affected by the diagnosis of cancer some time after initial treatment, as well as at the point of diagnosis. Continuity of patient care is invaluable and the role of the breast care nurse will continue to influence that care for the women who attend the programme.

Ward Nurses

Nurses on a general ward may be asked about the programme, as women in the ward for other clinical problems may be unable to attend their screening appointment. The ward nurse can provide information on how to rearrange this appointment after the current episode of care is complete.

Nurses in General Practice

Nurses in all areas of practice can be a source of valuable information on the NHSBSP. The Practice Nurse needs to be well informed so that she can discuss the programme with women who attend nurse-led clinics. She can provide them with information on the suitability of the programme for them, and why the NHSBSP is aimed at this group and not others. In addition, she can encourage those who have not attended on invitation to reconsider their decision.

When women are recalled for assessment the nurse may be approached for information on why this is the case. The nurse can explain that being recalled may not signify the presence of malignant disease but simply that the situation is unclear.

References

Aro AR, de Koning HJ Absetz P, Schreck M (1999) Psychological predictors of first attendance for organised mammography screening. Journal of Medical Screening 6(2): 82-8.

Aro HR, Polvikki Absetz S, van Elderen TM, van der Ploeg E et al. (2000) False positive findings in mammography screening induces short-term distress - breast cancer specific concern prevails longer. European Journal of Cancer 36(9): 1089-97.

Austoker J (1999) Gaining informed consent for screening. Is difficult - but many misconceptions need to be undone. British Medical Journal 319(7212): 722-2.

Austoker J, Ong G (1994) Written information needs of women who are recalled for further investigation of breast screening: results of a multi-centre study. Journal of Medical Screening 1(4): 238-44.

Baum M (1996) The breast screening controversy. European Journal of Cancer 32A(1): 9-11.

Baum M, Querci della Rovere G, Benson JR, Warren R et al. (1995) Screening for breast cancer, time to think-and stop? Lancet (North American Edition) 346(8972): 436-9.

Blanks RG (2000) Effect of the NHS breast screening programme on mortality from breast cancer in England and Wales, 1990-8: comparison of observed with predicted mortality. British Medical Journal 321(16 September): 665-9.

Blanks RG, Given-Wilson RM, Moss SM (1998) Efficiency of cancer detection during routine repeat (incident) screening: two view versus one view mammography. Journal of Medical Screening 5(3): 141-5.

Blanks RG, Moss SM, Wallis MG (1997) Use of two view mammography compared with one view in the detection of small invasive cancers: further results from the National Health Service breast screening programme. Journal of Medical Screening 4(2): 98-101.

Brett J, Austoker J, Ong G (1998) Do women who undergo further investigation for breast screening suffer adverse psychological consequences? A multicentre follow-up study comparing breast screening result groups five months after their last screening appointment. Journal of Public Health Medicine 20(4): 396-403.

Calman K, Hine D (1995) A Policy for Commissioning Cancer Services. A Report by the Expert Advisory Group on Cancer to the Chief Medical Officers of England and Wales. London: Department of Health.

Department of Health (1992) The Health of the Nation: A Strategy for Health in England. London: HMSO.

Department of Health (1998) The New NHS: Modern and Dependable. A National Framework for Assessing Performance. London: DoH.

Department of Health (2000a) The NHS Cancer Plan. A Plan for Investment, A Plan for Reform. London: DoH.

Department of Health (2000b) The NHS Plan. A Plan for Investment, A Plan for Reform. London: DoH.

Ellman R, Angeli N, Christians A, Moss S, Chamberlain J, Maguire PP (1989) Psychiatric morbidity associated with screening for breast cancer. British Journal of Cancer 60: 781-4.

Fallowfield LJ, Rodway A, Baum M (1990) What are the psychological factors influencing attendance: non attendance and attendance at a breast screening centre. Journal of the Royal Society of Medicine 83(9): 547-51.

Forrest APM (1986) Breast Cancer Screening: Report to the Health Ministers of England, Wales, Scotland and Northern Ireland. London: HMSO.

Lee L, Stickland V, Roebuck EJ, Wilson ARM (1995) Fundamentals of Mammography. London: WB Saunders.

McCann J, Britton PD, Warren RML (2001) Radiology peer review of interval cancers in East Anglian breast screening programme: what are we missing? Journal of Medical Screening 8(2) 77-85.

Moss SM, Brown J, Garvican L, Coleman DA, Johns LE, Blanks RG, Rubin G, Oswald J, Page A, Evans A, Gamble P, Wilson R, Lee L, Liston J, Sturdy L, Wardman G, Patnick J, Winder R (2001) Routine breast screening for women aged 65-69: results from evaluation of the demonstration sites. Journal of Cancer 85(9): 1289-94.

Ong G, Austoker J (1997) Recalling women for further investigation of breast screening: women's expediencies at the clinic and afterwards. Journal of Public Health Medicine 19(1): 29-36.

Ong GJ, Austoker J, Brett J (1997) Breast screening: adverse psychological consequences one month after placing women on early recall because of a diagnostic uncertainty. A multicentre study. Journal of Medical Screening 4(3): 158-68.

Pisano ED, Earp J, Schell M, Vakaty K, Denham A (1998) Screening behaviour of women after a false positive mammogram. Radiology 208: 245-9.

Pritchard Report (1988) Quality Assurance Guidelines in Mammography. NHSBSP

Rimer BK, Bluman LG (1997) The Psychological Consequences of Mammography. Journal of the National Cancer Institute Monographs No 22.

Scaf-Klomp W, Sanderman R, van de Wiel HBM, Otter R, van den Heuval WJA (1997) Distressed or relived? Psychological side effects of breast cancer screening in the Netherlands. Journal of Epidemiology and Community Health 51(6): 7705-10.

Shapiro S, Venet W, Strax P, Venet L (1982) Ten- to fourteen-year effect of breast screening on mortality. Journal of the American Cancer Institute 69: 349-55.

Steggles S, Lightfoot N, Sellick SM (1998) Psychological distress associated with organised breast cancer screening. Cancer Prevention and Control 2(5) 213-20.

Sutton S, Saidi G. Bickler G, Hunter J (1995) Does routine screening for breast cancer raise anxiety? Results from a three wave prospective study in England. Journal of Epidemiology and Community Health 49: 413-18.

Tabar L, Fagerburg CJ, Gad A, Baldentorp L Holmburg LH, Grontoft O et al. (1985) Reduction in mortality from breast cancer after mass screening with mammography. Randomised trial from the breast cancer screening working group of the Swedish National Board for Health. Lancet i: 829–32.

Wald N, Murphy P, Major P, Parkes C, Townsend J, Frost C (1995) UKCCCR multicentre randomised controlled trial of one and two view mammography in breast cancer screening. British Medical Journal 311: 1189–93.

Wilson JMG, Junger G (1968) Principles and Practice of Screening for Disease, WHO Public Health Paper 34. Geneva: World Health Organisation.

NHSBSP Publications

NHSBSP (2001a) Breast Screening: The Facts. Health Promotion England in Conjunction with NHS Cancer Screening programmes.

NHSBSP (2001b) Breast Screening Programme: Annual Review .

NHSBSP (2001c) Clinical Guidelines for Breast Screening Assessment, Publication No 49.

NHSBSP (1998) Quality Assurance Guidelines for Nurses in Breast Screening, Publication No 29.

CHAPTER 5

Surgery as a Treatment for Breast Cancer

VICTORIA HARMER

Introduction

The treatment of breast cancer often involves lengthy and complex procedures that require a high level of holistic nursing care. During cancer treatment patients face a number of challenges, both physical and emotional, some of which can be ameliorated through the use of the appropriate techniques (Harmer, 2000a).

All patients should be discussed at multi-disciplinary team (MDT) meetings to ensure the treatment suggested is the result of an informed consensus.

Most management plans for breast cancer will involve some form of surgery for local control of the disease (Harmer, 2000b). Surgery may be the first treatment modality used, or it can follow systemic treatments, chemotherapy or hormone therapy. Surgery can also be performed after radiotherapy has been given, although this may mean that postoperative healing will be slower.

There are clinical and pathological features of breast cancer that influence the type of surgery used. These features include the position and size of the cancer, the size of the host breast, the completeness of any initial excision, the histological grade, a young patient (under 35 years), the presence of an extensive in situ component, and lymphovascular invasion (Sainsbury et al., 2000).

Breast-conserving Surgery

Breast-conserving surgery is considered to be a more complex treatment than a mastectomy for breast cancer. This is because a separate incision is required for axillary lymph node dissection and postoperative radiotherapy is always recommended (Butler Nattinger et al., 2000).

Even if a cancer is suitable for breast-conserving surgery, a patient should be given a choice of operation. Survival rates are equal whether a patient has a mastectomy or breast-conserving surgery followed by a course of radiotherapy, (providing certain pathological criteria are met), in order to sterilize the tumour bed. Some people prefer to have the whole breast removed and therefore may not require daily radiotherapy lasting for many weeks. For others, the thought of losing their breast when it is not necessary would seem totally alien.

Women treated for breast cancer by breast-conserving surgery who do not have radiotherapy have local recurrence rates of 35% after twelve years (Fisher et al., 1995).

Excision Biopsy (see Fig 5.1a)

If a patient has a suspicious but non-conclusive triple assessment examination (clinical examination, imaging, cytology and/or core biopsy) of a breast lump, an excision biopsy may be required, which entails removal of the lump under general anaesthetic. The specimen can then be sent to the histology

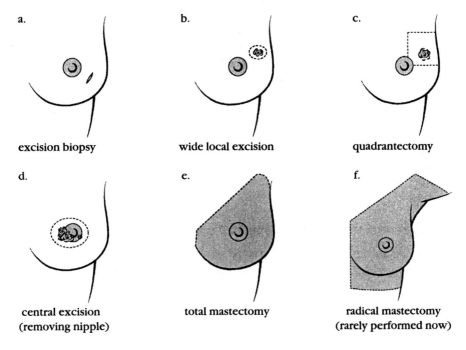

| a. | b. | c. |
| excision biopsy | wide local excision | quadrantectomy |

| d. | e. | f. |
| central excision (removing nipple) | total mastectomy | radical mastectomy (rarely performed now) |

Axillary procedures may or may not be carried out with any of the above breast procedures except radical mastectomy, which always includes axillary clearance

Figure 5.1: Operations for breast cancer.

department and analysed. If the lump is confirmed as breast cancer, a second operation is usually necessary so that good margins can be taken from around the lump, and some form of axillary lymph node surgery takes place.

Needle Wire Localization for Impalpable Breast Lumps

Some cancers are detected through screening investigations. The percentage of these screen-detected non-palpable breast cancers has risen from 5% in the early 1980s to 30% presently. This is due to the NHS Breast Screening Programme, which followed the Forrest Report (1986) and the fact that diagnostic methods have become more refined (Costa and Zurrida, 1998).

To assist in the surgical removal of these cancers (usually the first modality of treatment for screen-detected breast cancers), needle wires need to be placed to identify the location of these impalpable breast lesions. Thus the wire can guide the surgeon to the area to be removed.

A few hours pre-operatively, a radiologist will identify the location of the breast cancer using either ultrasound waves or X-rays. Local anaesthetic will be injected into the skin of the breast, so the procedure is minimally painful. The tip of the needle wire will then be inserted into the centre of the breast cancer, with the wire long enough to come out of the skin. The accurate placement of the wire is crucial. The radiologist will have been guided by micro-calcification seen on the mammogram or a suspicious shadow on ultrasound. The wire is then securely taped and the patient can return to the ward until the operation takes place.

The needle wire can then guide the surgeon and the correct piece of breast tissue can be removed. A specimen X-ray should be taken post-operatively, showing the tip of the wire and the cancer. Many screening units require a copy of this X-ray for their files.

Some breast units localize impalpable cancer by injecting it with a radioactive isotope (Luini et al., 1999).

The Importance of Clear Margins in Breast Cancer Surgery

In order for breast-conserving treatment to be successful, a margin of about 1 cm of normal breast tissue around the cancer must be excised. If there is in situ or invasive disease at the margin of the specimen removed from the breast, the local recurrence rate is increased. The completeness of excision is the most important factor influencing local recurrence after breast conservation surgery (Sainsbury et al., 2000).

In some cases, a patient may require a second operation once the histopathologist has examined the specimen if the margins of normal tissue are too small. This usually involves the surgeon opening the original excision wound, and excising a sliver of breast tissue from the margin required.

In a minority of cases the surgeon may realize that much more breast tissue needs to be removed in order to completely excise the cancer with good margins. A mastectomy may then be recommended to the patient.

There are studies at present discussing the value of magnetic resonance imaging (MRI) in determining clear margins for breast cancers. Some hospitals, within trial conditions, perform an MRI scan after the wide local excision while the patient is still anaesthetized. By doing this, it is hoped that where cancer or in situ disease persists in the breast at the margin of the excision, this will show up during the scan and the surgeon can therefore remove a sliver more from that margin. It is hoped this will stop the need for a second operation.

Wide Local Excision (Figure 5.1b and Figure 5.2)

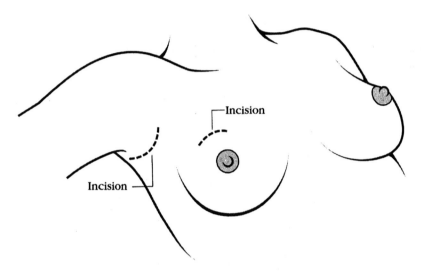

Figure 5.2: Appearance after wide local excision and axillary lymph node dissection.

This is the removal of the cancer with its surrounding tissue. Although there is no size limit for breast-conserving surgery, breast units tend not to offer this surgery to women with cancers over 4 cm because of poor cosmetic outcomes. In addition, randomized trials comparing breast-conserving surgery with mastectomy as treatments for breast cancer have never included breast cancers over 4 cm; some surgeons therefore suggest that breast-conserving surgery has not been adequately tested in larger tumours.

There is no age limit for breast-conserving surgery, although radiotherapy must always be given to the remaining breast tissue (Sainsbury et al., 2000). Possible exceptions for giving radiotherapy include small low-grade node-negative cancers that have been excised with good margins, or tumours in older women (> 55 years) who have undergone quadrantectomy rather than wide local excision.

If the cancer is found directly behind the nipple this operation is referred to as a central excision, which often includes removal of the nipple thus giving a poorer cosmetic result but one that the patient may still prefer to mastectomy (Figure 5.1d).

Quadrantectomy (Figure 5.1c)

When a quadrant of breast tissue is removed, cosmetic results are poorer. The resulting deficit is bigger than that following wide local excision, so a patient may be given the option of a mini-flap reconstruction. This reconstructive operation usually takes place one week after the quadrantectomy, to ensure surgical margins are checked and cancer free.

During this second reconstructive operation, part of the latissimus dorsi muscle is accessed and turned with its blood supply to the front to fill breast volume.

An axillary node clearance should accompany a quadrantectomy, and this may take place at the time of the mini-flap operation as it is thought to be technically easier.

Contraindications to Breast-conserving Surgery

Breast-conserving surgery may not be recommended by the medical team. This may be due to many factors:

- if there is a large breast cancer volume to breast volume ratio, which would result in a poor cosmetic result and noticeable breast asymmetry;
- if radiotherapy has been given to that breast previously;
- if there are diffuse, suspicious micro-calcifications over a large area of the breast;
- if the disease is multi-focal (i.e. there is more than one breast cancer in the same breast);
- if the breast cancer were located centrally to the breast, as the cosmetic result of breast-conserving treatment would be poor;
- if the patient with breast cancer was in the first half of pregnancy, as radiotherapy cannot be given as adjuvant treatment.

Treatment plans should always be discussed in partnership with the patient so that an agreed trajectory can be established.

Table 5.1: Characteristics of breast cancers that indicate an increased risk of local recurrence post breast conservation surgery

Feature	Description
Extensive component in situ (EIC)	In situ component forming > 25% of main tumour mass
Involved excision margins	Histological evidence that the surgeon has cut through the cancer when excising the lump
Presence of vascular and/or lymphatic invasion	Histological evidence of cancer within the blood vessels or lymphatic system
Young age	Being diagnosed with breast cancer under the age of 40 increases the chance of local recurrence

Source: Adapted from Leinster et al. (2000).

Mastectomy (Figures 5.1e and f and Figure 5.3)

About 30% of all breast cancers are unsuitable for breast-conserving surgery and require a mastectomy. Some women opt for a mastectomy rather than for the 'package' of breast-conserving surgery and radiotherapy, as they feel daily hospital treatments interfere too much with the activities of daily living, either the travelling distance to the radiotherapy centre is too great, or they want to avoid the chance of a re-excision in order to clear margins.

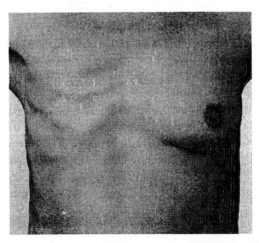

Figure 5.3: Appearance after a total mastectomy. Photo by Richard Davies.

Radiotherapy is, however, sometimes required post-mastectomy. Criteria for post-mastectomy radiotherapy vary between different centres, but generally include high-grade, large cancers with vascular involvement, and/or positive lymph nodes (particularly a high number of positive lymph nodes).

A mastectomy is usually the recommended surgical option for men diagnosed with breast cancer because the breast is small and clearance more difficult.

The most common mastectomy is the total mastectomy. This refers to the total removal of breast tissue, including the tail of Spence, which extends into the axillary space (Roses, 1999). It incorporates an ellipse of skin that includes the nipple.

In a modified radical mastectomy, the pectoralis minor muscle is removed or divided to enable the surgeon to clear the axillary nodes fully (see Figure 5.4 for anatomy and physiology breast revision diagram).

A subcutaneous mastectomy that leaves the nipple intact may be performed, especially as part of a reconstructive operation. If this is the case, there can be no guarantee that all of the breast tissue has been removed. The procedure is therefore not commonly recommended for most breast cancer patients (Leinster et al., 2000).

Mastectomy for invasive breast cancer should always be combined with some axillary node surgery.

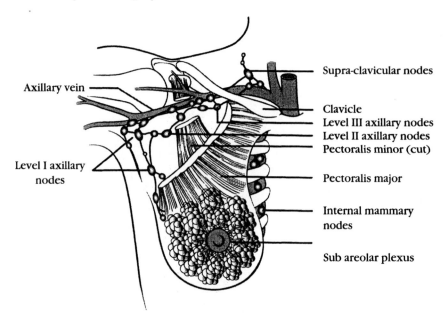

Figure 5.4: Anatomy and physiology breast revision.

Neoadjuvant Chemotherapy

Chemotherapy may be offered as the first treatment modality if the primary breast tumour is thought to be large (above 3 cm).

Following chemotherapy, there may be a sufficient reduction in the size of the breast cancer to then offer breast-conserving surgery and radiotherapy rather than mastectomy.

Trials have shown that neoadjuvant chemotherapy does not improve survival compared with patients who receive chemotherapy post-operatively but can downstage the tumour allowing more patients to have breast-conserving surgery which appears to be safe, effective and improves a person's quality of life (Stebbing and Gaya, 2001).

Breast Cancer Recurrence

If a patient has previously had breast-conserving surgery and develops a local recurrence, a mastectomy would usually be advised as treatment. The breast cancer has shown itself to be aggressive and resistant to treatment and should be dealt with accordingly. Wound healing may take longer if radiotherapy has previously been given.

If the patient has previously had a mastectomy and develops a local recurrence, radiotherapy can be used to the skin flaps in addition to further surgical resection. However, radiotherapy can only be used radically once, so if it has been used previously a re-excision of the skin flaps and systemic treatment may be offered. If the breast cancer has recurred extensively within the skin flaps a skin graft may be required when re-excision takes place.

Extensive skin recurrence is a potentially serious situation and may herald systemic disease.

The Axilla

How the axilla is treated has remained controversial for the last 50 years, and treatment has varied from hospital to hospital with lymph nodes being sampled, cleared or irradiated.

It is probable that all surgery for breast cancer will include surgery to the axillary lymph nodes. There are about 20–30 axillary lymph nodes in each armpit, which form part of the lymphatic system draining fluid and infection from the breast. The lymph nodes do not serve as an adequate anatomical barrier to the spread of cancer and are often the first place where breast cancer metastasizes (Harmer, 2000b). However treated, the cancer status of the lymph node remains the single most important and powerful prognostic factor, and one on which to base treatment decisions as it shows the potential

of the disease to metastasize (Bundred et al., 2000; Reintgen et al., 2000; Whitworth et al., 2000).

Lymphatic Mapping and Sentinel Node Biopsy in Breast Cancer

The process of sentinel node biopsy was first reported in breast cancer by Krag et al. (1993) using a radioactive isotope. Giuliano et al. (1994) used a blue dye to map this process, and with its development the success at finding the sentinel node has reached well over 95%.

The sentinel node is identified as the lymph node that drains and receives fluid first from the area of the breast that has the tumour. It is the most likely lymph node to contain metastatic cancer (Figure 5.5 shows sentinel node spread).

A sentinel node biopsy is minimally invasive, and its examination by frozen section is thought to be an accurate and reliable predictor in determining axillary lymph node cancer status at the time of operation (Jansen et al., 1998; Rodier et al., 2000; Badwe and Mittra 2001; Veronesi et al., 2001). By using this technique, it is thought that many women with primary breast cancer could avoid being over-treated by an axillary node clearance bearing in mind the morbidity this carries with it (Beechey-Newman, 2002).

Two hours prior to surgery, or thereabouts, a radioactive isotope is injected around the breast cancer by the surgeon. A blue dye is also injected 5–10 minutes prior to axillary exploration. The optimal technique is the use of this combination (McIntosh and Purushotham, 1998). The theory is that, once injected, the dye and radioactive material will be drawn through the breast to the lymph nodes downstream. Thus when the surgeon opens the

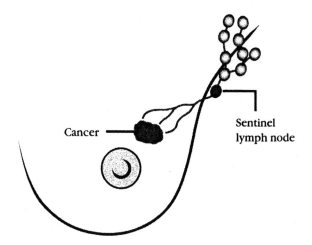

Figure 5.5: Sentinel node spread.

axilla during the operation, a blue lymph node will be visible, which also concentrates the radioactive particles by phagocytosis. This node is the sentinel node: the first lymph node to receive fluid from that area of the breast where the breast cancer is. This sentinel node can then be removed and sent to the histopathology laboratory for analysis as a frozen section. The surgical team, in the meantime, can be operating on the breast until they are given the pathology findings on whether cancer was found in the node. Many surgeons choose to wait until the sentinel node is examined by paraffin section as this may entail further surgery if the results are positive.

If there is cancer found in the sentinel node, the surgeon may choose to perform an axillary node clearance or give radiotherapy to the axilla.

Post-operatively some care should be taken with the arm which has had the nodes sampled, to avoid trauma and prevent infection, although this needs not be as meticulous as if the patient had all the lymph nodes removed.

If cancer is not found in the sentinel node, the surgeon may remove a further three lymph nodes from around that area.

Pre-operatively the patient must give her/his consent for both procedures.

Nurses should be mindful if a patient has returned from a sentinel node frozen section and has required an axillary node clearance. Once patients realize their cancer has spread to the lymph nodes, depression and distress may well occur because if lymph nodes contain cancer, chemotherapy is often offered as a treatment modality.

The downside to the sentinel node biopsy technique is that it demands a close working relationship between the clinical physics department, the surgical team and the histopathologist. This may not be a realistic situation in some hospitals. The probe used to detect radioactivity is expensive and requires use from a skilled operator constantly performing the technique to ensure confidence and competence.

The sentinel node biopsy remains a relatively new technique, and one that is ultimately successful in identifying the 'first station' lymph node in 98.4% of patients and has a false-negative rate of 4.4%, when metastastic lymph nodes will remain untreated in the axilla (Krag et al., 2001). It must also be noted that there is a variation in the institutional, and individual surgeon's, ability to define and identify sentinel lymph nodes. A learning curve can be illustrated.

Breast cancers that present in the inner quadrant of the breast may drain and therefore metastasize first to the internal mammary nodes. If this is the case, excising the axillary lymph nodes may not result in complete staging.

Although currently thought to be state-of-the-art, it is expected that sentinel node biopsy will take its place as standard treatment in future years (Whitworth et al., 2000). It offers a major advance in treating the node-negative population who therefore escape possibly needless axillary surgery

(Reintgen et al., 2000). However, many controversial issues need be resolved prior to this happening.

In the era of non-palpable screen-detected breast cancers, this technique allows treatment and assessment of the axilla while sparing the potential problems associated with an axillary clearance, as most women with screen-detected breast cancers do not harbour metastasis in the downstream lymph nodes (Badwe and Mittra, 2001).

There should be a careful selection process for patients undergoing sentinel node frozen sections. People with larger sized or multi-focal breast cancers may not be appropriate for this technique. Treatment must be individualized.

Axillary Node Clearance

Axillary lymph node clearance is usually indicated if a patient has a large or multi-focal breast cancer.

Axillary clearance may be to any of the three levels of lymph nodes (see Chapter 1 and Figure 5.4). A clearance should strip the fascia from the walls of the axilla below the axillary vein, while preserving the long thoracic nerve and thoracodorsal bundle. With a level three clearance the chance of significant lymphoedema is 10% (Leinster et al., 2000).

If an axillary node clearance has been performed, the patient should be informed that care should be taken against infection and trauma of that arm for the rest of her/his life, in order to reduce the chance of lymphoedema.

It is emerging that lymphoedema is a lifelong risk for patients who undergo axillary surgery with or without radiotherapy, rather than a sequela of treatment, which develops soon after initial surgery or radiotherapy (MacLaren and Harmer, 2002).

Nurses can assist greatly with a patient's compliance with 'arm care' by reinforcing the following recommendations. For instance, after a clearance, a patient should not have blood pressure taken on the affected arm nor should blood be taken from the arm, venflons inserted or injections into it. Nurses can make things easier for patients by having the knowledge of what to do and what not to do. Some hospitals give patients who have had this surgery 'credit cards', which state why invasive procedures cannot be carried out on affected arms. This is a helpful reminder and piece of teaching apparatus for healthcare professionals.

For many patients who experience the development of lymphoedema, it heralds a lifetime of ongoing management and attention to a medical condition, which can be disruptive to daily activities (MacLaren and Harmer, 2002). It is therefore vital to try to prevent it.

More information on lymphoedema and 'do's and don'ts' of post-axillary node clearance is available in Chapter 11.

Axillary Recurrence

An axillary recurrence following previous surgery should be rare. If it does happen, repeat surgical axillary intervention should take place. Adjuvant systemic treatment can be appropriate, although reported experience is limited (Roses, 1999). Radiotherapy can also be given, although the addition of radiation to axillary surgery increases the risk of subsequent lymphoedema.

Complications of Breast Surgery

Seroma Formation

It is normal for haemo-serous fluid to collect post-operatively at the site of excision. Fluid collects where there is a space following tissue removal and it will continue to do so until the underlying tissues adhere. This is why post-operative closed suction drainage is used. The appropriate drains are inserted if a patient has had an axillary clearance, a wide local excision or a mastectomy. They are removed at various post-operative intervals according to hospital policy, surgeon's preference, and the volume they have drained over a 24-hour period. It is quite usual, however, for serous fluid to collect after removal of the drain. Depending on the amount that has collected, a surgeon or specialist nurse may aspirate this fluid on a regular basis, before the body then reabsorbs it. Undrained seromas could become infected and are uncomfortable. The nurse should explain that these seromas are common and, apart from the inconvenience of drainage, are not important.

Infection

As with all surgery, there is the possibility of infection after breast surgery, although this is rare. This should be treated according to hospital policy and antibiotics prescribed. Care should be taken if this occurs as patients may experience psychological problems in addition to pain and fever, reacting to how their body image is affected by such a personal part of the body becoming infected.

Flap Necrosis

This occurs when the skin flaps post-mastectomy become necrotic and may follow if the skin is pulled too tight on closure. It is rare and more often occurs in heavy smokers or older patients. The necrosis due to impaired blood supply may resolve with regular dressings but occasionally the necrotic skin may need to be excised, and there is the additional possibility of skin grafts being required.

Cording

This may occur post-lymph-node surgery due to fibrosis or thickened lymph or blood vessels. Cording causes pain and a decrease in arm mobility. It is through exercise that cording can be treated (see Chapter 6).

Timing of Surgery Treatment for Primary Breast Cancer in Relation to the Menstrual Cycle

There have been many retrospective studies over the last 13 years to assess whether there is any relationship between the menstrual phase and the timing of the surgical intervention for primary breast cancer that will impact on disease-free and overall survival rates.

Some evidence suggests that survival is improved if surgery is performed during the luteal phase of the cycle (Veronesi et al., 1994).

Much of the literature is contradictory, and there are shortcomings in the data, but there is still no conclusive evidence to lead us to time breast surgery according to the phase of the menstrual cycle (Hortobagyi ,2002).

Nursing Care

Pre-operatively

Ward nurses play a vital role in the patient's surgical experience. They must assess the health needs of the individual and form a foundation for all decision-making and problem-solving activities concerned with care.

Nurses must continually assess how the patient's state of health may be influencing her/his level of dependence, giving the ability to pitch nurse intervention at the correct level.

The nurse's main aim pre-operatively must be to ensure a safe environment for the patient. This means identifying any allergies and administering regular required medication according to the prescription chart. The nurse must also ensure baseline observations (temperature, blood pressure, pulse, respiration, oxygen saturation) are recorded, detecting any abnormalities that may delay the operation.

Hospitals will have a pre-operative integrated care pathway that should be followed and noted. This will ensure, among other things, that the patient is correctly dressed for the operation; that nail varnish, jewellery and prostheses are removed; and that the correct size of anti-thrombotic stockings is worn. These stockings decrease the chance of a deep vein thrombosis, a potential problem for patients undergoing surgery. They give legs graded compression to encourage the complete emptying of vein segments, thereby decreasing pooling and venous stasis.

Nurses must also ensure a patient undergoes a period of starvation and fluid deprivation, which is a medical and legal requirement prior to an anaesthetic, except in cases of emergency.

Boore (1978) demonstrated that the provision of information before surgery lowers anxiety levels, reduces stress, decreases pain and promotes a better and quicker recovery. A nurse must appreciate this and assist to her/his best ability.

Post-operatively

The post-operative period contains the potential for many problems. The most important task is to check that the patient's airway is clear and that oxygen is given if prescribed. Mouth care is extremely important for patient safety and comfort. Blood is often present after an endotracheal intubation. If the patient is unable to drink water, the nurse should use mouthwash and foam sticks to sweep the mouth, gums and teeth, removing any blood or debris. Petroleum jelly should be applied to dry, rough or chapped lips.

Observations (temperature, pulse, blood pressure, respiration and oxygen saturation) should be performed regularly and according to hospital policy. Any abnormalities should naturally be reported.

Pain should be assessed regularly and analgesia administered swiftly.

Dressings should be checked regularly for post-operative bleeding and any blood on the dressing marked and monitored. Vacuum suction drains should be labelled and checked regularly. These drainage bottles will be removed in time, according to the amount drained, the surgeon's preference and hospital policy.

Nurses should ensure that patients are safe, clean and comfortable while dependent. As a patient becomes less dependent, nurses should be guided by her/him as to what care is required.

It must be remembered that the nurse does not only care for the patient, although this must be the focus. Post-operatively it is vital that the nurse informs the patient's chosen family and friends of patient progress.

When a patient comes to a post-operative outpatient clinic the nurse should be sensitive, as the patient may not have looked at the breast following surgery. The nurse must also be aware that the patient may be awaiting pathology results and discussions regarding the next step in the treatment trajectory. The breast specialist nurse should be informed of any unseen events.

Breast Prosthesis

It is important for every woman who has had a mastectomy to be fitted with a breast prosthesis prior to discharge home so that her dignity and confidence is maintained.

Temporary Prosthesis

The first prosthesis a woman will be fitted with is a soft, foam breast form. This will be gentle next to the skin while healing takes place. These prostheses either sit inside the empty cup of a bra or, because they have a cloth cover, they may be pinned at the appropriate level to the inside of a vest or shirt.

The temporary breast prosthesis is often called a 'comfy' or 'softy'. It is obviously lighter than the natural breast, so symmetry is often a problem, and bra straps may need to be adjusted to compensate for this. The bra strap on the side of the bra with the natural breast should be tightened so that the breast is lifted and aligned with the lighter side where the prosthesis is situated.

Permanent Silicone Breast Prosthesis

Eight weeks after mastectomy, an appointment is usually made for the patient so the breast care nurse can fit a more natural-looking prosthesis. A permanent silicone prosthesis is heavier than the temporary one, so when it is in the bra it looks more natural.

The patient should bring a correctly fitting cotton bra, preferably a sports bra, and a plain-coloured, tight-fitting T-shirt, so that the profile can be seen and a good match to the natural breast found (bras and swimwear will be discussed later in this chapter).

Thankfully there are many manufacturers of breast prostheses, so the range is wide. Different companies produce different-shaped prostheses, some more ptotic, some with extra silicone at the sides to fill any deficit of tissue and some that adhere to the chest wall.

Adhesive prostheses can be used six months post-mastectomy, or six months post-radiotherapy to the chest wall. Although they are recommended for use with a bra, some smaller breasted women feel able to use them without a bra. The chest wall first needs to be prepared by using a toning liquid to remove dead skin cells and thus provide a good surface for the prosthesis to stick to. When the prosthesis loses its adhesion (some say up to three days later) it is removed and cleaned with a special cleanser and brush. Some companies have developed a system of stickers to adhere the prosthesis to the chest wall. Once the adhesion has gone, the sticker needs be removed and replaced with another sticker. These adhesive prostheses are especially useful for women who enjoy healthy physical lives.

Breast prostheses are available in different colours, and this subject must be approached with care. Some women are most offended when faced with a brown breast form, and others upset if faced with a prosthesis for Caucasian-coloured skin. It is a sensitive subject and one that can be most surprising.

The prosthesis appointment presents an ideal opportunity to assess the patient's body image, coping mechanisms and support network. Each time a woman has a breast prosthesis appointment, it is a perfect time to reassess her psychologically and socially.

Permanent breast prostheses should last for at least a year; however, if a woman's weight fluctuates she will need to be refitted.

Made-to-measure Silicone Prosthesis

If a woman's chest wall is notably uneven, possibly as a result of a previous infection, a made-to-measure prosthesis may be required. An appointment will be made with a specialist from the company at which a 'normal' prosthesis will be fitted and measurements and notes of areas where extra silicone is needed will be made. This can be effective in 'filling in' or 'building up' parts of the chest wall. The end result is a prosthesis which has added parts that should fit the wearer comfortably and safely. These prostheses are more expensive than others and take about three months to be made.

Prosthetic Nipples

Although all breast prostheses have a nipple built into them, some women prefer to wear a prosthetic one. These can be bought from specialist companies, or made in some hospital surgical appliance departments. Those from companies tend to look generic and are stuck on to the breast form using special adhesive. The nipples that are made in hospital departments look much more realistic, although the process of making them can sometimes be thought to be distressing. First, a plaster cast of the natural nipple is taken and silicone used to make the shape of the nipple. The nipple will then be painted to match the natural side. These are also stuck on using adhesive.

Nipples can also be tattooed or reconstructed (see Chapter 7).

Choosing a Bra after Breast Surgery

The breast care nurse should give bra advice to women who have had breast surgery. Some feel they could not bear to wear a bra after breast surgery; others feel a bra is very supportive. There are no rules for this and each woman should do what is comfortable for them.

It is advisable for women to be measured correctly and fitted by a trained bra fitter. This should ideally take place pre-operatively, although if time does not allow for this some department stores have fitters trained to measure women for bras after breast surgery. An easy solution is to advise the purchase of a bra one size larger around the girth. This will compensate for any swelling that may occur, and ensures that the bra is not too tight where it may be painful.

Underwired bras are really not advised, as the wire may dig into skin around the operation site, which may be numb. Underwired bras are also not advised if radiotherapy is to be given, as a reaction may be caused if the wire irritates fragile skin.

The best choice of bra is a soft cotton sports bra. The bra should ideally have wide, padded, adjustable shoulder straps, a high neckline, a wide rib band underneath the cups, at least two hook fastenings, and good separation between the cups. This not only gives support to women who have had parts of their breast removed but can also contain a breast prosthesis safely.

A long-line bra or corselette is suitable after breast surgery.

Pocketed Bras and Swimwear

The majority of women find that following mastectomy they are able to wear an ordinary well-fitting bra. Some prefer the security of a pocketed bra, especially if they have a very active lifestyle.

Swimwear is slightly different. If a woman uses a breast prosthesis for swimming she needs pocketed swimwear. There is enough competition, so the swimwear can be elegant and fashionable. Some high street stores are also introducing a range of pocketed swimwear. Although the front of the costume/bikini needs to be firm and supportive, the back can be stylish and flattering.

Breast prostheses used for swimming are usually of the lighter variety, so that the weight of the water behind the prosthesis does not pull the costume.

Adapting Bras

Women who prefer the security of a pocketed bra can adapt their own current bras. They can buy and sew in soft cotton pockets bought from department stores.

Bias binding or ribbon can adapt a bra, with strips sewn from top to bottom of the cup and the prosthesis sitting behind.

It is important for nurses to discuss this information with patients. The patient must be empowered and confident in the way she dresses as well as feeling secure and comfortable.

Palliative Surgery

If a patient has a systemically advanced or locally advanced breast cancer, surgery may still be required. This is mainly the case for patients with fungating lesions. These are breast cancers that have grown extensively, ulcerating the breast with usually little systemic spread. Mastectomy is the operation of choice, although skin-flap coverage is often an issue as much of the skin of the breast will need to be removed. Clearance of the cancer by mastectomy for a fungating lesion is usually short lived, as recurrence may quickly occur on the chest wall. Radiotherapy may be an option at this point. The relief from debulking a fungating lesion is intense, preventing bleeding, smelling and the necessity for dressings. (More information on fungating wounds can be found in Chapter 12.)

Psychological Issues and Breast Cancer Surgery

There are many potential psychological issues that someone with a breast cancer diagnosis could experience at any time during her/his cancer journey. Care and support should be given to enable patients to cope with this huge, potentially life-threatening diagnosis, as well as with the treatment modalities and their side effects.

There is much literature that is confusing and contradictory regarding the psychological issues of surgery for breast cancer. Women may feel disfigured after surgery, or may feel euphoric that treatment has begun and see life in a different way having had a 'brush' with death.

There is also contradicting information at play in some cases: women who have breast-conserving surgery may be less affected psychologically and quicker to resume sexual relationships than those who have had a breast removed. Other research shows no difference in psychological issues between women who have had breast-conserving surgery and those post-mastectomy, underlining the fact that survival from cancer is the major concern.

Women can be extremely worried about the response of their partner to their surgery. Partners are also anxious about how they will respond. On the one hand, a partner may want to initiate sex and this may be considered insensitive, whereas if a partner does not initiate sex the person with breast cancer may feel unattractive and undesirable (Love, 2000).

In spite of the varied responses, nurses can help people psychologically following surgery for breast cancer. There is no way of telling when people with breast cancer will choose to voice their deepest concerns, although strangely they sometimes confide in the most junior nurses who lack experience. The nurse must know her limitations and that expert help is available.

It is hoped that this chapter, along with Chapter 15 (Psychological Issues for the Person with Breast Cancer) will give information to nurses about this treatment modality and its possible effects.

Surgery has a crucial role in the treatment of breast cancer. All practitioners should be continually striving to achieve the highest possible standard in the delivery of care. It is with the involvement of the multidisciplinary team that the individual treatment trajectory is planned and executed in partnership with the patient and carers.

Nurses must be vigilant and offer appropriate support throughout this treatment as its effects can have tremendous personal impact.

References

Badwe RA Mittra I (2001) Sentinel node biopsy in breast cancer. Lancet 357(23 June): 2054.

Beechey-Newman N (2002) Sentinel node biopsy in primary breast cancer. International Journal of Clinical Practice 56(2): 111-15.

Boore J (1978) Prescription for Recovery. London: Royal College of Nursing.

Bundred NJ, Morgan DAL, Dixon JM (2000) Management of regional nodes in breast cancer. In Dixon JM (Ed) ABC of Breast Cancer, 2nd edn. London: BMJ Publishing.

Butler Nattinger A, Hoffmann RG, Kneusel RT, Schapira MM (2000) Relation between appropriateness of primary therapy for early-stage breast carcinoma and increased use of breast-conserving surgery. Lancet 356 (34 September): 1148-53.

Costa A, Zurrida S (1998) The future of breast cancer surgery. Oncology in Practice 3: 8-10.

Fisher B, Anderson S, Redmond C, Wolmark N, Wickerham DL, Cronin WM (1995) Re-analysis and results after 12 years of follow-up in a randomized clinical trial comparing total mastectomy with lumpectomy with or without irradiation in the treatment of breast cancer. New England Journal of Medicine 333: 1546-61.

Forrest APM (1986) Breast Cancer Screening: Report to the Health Ministers of England, Wales, Scotland and Northern Ireland. London: HMSO.

Giuliano AE, Kirgan DM, Guenther JM, Morton DL (1994) Lymphatic mapping and sentinel lymphadenectomy for breast cancer. Annals of Surgery 220(3): 391-8.

Harmer V (2000a) Symptom control for breast cancer. Nursing Times 96(50): 38-9.

Harmer V (2000b) The surgical management of breast cancer. Nursing Times 96(48): 34-5.

Hortobagyi G (2002) The influence of menstrual cycle phase on surgical treatment of primary breast cancer: have we made any progress over the past 13 years? Journal of the National Cancer Institute 94(9): 641-3.

Jansen L, Nieweg OE, Valdes Olmos RA, Rutgers E J, Peterse JL, de Vries J, Doting MH, Kroon BB (1998) Improved staging of breast cancer through lymphatic mapping and sentinel node biopsy. European Journal of Surgical Oncology 24(5): 445-6.

Krag DN, Weaver DC, Alex JC, Fairbank JT (1993) Surgical resection and radiolocalization of the sentinel lymph node in breast cancer using a gamma probe. Surgical Oncology 2(6): 335-9.

Krag DN, Harlow S, Weaver D, Ashikaga T (2001) Radiolabelled sentinel node biopsy: collaborative trial with the National Cancer Institute. World Journal of Surgery 25(6): 823-8.

Leinster SJ, Gibbs TJ, Downey H (2000) Shared Care for Breast Disease. Oxford: Isis Medical Media.

Love SM (2000) Dr Susan Love's Breast Book, 3rd edn. USA: Perseus.

Luini A, Zurrida S, Paganelli G, Galimberti V, Sacchini V, Monti S, Veronesi P, Viale G, Veronesi U (1999) Comparison of radioguided excision with wire localization of occult breast lesions. Br J Surg 86(4): 522–5.

MacLaren J, Harmer V (2002) Breast cancer related lymphoedema: a review of evidence based management. CME Cancer Medicine 1(2): 56–60.

McIntosh SA, Purushotham AD (1998) Lymphatic mapping and sentinel node biopsy in breast cancer. British Journal of Surgery 85(10): 1347–56.

Reintgen D, Giuliano R, Cox CE (2000) Sentinel node biopsy in breast cancer: an overview. Breast Journal 6(5): 299–305.

Rodier JF, Routiot T, Mignotte H, Janser JC, Bremond A, David E, Barlier C, Ghnassia JP, Treilleux I, Chassagne C, Velten M (2000) Lymphatic mapping and sentinel node biopsy of operable breast cancer. World Journal of Surgery 24(10): 1220–5.

Roses DF (1999) Breast Cancer. Philadelphia, PA: Churchill Livingstone.

Sainsbury JRC, Anderson TJ, Morgan DAL (2000) Breast cancer. In Dixon JM (Ed) ABC of Breast Diseases, 2nd edn. London: BMJ Publishing.

Stebbing JJ, Gaya A (2001) The evidence-based use of induction chemotherapy in breast cancer. Breast Cancer 8(1): 23–37.

Veronesi U, Galimberti V, Zurrida S, Pigatto F, Veronesi P, Robertson C, Paganelli G, Sciascia V, Viale G (2001) Sentinel lymph node biopsy as an indicator for axillary dissection in early breast cancer. European Journal of Cancer 37(4): 454–8.

Veronesi U, Luini A, Mariani L, Del Vecchio M, Alvez D, Andreoli C, Giacobone A, Merson M, Pacetti G, Raselli R, Saccozzi R (1994) Effect of menstrual phase on surgical treatment of breast cancer. Lancet 343(8912): 1545–7.

Whitworth P, McMasters KM, Tafra L, Edwards MJ (2000) State-of-the-art lymph node staging for breast cancer in the year 2000. American Journal of Surgery 180(4): 262–7.

CHAPTER 6

Physiotherapy for Patients with Breast Cancer

HELEN MACLEOD AND PAULINE KOELLING

Introduction

This chapter will look at the role of the physiotherapist in the management and treatment of the patient with breast cancer. Particular attention will be paid to the input the physiotherapist has in the acute phase following certain types of breast surgery, and the latter part of this chapter will focus on physiotherapy for patients with metastatic breast disease.

Physiotherapists may be involved in the treatment of breast cancer patients at any stage of their disease. Newly diagnosed patients are often treated with a combination of surgery, radiotherapy and chemotherapy. As a result of this, patients frequently require physiotherapy intervention. Following breast surgery patients can experience problems with pain, limited shoulder movement and lymphoedema. Radiotherapy to breast tissue can cause soft tissue fibrosis, resulting in movement limitation and lymphoedema. Chemotherapy can lead to general debility. Physiotherapists' knowledge of anatomy and normal movement makes them ideally suited to treating this group of patients.

Progressive breast disease can result in bone, brain, lung or liver metastases. Patients present with a variety of symptoms affecting their mobility and respiratory function, and may benefit from assessment and treatment by a physiotherapist. Again, they may undergo a combination of treatments as they enter the palliative phase of their disease, and the physiotherapist should take a holistic approach towards the patient.

Physiotherapy and Breast Surgery

Referral Criteria

Not every patient undergoing breast surgery will need to be seen by a physiotherapist, as more minor surgery is unlikely to cause problems.

Appropriate referrals include:

- axillary intervention, i.e. axillary lymph node dissection, axillary sampling and sentinel lymph node biopsy;
- mastectomy, i.e. simple, modified radical and subcutaneous;
- reconstructive surgery, i.e. myocutaneous flap repair and tissue expander.

Inappropriate referrals include:

- lumpectomy, wide local excision without axillary dissection;
- wire localization and excision biopsy;
- implant exchanges;
- mastopexy.

Patients are usually seen by the physiotherapist from the first post-operative day, although pre-operative assessment would be useful in some cases, e.g. patients with pre-existing mobility or shoulder problems. This may be difficult, however, due to limited access to patients pre-operatively and limited resources in staffing levels. Seeing patients at pre-admission clinics would be ideal, as this would allow the physiotherapist an opportunity to assess the patient's pre-operative range of shoulder movement and discuss any history of joint problems and their current level of function. This might necessitate early referral to other members of the multidisciplinary team if there are issues relating to safe discharge planning following surgery.

It appears to be well documented that 'After surgical intervention for breast carcinoma, the most frequent problems are oedema of the ipsilateral upper extremity and shoulder dysfunction' (Wingate, 1985). This is particularly the case when radiotherapy is also given as part of the patient's treatment regime. However, there is even less literature to support the role of active physiotherapy in the prevention and treatment of problems following radiotherapy. It is an area in need of further investigation, and this chapter is based on the current practice of the physiotherapy service at the Royal Marsden Hospital in London and Surrey.

Aims of Physiotherapy following Breast Surgery

Post-operative physiotherapy should seek to:

- minimize pain;
- increase shoulder range of movement;
- maintain soft tissue extensibility;
- return the patient to her/his pre-operative level of function.

Arm Exercise Regime

- Set A – from day 1, short lever exercises (to minimize the stress placed on the surgical incision during the movement).

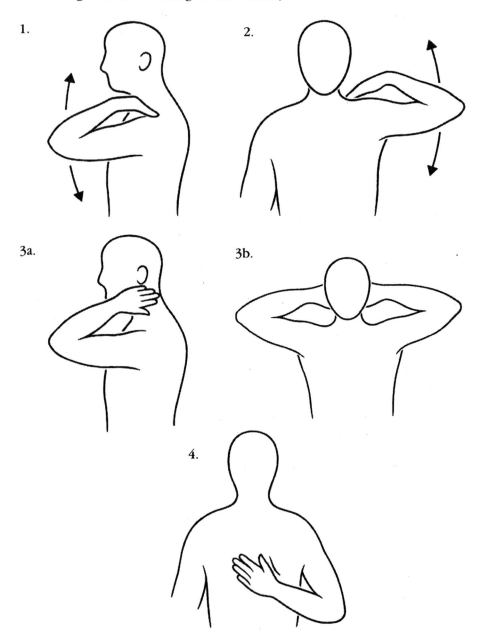

Figure 6.1: Set A arm exercises.

- Set B - following removal of drains, long lever exercises (to increase shoulder range of movement).
- Set C - (page 106) following removal of sutures/clips or at 10-14 days if sutures are dissolvable, end of range sustained stretches in supine (to stretch the soft tissues around the shoulder and chest wall).

These exercises should be performed within a pain-free range.

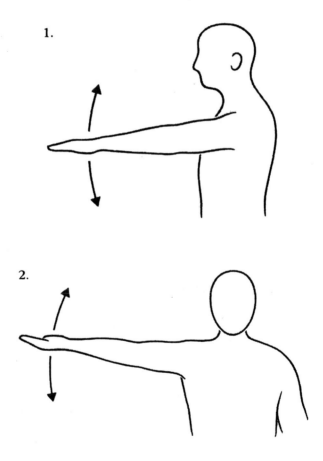

Figure 6.2: Set B arm exercises.

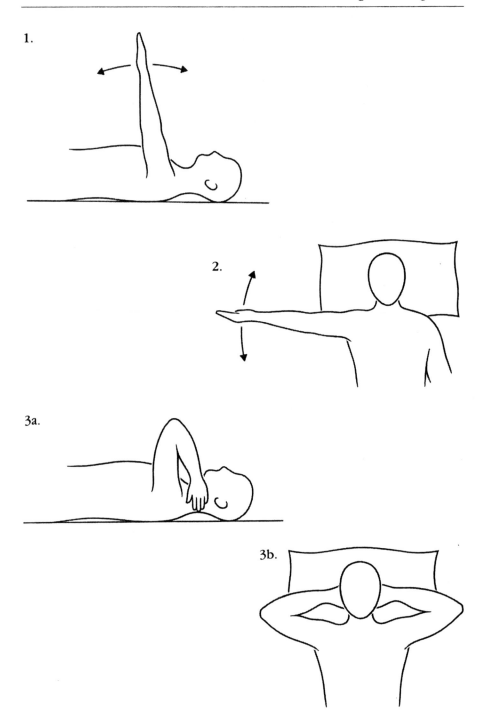

Figure 6.3: Set C arm exercises.

First Post-operative Day

Assessment

The physiotherapist's initial assessment of the patient will include a review of respiratory status, the number and position of drainage tubes, the wound dressing and analgesia. Questioning of the patient will establish hand dominance, any previous history of shoulder problems, occupational and leisure activities, and level of pain control. An explanation of the effects of the surgery will introduce the need for an exercise regime.

Exercises

Patients are taught Set A exercises and encouraged to perform these three times a day within their limits of comfort. It is useful at this stage to correct their posture, as patients can easily adopt a position where the shoulder on the affected side is elevated and protracted in response to pain. They can also develop poor patterns of movement to minimize discomfort and should be encouraged to move their affected arm as normally as possible.

General advice

Patients are provided with written information regarding the general use of their arm following breast surgery.

- Lifting and housework – for the first 4–6 weeks following their operation patients are advised to lift only light objects with their affected arm. They are also encouraged to use their unaffected arm for heavy or repetitive tasks such as vacuum cleaning, ironing and window cleaning.
- Driving – patients are advised not to drive until after the first outpatient appointment following their operation. They should only resume driving once they feel confident to do so, and should start with short distances. If they have also undergone abdominal surgery it is sensible to wait six weeks before driving again.
- Sport and leisure activities – swimming may begin once good shoulder movement is regained and the operation scar has healed (usually after 4–6 weeks). If they are currently having radiotherapy they need to check with their radiographer that swimming will not damage fragile skin. Most other sporting activities can be restarted within two months of surgery.

Discuss complications

Patients are informed of the particular complications that are usually associated with axillary intervention, e.g. altered sensation, seroma formation, cording and lymphoedema. These will be discussed later in the chapter.

Pre-discharge

Patients usually stay in hospital until their drains are removed, although some are now able to go home with them still in situ. (If a patient goes home with drains in, she/he is advised to continue Set A exercises, and to make an appointment to see the physiotherapist when the drain is removed.)

Following the removal of drains, Set B exercises are taught and the range of movement is checked. At this stage patients should be able to elevate their affected arm to about 90 degrees and they are encouraged to progress their range, within their limits of comfort. Set C exercises are demonstrated to them and the physiotherapist will discuss the importance of these stretches. Many patients will go on to have adjuvant radiotherapy as part of their treatment. For this patients are required to lie supine with both arms elevated and externally rotated above their head. The Set C exercises will help them achieve and maintain this position.

The physiotherapist may arrange to see the patient at the first outpatient appointment, or alternatively invite her/him to attend a 'Drop-in Clinic' run by the physiotherapy service.

First Outpatient Appointment

Patients attend for their first outpatient appointment at about 7–10 days.

At this point, the physiotherapist may assess for signs of seroma, infection or haematoma. The patient's range of movement and level of pain are reviewed, and the axilla and arm inspected for signs of early cording.

Patients should be able to perform their exercises correctly and have a good understanding of the need for an ongoing exercise regime. It is important to correct posture and ensure poor movement patterns are not developing.

From this assessment the physiotherapist will be able to decide if any patients require further physiotherapy input.

Reconstructive Surgery

Women may have reconstructive surgery at the time of their cancer surgery, or they may delay this to a later date.

Latissimus Dorsi Flap Reconstruction

Following this procedure patients are instructed in the set A, B and C exercises, although progress is slower and it may take longer for them to resume their normal activities. Particular attention should be paid to posture and they will benefit from additional exercises to stretch the scar on their back.

Transverse Rectus Abdominus Flap Reconstruction

The large abdominal wound increases the potential for respiratory complications in the early post-operative stage. The physiotherapist will assess respiratory function and advise on breathing exercises and supported cough techniques. Set A, B and C exercises are followed within the patient's level of comfort. Abdominal strengthening exercises are usually started once the patient is more mobile and pain controlled, and back-care and lifting techniques are discussed to minimize strain on the abdominal muscles.

Patients are advised to delay driving until six weeks after their operation.

Radiotherapy Class

Some hospitals run a multi-professional information class to any patient undergoing radiotherapy to the breast and/or axilla. This is usually run jointly by the physiotherapist, lymphoedema nurse specialist and therapy radiographer. The aim of the class is to increase patients' awareness of the potential long-term effects of radiotherapy relating to shoulder movement and lymphoedema (Hammick et al., 1996).

Information includes an explanation of the effects of radiotherapy, the need for a continued exercise regime, lymphoedema advice and post-radiotherapy skin care advice.

Complications Following Surgery

Cording

Cording is frequently seen in patients who have had axillary surgery and can start to form about a week post-operatively. In an unpublished study (Williams, 1994) 83% of patients had cording after axillary surgery. It is seen as a tight band-like structure of varying thickness arising from the axilla and stretching down the inner aspect of the upper arm when the arm is stretched (Figure 6.4). In some cases thinner string-like cords can be felt at the inner aspect of the elbow, or even wrist. Cording may limit arm movement when stretched, and can vary between feeling tight and being very painful. Some patients also feel tightness over the front of the ribs below the breast, and cording can, more rarely, be present here. Although a result of axillary surgery, it is not known which tissue is involved. Although there is little research on the subject, hypotheses suggest it may be thickened lymph or blood vessels, or fibrosis in the fascial planes caused by scarring. We do

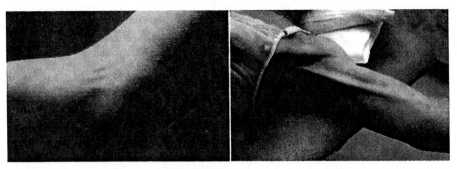

Figure 6.4: A patient with cording at the elbow and in the axilla after axillary node surgery.

know, however, that cording will stretch out with exercises. Normal range of movement (ROM) is usually regained within three months if no other complications are involved. Those women who have had reconstruction of the breast mound may find that recovery takes longer. When done regularly, the exercises outlined above should restore ROM, but a physiotherapist can treat the cords using soft tissue mobilizations to speed up recovery. Patients are encouraged to use the arm as normally as possible but are advised not to lift or carry heavy objects for 4-6 weeks. If pain persists or movement remains limited after this time, the patient should be referred to a chartered physiotherapist for assessment and treatment.

Seroma

Seroma formation after axillary surgery is considered the most common complication (Schulz et al., 1997). Controversy surrounds the issue of whether early mobilization of the shoulder is linked to seroma formation, and current research on the matter remains inconclusive. Some research (e.g. Rodier et al., 1987) suggests early exercise in order to avoid shoulder stiffness caused by scar tissue formation. Early exercise is also thought to encourage normal lymphatic, arterial and venous circulation (Miller, 1998) in a limb predisposed to lymphoedema. Schultz et al. (1997) advocate avoidance of early exercise in order to minimize complications with seroma. Even those studies that delayed exercise allowed normal activities of the affected limb immediately post-operatively, and did not restrict shoulder movement completely. The difficulty in assessing the research is the large number of variables that could influence outcome, for instance: type and extent of surgery, age of patient, surgeon involved, number of nodes removed, number of days with drain, number of positive nodes, level of pain, patient's normal activity levels, etc.

Axillary seroma can be uncomfortable, and the resulting limitation of ROM at the shoulder will not be altered by exercise. Often the fluid can be aspirated and the exercises resumed. Some patients present with seroma of the anterior chest wall, or under the scar of the latissimus dorsi flap on the posterior thorax. Both these can limit shoulder movement. If patients present with seroma, they are advised to continue Set A exercises within the limit of their discomfort, and are reviewed by a doctor for possible aspiration of fluid. Unfortunately, once removed the fluid can reaccumulate over a few days, and the procedure may need to be repeated several times before the seroma settles.

Altered Posture

Resuming normal posture is critical post-breast surgery. It is natural to hunch forward to avoid stretching the wound and to protect the sensitive area in front. If the wounds heal with the shoulder girdle in a protracted or forward position, the patient is much more likely to get shoulder problems later. This is because the shoulder joint is being worked out of alignment and certain muscles are being stretched while others are shortened. Even after a few days of shortening the pectoral muscles are overworked and painful, while the scapular muscles are stretched and weakened. This can lead to impingement problems in the shoulder joint or neck problems later on. Even if a patient had good posture pre-operatively, the whole cancer and hospital experience can quickly alter habits, and nearly all patients use 'trick' movements to avoid the stretch if it is uncomfortable. From the beginning, simply lying flat on the floor and pushing both shoulders back and down onto the floor will help stretch out the anterior scar and relax the pectoral muscles. This is especially important in those women who have elected to have immediate reconstruction (with or without implant), as the pectoral muscles are more likely to be tight and sore.

Altered movement patterns can be identified and corrected by a chartered physiotherapist. After days or weeks of poor positioning myofascial trigger points can be found within the affected muscles, exacerbating the pain cycle. A trigger point is defined as a 'hyperirritable locus within a taut band of muscle, located in the muscular tissue and/or its associated fascia. The spot is painful on compression and can evoke characteristic referred pain and autonomic phenomena' (Travell and Simons, 1992). The main culprits tend to be the pectoral muscles, latissimus dorsi, upper trapezius and infra-spinatus. These muscles can be responsible for referring pain into the shoulder or arm, and can limit movement of the shoulder. The more complications to do with wound healing or pain, the more likely trigger points will be found in these areas. Release of the tension here can ease pain and regain the patient 20–30 degrees more movement in one treatment session.

Scar Sensitivity

Some women are reluctant to look at the scar and touching it can be a very emotional issue, not just because of changes in body image but for fear of damaging the wound or, if they have had a reconstruction, moving the implant. Once the scar has healed and infection is not a risk, it is useful to encourage touch and gentle massage of the area, especially if it is very sensitive or tight. Superolateral movement of the soft tissues across the chest wall is necessary for the arm to move into full elevation, and tethering of post-operative scarring and exudate in the soft tissues will impair movement and cause discomfort. It is useful to encourage the patient to massage the scar gently so that it becomes more supple and it helps the patient to reacquaint her/himself with the numb and 'odd feeling' chest wall. Very sensitive scarring can be gradually desensitized in this way, although this would not be advocated during radiotherapy treatment when the skin is more fragile. Once healed, if soft tissue stiffness remains that is painful and limits movement, myofascial release techniques used by a chartered physiotherapist can be useful to lengthen tissues and enable them to move more freely over the chest wall as the arm moves into flexion or abduction.

Nerve Damage

There are three nerves that are at risk of damage during axillary surgery. The most commonly disturbed is the intercostobrachial nerve. Division or damage of this nerve causes numbness of the medial arm from the axilla to the elbow. If it has only been bruised (neuropraxia) patients may complain of an uncomfortable tenderness that keeps them from putting the arm by their side, and they may even present standing with their hand on their hip so the skin is not disturbed. Some people cannot even bear the feeling of clothing on the skin, but over a period of weeks or months this feeling should gradually fade.

The long thoracic nerve supplies the serratus anterior muscle. When this is damaged there will be poor control of the scapula, and it will wing out from the chest wall along its medial border. This results in limited strength and ROM of the arm and a decrease in stability of the shoulder girdle. The thoracodorsal nerve supplies the latissimus dorsi muscle. If this is damaged, obvious deformity does not result but there is weakness of medial rotation and adduction of the arm. In either case, referral should be made to a physiotherapist to advise on strengthening of the muscle as the nerve regains function, and on how to avoid further soft tissue damage if weakness is permanent. Needless to say damage of these two nerves is rare but, if it does arise, is normally a neuropraxia, which will resolve within weeks or months.

Wound Problems

Delayed wound healing in the axilla or on the chest wall due to haematoma or infection will usually cause restriction in arm movement because of pain.

Exercises should be kept to a minimum during this phase using the limb in the pain-free range only. Strong stretches over a troublesome wound must be avoided or healing may be further delayed. Once healing has occurred, movement may be limited due to fibrosis of scar tissue but exercises can be resumed as pain allows under the guidance of a chartered physiotherapist. The therapist will need to ascertain which, if any, structures are causing the pain and why. She/he will also need to assess which structures around the chest wall and shoulder are tight, in order to give the right treatment and advice.

Radiotherapy Side Effects

Those patients who need radiotherapy as an adjunct to treatment are more likely to notice problems with the ipsilateral arm (Bentzen and Dische, 2000; Isaksson and Feuk, 2000). Radiotherapy damages the soft tissues within the field of treatment and in the short term can cause acute inflammatory changes such as redness, sensitivity and desquamation of the skin. Strong stretches of the shoulder will be uncomfortable and massage of the skin is not recommended until healing has taken place. Later, skin changes include pigmentation and telangiectasis. Subcutaneous fibrosis of soft tissues is commonly seen by the end of treatment, and can continue to form gradually years after treatment (Rytov et al., 1983; Kurtz, 1995). This causes a fibrous band of tissue at the anterior axillary fold from the anterior chest wall along the band of pectoral muscle. The physiotherapist will instruct the patient to continue putting the shoulder through a full range of movement, stretching out once a day when full movement is regained, just to ensure stiffness does not recur. Our experience at the Royal Marsden Hospital suggests that patients tend to forget to continue stretches, and as normal daily routines do not put the shoulder through a full range of movement, stiffness goes unnoticed until it starts producing arm symptoms later on. Patients sometimes come back to clinic perhaps a year after radiotherapy has finished, complaining of symptoms either directly or indirectly related to their breast cancer surgery and radiotherapy, with or without any signs of lymphoedema. It is worthwhile highlighting the need to continue stretches for years after radiotherapy, as research suggests fibrosis may progress at least up to 10 years (Kurtz, 1995).

Brachial plexus lesions due to radiotherapy are much less common with modern radiotherapy techniques. Patients who were treated with higher doses and larger fields in the past, however, may develop a progressive weakness in the ipsilateral arm if the radiotherapy field encompassed the nerves lying under the supraclavicular fossa. This can cause profound weakness and atrophy of the arm, and, both physically and psychologically, the effects can be devastating. Brachial plexus damage is irreversible but assessment by a chartered physiotherapist and an occupational therapist can be helpful to advise on symptom control and maximizing function. Active exercise and gentle stretches may help to prevent tightening and stiffening of the joints and soft tissues involved. Splinting of the hand and wrist may be appropriate to protect the joints and minimize pain. No amount of exercise will regain lost muscle power. This is because the damage is to the nerve supply, not the muscle itself. Ill-advised exercise can lead to an increase in symptoms and is best avoided.

Other side effects worth bearing in mind for the physiotherapist treating this patient group are radiation-induced malignancy, pulmonary fibrosis and lymphoedema of the arm (Wallgren, 1992). Lethargy is a commonly experienced effect, which can limit the patient's capacity for exercise and slow her/his progress with rehabilitation. This is normally experienced towards the end of treatment and over the next month after treatment has finished. It is often helpful to spend time explaining in detail the effects of the treatment and the rationale for stretches, and to tailor the exercise plan to the individual's ability at the time.

Lymphoedema

This can be a big concern to patients who have undergone lymph node removal and/or radiotherapy to lymphatic structures but sensible precautions will limit the risk of it occurring, and it is usually possible to treat the limb and prevent it from becoming a significant problem. Clinical nurse specialists or physiotherapists should be notified of hand, arm or trunk swelling early on, and gentle exercises and advice on activities and control of the condition will be given. In some cases elastic support sleeves and gloves or manual lymph drainage can help. Interestingly, although traditionally we warn women with axillary dissections, with or without radiotherapy, to avoid strenuous and prolonged upper limb activity in order to decrease the risk of lymphoedema, a recent study (Harris and Niesen-Vertommen, 2000) suggested this is unsubstantiated by research and places unnecessary limits on a woman's activities. Harris's study shows it may be quite safe to exercise vigorously and not develop arm swelling, and makes a plea for further research in this area which would enhance quality of life for those people wishing to return to more strenuous recreational activities.

Heavy lymphoedematous arms are uncomfortable and difficult to carry, causing changes in posture at the shoulder girdle, back and neck. Shoulder, elbow and hand joints can become tight, causing more discomfort. Physiotherapy can be useful in maintaining function of the limb, and easing secondary neck, back or other joint pain.

The lymphoedema chapter in this book will explain in more detail the causes of and treatments for the problem.

Muscle Weakness

Weakness can be caused by surgery for breast cancer for several reasons:

- Pain can inhibit strong muscle contraction (Guymer, 1997). It also means that women avoid using the painful body part, and the muscles weaken progressively from under-use.
- Pain can also elicit raised tone in the muscle concerned, or irradiate to surrounding muscles (Guymer, 1997).
- Muscle action can be limited by nerve damage, as discussed above.
- Muscles on excessive stretch are working at a mechanical disadvantage and can be weakened. For example, the submuscular implants placed underneath the pectoralis major put the muscle on stretch, and make it harder to contract.
- TRAM flaps harvested from the rectus abdominis muscle, both pedicled and free flaps, cause weakness of the abdominal wall. This can lead to abdominal herniation and decreased trunk stability when the patient is faced with functional activities.

Recent innovations in plastic surgery have meant that some surgeons are performing the DIEP (deep inferior epigastric perforator) flap in reconstructions rather than taking rectus abdominis muscle in a TRAM (transverse rectus abdominis myocutaneous) flap to rebuild the breast mound. It is hoped this will decrease the risk of abdominal herniation and muscle weakness, which can predispose to trunk instability and low back pain. Futter et al. (2000) found that while no muscle was removed in the DIEP flaps there was still a strength deficit, although not as marked compared with the TRAM flap. Blondeel et al. (1997) found that not only was there a deficit in trunk flexion strength following the TRAM flap surgery but that the oblique muscle function was also impaired, weakening rotation. The abdominal muscles work not only concentrically to flex the trunk but also eccentrically and statically to stabilize the lumbar spine and the pelvis and the rib cage, allowing the limbs to move freely. Futter et al. found that those women expressing difficulty carrying out activities such as lifting heavy objects or shopping, vacuuming, moving furniture, etc. were those who demonstrated weak trunk muscles post-operatively. This means that the TRAM flaps can cause weakness in the abdominal muscles and also impair normal daily functional activities. Therefore, patients undergoing this type of surgery should be referred to a physiotherapist to be taught appropriate strengthening exercises and back care advice before going home and may need to be seen on an outpatient basis once discharged.

Pain

Once the initial surgical pain has faded, patients can present with pain for a number of reasons. For example, nerve damage, swelling, altered movement patterns due to stiffness, etc. Many women interpret their pain as disease recurrence, and it is often necessary to reassure them that their discomfort is an unfortunate side effect of necessary treatment rather than a sign of returning cancer. If there is any possibility that metastases are present the doctors concerned should be consulted, and manual physiotherapy techniques to the area abandoned until investigations prove otherwise.

Physiotherapists can help relieve pain caused by muscle spasm, postural changes, joint stiffness, altered biomechanics, scar tissue, cording, or weakness by assessing the probable cause and using various mobilizing and soft tissue techniques. Electrotherapy is contraindicated over any area that may contain cancerous cells, although transcutaneous electrical nerve stimulation (TENS) machines (small, portable electrical nerve stimulators) may be useful in some cases to help with pain relief (Forster and Palastanga, 1981).

It is estimated that around a quarter of women go on to develop post-mastectomy pain syndrome (PMPS) (Wallace et al., 1996; Smith et al., 1999). One study (Tasmuth et al., 1996) found that one year after surgery 80% of women had treatment-related symptoms. These symptoms range from infrequent mild problems to pain that constantly disturbs daily activities and sleep. PMPS is a poorly recognized and poorly treated chronic pain condition following breast surgery where women complain of tight, burning, constricting pain, and loss of sensation in the anterior chest wall, axilla and posterior aspect of the upper arm in the distribution of the intercostobrachial nerve (Granek et al., 1984). They may also demonstrate loss of movement and arm weakness with postural changes. Wallace et al. (1996) found a higher incidence of PMPS with patients who had had mastectomy and reconstruction. Smith et al. (1999) found that the main contributing factors to PMPS in their group of patients were surgery and age. Heavier and taller patients in this study seemed more likely to develop pain, and those reporting PMPS were more likely to have had chemotherapy, post-operative radiotherapy and tamoxifen. Tasmuth et al. (1996) found a correlation between anxiety levels and depression with PMPS. Causes of PMPS remain uncertain, although work by Gottrup et al. (2000) suggests a neurological central sensitization of pain mechanisms similar to that seen in other neuropathic pain patients. Neuropathic pain has been shown to be effectively treated by drugs acting on the nervous system, such as amitriptyline (Kalso et al., 1996). Owing to the complexity of the problem, it may be best treated using a multidisciplinary approach, using pharmacological and physical modalities such as analgesia, physiotherapy, massage, exercise, acupuncture, TENS and psychological help, e.g. cognitive behavioural strategies to cope with chronic pain. Robb (Robb and Newham, 2002) showed that a combination of physiotherapy and psychology interventions helped patients to recognize the many factors contributing to their pain and improve their ability to cope with these factors.

PMPS is a condition that is more prevalent than previously thought and is still under-diagnosed and poorly understood. Further research is needed to improve our understanding of its aetiology and treatment. A wide range of treatment modalities may help, and more research is needed to examine the effects of holistic approaches to treatment.

Chemotherapy

Primary chemotherapy for early stage breast cancer may result in neutropenic episodes requiring hospital admission. The patient may present with a respiratory infection and difficulty expectorating. Appropriate chest physiotherapy techniques may be of benefit. General muscle weakness and loss of mobility may also be a symptom in this group of patients, and a graduated exercise programme will encourage a return to normal function. Patients could become involved in an outpatient circuit exercise programme following the completion of their chemotherapy. This would encourage an increased feeling of well-being and confidence to undertake other forms of exercise such as joining their local gym.

Physiotherapy and Metastatic Disease

When considering the patient with metastatic breast disease the physiotherapist rarely works in isolation and liaises closely with occupational therapists, social workers, community liaison nurses, lymphoedema nurses, doctors and other members of the multidisciplinary team. Good communication within the team and with the patient and her/his family is vital to ensure that everyone is working towards the patient's goals. This may mean helping the patient continue to care for the family at home, or to adjust to the terminal phase of the disease and find the most appropriate setting for them.

Breast cancer metastasizes primarily to bone, lung, liver and brain. Patients may present with a multitude of problems, i.e. pain, fractures, spinal cord compression, hypercalcaemia, chest infections, dyspnoea, pleural effusions, lymphangitis, abdominal ascites, hemiplegia, ataxia, etc. Physiotherapy assessment and treatment can begin once the patient is medically stable.

Bone Metastases

Depending on the site of bony involvement, patients will usually present with pain and limited mobility. Some patients will require an orthopaedic assessment. Once the patient is adequately pain controlled and there is minimal risk of pathological fracture according to the doctors, the physiotherapist will assess the range of movement of the affected joints, look for signs of muscle wasting and weakness and, where appropriate, analyse the patient's gait pattern.

Treatment may involve teaching the patient maintenance and strengthening exercises and possibly providing a walking aid to encourage a more normal gait. Gait re-education is important to facilitate the patient's return to normal functional independence. Daily physiotherapy sessions may be appropriate in the initial stages of the patient's treatment and the physiotherapist will then monitor progress. Prior to any discharge planning, the physiotherapist will review the patient's function, i.e. can she/he transfer independently from a lying to a sitting position, from sitting to standing, maintain a safe standing balance, walk with or without a walking aid and climb stairs?

Pathological Fractures

Bony metastases that have resulted in pathological fracture may require orthopaedic intervention depending on the fracture site. Upper limb fractures are not always surgically stabilized and may require some form of arm support, for example a polysling. Exercises are begun under the guidance of the physiotherapist and particular attention is paid to functional activities.

Lower limb fractures are often surgically fixated allowing the patient to weight-bear again. It is important to encourage early exercises of the affected and unaffected limbs to maintain muscle strength. The patient should be provided with the appropriate walking aid as soon as possible and encouraged to resume weight bearing as pain and stability of the fracture site allow. The physiotherapist will assess and re-educate her/his gait pattern, and teach the patient how to manage stairs and other functional activities with a walking aid if appropriate.

Spinal Cord Compression

This is an oncological emergency, and immediate medical attention is vital to limit the amount of permanent neurological damage. Spinal cord compression is caused by invasion of the epidural space with involvement of the spinal cord or nerve roots at any level, and is characterized by sensory and/or motor impairment and pain. It may also be accompanied by bladder and bowel symptoms (Lindsay and Bone, 1997). Radiotherapy is the treatment of choice, although surgical intervention may be useful to decompress the nerves or cord or to stabilize bony collapse. In the acute phase a physiotherapist may be involved in assessing respiratory status if the respiratory system is compromised. Once the lesion is known to be stable, further assessment by physiotherapists and occupational therapists will determine the extent of the patient's functional deficit and potential for rehabilitation, which may be restorative or palliative. The goal of therapy is maximum independence and quality of life, whether the patient is walking or restricted to a wheelchair.

Hypercalcaemia

Patients with bony metastatic disease may develop hypercalcaemia where there is a rise in serum calcium levels. The main symptoms include confusion, nausea, vomiting and lethargy. Following medical intervention, patients may be referred to the physiotherapist to increase their general mobility prior to discharge home.

Lung Metastases

Respiratory infections and progressive breathlessness are common features of lung involvement. As a result of this the patient's general mobility may become limited, which can lead to a decrease in exercise tolerance and function.

Chest physiotherapy techniques may be appropriate for patients who have a productive chest infection with difficulty expectorating sputum. The physiotherapist should be cautious, however, if there is evidence of metastatic rib disease, as some techniques may cause fracture. Advice on positioning, relaxation and breathing control may be useful adjuncts for these patients. The physiotherapist will encourage the patient to increase her/his mobility gradually, and advise on pacing. The provision of a walking aid may help to increase stability and conserve energy.

Pleural Effusions and Lymphangitis

Both of these conditions require medical intervention. Advice on positioning of the patient may be useful.

Liver Metastases

Physiotherapists may be involved with patients suffering from abdominal ascites and/or lower limb lymphoedema. Appropriate walking aids may be provided, and strategies taught for moving in bed or transferring from bed to chair. Positioning may help with shortness of breath resulting from abdominal swelling, which compromises diaphragmatic excursion.

Brain Metastases

Brain metastases can cause a variety of impairments, such as movement, speech, cognitive or visual problems. Physiotherapists, occupational therapists, and speech and language therapists work together in assessing these deficits, providing support for patients and their families. Hemiplegic patients present with limb weakness, alteration in muscle tone, and varying degrees of difficulty in functional movement of upper and/or lower limbs. Ataxic patients have difficulty in coordinating movement and have impaired balance reactions. Physiotherapy can help normalize tone, improve mobility and provide strategies for maximizing function.

Fatigue

Fatigue is a symptom of the disease or of the treatment used. Physiotherapists can be involved in providing exercise, and maintaining stamina and fitness tailored to each patient's potential.

Pain

Pain caused directly by the disease is well controlled by drugs but some pain can be relieved by the physiotherapist, particularly if it is positional, muscular, caused by stiffness, or due to abnormal posture or movement. TENS has been shown to be beneficial with some patients, and patients may be loaned a TENS machine on the ward or to take home. This machine is a small, portable electrical nerve stimulator, which can be purchased, although it is recommended to try one out before buying one, as some people do not find benefit.

Summary

Physiotherapists may be involved with breast cancer patients from diagnosis through to terminal stages of their disease. They may be involved in treating problems caused by the cancer itself or its treatment, most especially surgery and radiotherapy. Recurrence of breast cancer may present in a variety of ways and all health professionals must be vigilant. If recurrence is suspected the patient must be referred back to the oncologist or surgeon for appropriate treatment. Physiotherapists are often actively involved in providing symptom control and palliative care. This may be in a hospital, a hospice or in the patient's home.

References

Bentzen SM, Dische S (2000) Morbidity related to axillary irradiation in the treatment of breast cancer. Acta Oncologica (39)3: 337–47.

Blondeel Ph N, Boeckx W, Vanderstraeten G, Lysens R, Van Landuyt K, Tonnard P, Monstrey S, Matton S (1997) The fate of the abdominal muscles after free TRAM flap surgery. British Journal of Plastic Surgery (50): 315–321.

Forster A, Palastanga N (1981) Clayton's Electrotherapy: Theory and Practice, 9th edn. London: Baillière Tindall.

Futter C, Webster M, Hagen S, Mitchell S (2000) A retrospective comparison of abdominal muscle strength following breast reconstruction with a free TRAM or DIEP flap. British Journal of Plastic Surgery (53): 578–83.

Gottrup H, Andersen J, Arendt-Neilson L, Jensen T (2000) Psychophysical examination in patients with post-mastectomy pain. Pain (87): 275–84.

Granek I, Ashikari R, Foley K (1984) The Post-Mastectomy Pain Syndrome: Clinical and Anatomical Correlates. New York: Memorial Sloan-Kettering Cancer Centre.

Guymer A (1997) The neuromuscular facilitation of movement. In Wells, Frampton, Bowsher (Eds) Pain Management by Physiotherapy, 2nd edn. Oxford: Butterworth Heinemann.

Hammick M, Howard E, Macleod H, Smith J (1996) A multidisciplinary symptom control class for breast cancer patients. British Journal of Therapy and Rehabilitation 3(6): 333–6.

Harris S, Niesen-Vertommen S (2000) Challenging the myth of exercise-induced lympoedema following breast cancer: a series of case reports. Journal of Surgical Oncology (74): 95–9.

Isaksson G, Feuk B (2000) Morbidity from axillary treatment in breast cancer. Acta Oncologica 39(3): 335–6.

Kalso E, Tasmuth T, Neuvonen P (1996) Amitriptyline effectively relieves neuropathic pain following treatment of breast cancer. Pain (64): 293–302.

Kurtz JM (1995). Impact of radiotherapy on breast cosmesis. The Breast 4: 163–9.

Lindsay KW, Bone I (1997) Neurology and Neurosurgery Illustrated, Section IV. London: Churchill Livingstone.

Miller LT (1998) Exercise in the management of breast cancer-related lymphoedema. Innovations in Breast Cancer Care 3(4): 101–6.

Robb K, Newham D (2002) Non-pharmacological interventions in the management of chronic pain associated with breast cancer treatment. Unpublished.

Rodier JF, Gadonneix P, Dauplat J, Issert B, Giraud B (1987) Influence of the timing of physiotherapy on the lymphatic complications of axillary dissection for breast cancer. International Surgery (72): 166–9.

Rytov N, Blichert-Toft M, Madsen E L, Weber J (1983) Influence of adjuvant irradiation on shoulder joint function after mastectomy for breast carcinoma. Acta Radiologica Oncology 22(1): 29–33.

Schultz I, Barholm M, Grondal S (1997) Delayed shoulder exercises in reducing seroma frequency after modified radical mastectomy: a prospective randomized study. Annals of Surgical Oncology 4(4): 293–7.

Smith W, Bourne, D, Squair J, Phillips D, Chambers W (1999) A retrospective cohort study of post mastectomy pain syndrome. Pain (83): 91–5.

Tasmuth T, Von Smitten K, Kalso E (1996) Pain and other symptoms during the first year after radical and conservative surgery for breast cancer. British Journal of Cancer (74): 2024–31.

Travell J, Simons D (1992) Myofascial pain and dysfunction. In: The Trigger Point Manual. Philadelphia, PA: Lippincott Williams and Wilkins.

Wallace M, Wallace A, Lee J, Dobke M (1996) Pain after breast surgery: a survey of 282 women. Pain (66): 195–205.

Wallgren A (1992) Late effects of radiotherapy in the treatment of breast cancer. Acta Oncologica 31(2): 237–42.

Williams C (1994) Pain and upper limb function following breast surgery: an investigation into the effect of physiotherapy. Unpublished MSc Study.

Wingate L (1985) Efficacy of physical therapy for patients who have undergone mastectomies. Physiotherapy 65(6): 896–900.

CHAPTER 7

Breast Reconstruction

NICOLA WEST

Introduction

> Breasts are exalted as the epitome of all that is feminine and desirable in a woman. They are the basic stock in trade of the adman's art and the romantic novelist's passionate pen. (Faulder 1982)

It is hardly surprising that women undergoing treatment for breast cancer not only have the fear of a potentially life-threatening disease but also the worry of disfigurement and possible rejection following the loss of a breast with all its associated psychological and psychosocial problems (Kasper, 1995; Kissane et al., 1998). Indeed around 50 per cent of women undergoing mastectomy and wide local excision suffer high levels of anxiety and depression pre-operatively and one-third suffer from psychological problems up to one year post-operatively (Goldberg et al., 1992). Sexual problems occur in approximately 25 per cent of women regardless of the surgery received (Schover, 1991; Young-McCaughan, 1996).

The modern management of breast cancer aims to minimize chest wall deformity following all types of surgery. The cosmetic result is now given much more attention without compromising the well-being and safety of the patient.

Although mastectomy has been the standard treatment for breast cancer for almost a century, a wide local excision followed by radiotherapy is now the more modern form of treatment offered with the same long-term survival (Veronesi et al., 1981; Fisher et al., 1989). Where possible, women are now also given a choice in their treatment. In a small study conducted by Cotton et al. (1991) of those women offered a choice, approximately 50 per cent chose mastectomy and 50 per cent chose wide local excision. Morrow et al. (1998) reported that over 50 per cent of women chose mastectomy compared with wide local excision. Furthermore, in 1995 and 1996 more than 13 000 women in the UK were treated by mastectomy for their breast cancer (Department of Health 1996). Not all women, however, welcome this choice of treatment, and find having a choice stressful (Pierce, 1993; Fallowfield et al., 1994). There are also cultural differences in the choice process. Asian cultures, for example, place far less importance on the breast. They value role fulfilment and place greater importance on this rather than on physical characteristics as a sign of femininity and beauty. Roles such as manager and that of mother are far more significant than physical images to one's sense of self (Kagawa-Singer et al., 1997). In Japanese culture the nape of the neck and skin lightness are central to the foci of beauty and in Chinese culture deportment depicts the essential elements of beauty.

Having a choice of treatment depends, however, on the patient's view, the expertise and attitude of the surgeon, the position of the tumour in the breast and where a woman receives her treatment. For those women with large tumours, central tumours or multifocal disease a mastectomy is usually recommended, and breast reconstruction should therefore be an integral part of the patient's overall treatment. The surgeon's priorities, however, are obviously to eradicate the disease and decrease the potential for future recurrence.

Breast Reconstruction

Breast reconstruction is a term used to describe a range of surgical procedures with the aim of re-creating breast shape. It can be offered to women who have risk-reducing mastectomies, wide excisions where large amounts of tissue are removed, skin-sparing mastectomy, asymmetry of one breast and mastectomy. It can also be offered to women with Poland's Syndrome or congenital absence of a breast. It is not contra-indicated in patients who require adjuvant treatment and does not compromise further detection of disease.

The NHS Executive in 1996 recommended that all women undergoing mastectomy should be given the option of breast reconstruction, both immediate and delayed. Despite the availability and a consistent increase in demand for breast reconstruction in specialist units in the UK, less than half of the women offered it actually take it up (Watson et al., 1995). Significant variation also exists in the delivery of breast reconstruction in the UK and Ireland (Callaghan et al., 2002).

The age, workload and personal characteristics of the surgeon are important factors in determining reconstructive practice (Callaghan et al., 2002).

Overall, it is estimated that between 10 and 20 per cent of patients eventually take up the offer of breast reconstruction (Handel et al., 1990).

This figure is slightly higher in America where it is taken up by approximately 30 per cent of women undergoing mastectomy (cited in Rowland et al., 1995). Most women who choose mastectomy opt to wear an external prosthesis, which for some can be heavy, embarrassing, uncomfortable and inconvenient (Schain et al., 1985).

The purpose of breast reconstruction is to reconstruct a 'breast mound' in order to produce some symmetry of the size and contour of the lost breast. It has to be acknowledged that a reconstructed breast, however, does not have the function or physiological attributes of a natural breast (Ward, 1981). It should aim to match the remaining breast thus restoring feelings of attractiveness and wholeness.

Breast reconstruction techniques and results have improved considerably over the last decade. There has also been an increase in the number of specialist surgeons performing breast reconstruction, and an improvement in the quality of implants with the introduction of textured surface implants that now come in varying shapes and sizes. This is in contrast with the late twentieth century where attempts at breast reconstruction resulted in substantial scarring, failed procedures and poor results (Bostwick, 1990).

Types of Breast Reconstruction

With any breast reconstruction technique, various factors have to be taken into consideration. These include: patient's body shape, size of remaining breast and lost breast, skin condition, health status, patient choice, adjuvant therapy, previous surgery, lifestyle, occupation and finally expectations. The two main methods of breast reconstruction are implants and autologous tissue flaps.

Implant Surgery

Implants are either silicone gel or saline. They are placed sub-muscularly as opposed to subcutaneously because the cosmetic result is superior. Silicone implants were introduced in the 1960s (Bostwick, 1990) and since then major improvements have been achieved with the use of temporary expanders used since the 1970s, to gradually stretch the skin. Much of the controversy surrounding the safety of silicone implants has now been resolved with the conclusion that silicone is safe to use and does not cause further cancer, connective tissue disease or any life-threatening illness. Soya bean oil and trilucent implants, once thought to be safer than silicone implants, were removed from the UK market in 1999 because of their questionable safety with regard to toxic leaks. Polyurethane-covered implants were also removed in 1991 owing to concerns around safety (Department of Health, 1999). Implants can obscure breast tissue, making future mammography more difficult. Women who have had local excisions with implants therefore should inform the radiographer.

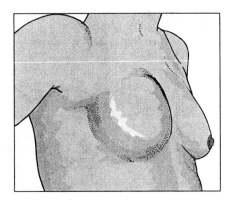

Figure 7.1: Implant surgery.

Tissue Expanders

Introduced in the 1970s, these may be temporary or permanent, smooth or textured. Expanders are used when there is insufficient skin to cover an implant and its purpose is to gradually create a submuscular space. Expanders are placed under the pectoralis major muscle and gradually expanded every few weeks. Temporary expanders are usually saline and are removed in a second operation, when the desired size is reached. Permanent expanders, e.g. a Becker expander, are left in place when the volume and desired shape have been achieved. The best results with implants are seen in those women who have small/moderate sized breasts, have little or no ptosis, have healthy skin to stretch, and have had no muscle removed during the mastectomy. Tissue expanders are not suitable for those women who have undergone radiotherapy because the skin will not stretch adequately.

Those women who are particularly keen on implant/expander breast reconstruction, however, and who have larger breasts, may also require reduction of the contralateral breast to produce symmetry (see Figures 7.2 and 7.3).

Both temporary and permanent expanders are inserted under the pectoralis major muscle and expanded gradually through a fill port every few weeks by injecting sterile saline. It is an aseptic technique carried out as an extended role by a clinical nurse specialist or a doctor. Temporary expanders are usually textured, round or anatomical and their availability

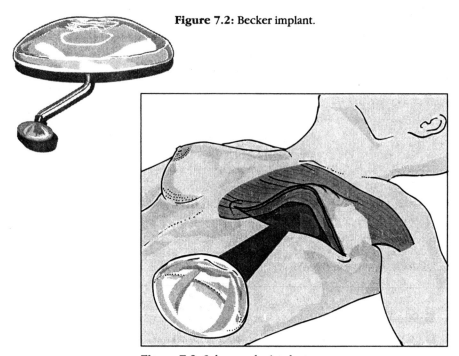

Figure 7.2: Becker implant.

Figure 7.3: Submuscular implant.

will depend on the hospital and surgeon involved. They are easier and less painful to expand than smooth-surfaced implants. Smooth-surfaced implants tend to cause more capsular contractures than textured implants and are nowadays being replaced by textured ones.

Once inflation has been achieved with a temporary expander and the 'reconstructed' breast is larger than the natural breast, the patient is given some months for the skin to adjust. When the permanent implant is then inserted, this will give a more natural look. The permanent implant is silicone or saline. A second operation is necessary to remove the inflatable implant and insert the permanent one. This method is useful for the patient with insufficient tissue after mastectomy and where the desired shape and size of the breast cannot be achieved with a single-stage procedure.

Permanent Expanders

Permanent expanders have a double lumen with an outer shell of silicone gel and a saline filled inflatable inner chamber. The implant is gradually expanded using sterile saline through a remote port connected to the inflatable chamber. Again, the implant is over-inflated but then deflated after a few months by removing some of the saline through the same fill port, with the aim of matching the contralateral breast. This deflation also attempts to achieve some ptosis. The port may then be removed at a later date under local anaesthetic in day surgery. Patients suitable for this method are small/moderate-size-breasted women who desire a simple reconstruction, have mild ptosis and realize it may not perfectly match the opposite breast.

Fixed Volume Implants

Where a woman has sufficient skin and is small breasted, a satisfactory result may be achieved in theatre with a fixed volume implant that is permanent. These are used for women who desire a simple, quick reconstruction.

Round versus Anatomical Devices

The first implants introduced were round but it was soon recognized that not all breasts are round and these early smooth round-surfaced implants showed little promise. The idea to produce implants with different base widths, heights and projections in the 1990s, and textured surfaces, therefore led to major improvements.

The advantages of any implant breast reconstruction compared with 'flap' surgery are that it is less invasive and relatively simple to do, patients have a quicker recovery, minimal scarring and the skin colour and texture are better (Beasley and Ballard, 1990) (Figure 7.4).

The disadvantages of implant surgery are that women may need surgery to the contralateral breast to achieve symmetry, the implant may need replacing at some time, infection may occur, and implant leakage or contracture formation are also potential complications, as is expander valve dysfunction. There is some discomfort after inflation and long term a patient may be displeased with the final result.

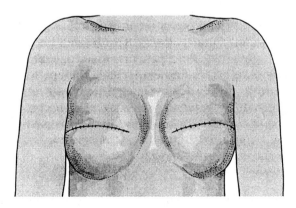

Figure 7.4: Bilateral mastectomy with implants.

There is still some debate as to the lifespan of implants. The general consensus is that an implant will need replacing at between 10 and 25 years but views on this vary and there is no evidence to support these figures. Implants are generally removed if there is a problem.

Summary of Potential Implant Complications

- Infection.
- Capsular contractures.
- Deflation – especially with a saline-only implant.
- Haematoma.
- Expander valve dysfunction.

It is not necessarily a medical problem if an implant shows signs of wear and tear, ruptures, or the gel leaks into the fibrous capsule. If the gel moves outside the shell and capsule, however, it can form a series of lumps causing local tenderness that may mimic cancer. Implants are only generally removed at the patient's request, when a capsular contracture forms or when aesthetic considerations predominate.

Capsular contracture, which is a later complication of breast implant surgery, is caused by fibrous tissue forming a band or capsule around the implant. As the fibrous tissue contracts it may become more uncomfortable, cause hardness in the breast and change the shape of the breast reconstruction. Surgery may be required to break or remove the capsule and replace the implant.

Dickson et al. (1987) reported increased capsular contracture in patients who had received post-operative radiotherapy with an implant. In addition Krueger et al. (2001) found increased expander implant failure in patients who received radiotherapy compared with non-irradiated patients. There have also been reports of implant failure leading to removal in patients undergoing radiotherapy (Barreau-Pouhaer et al., 1992). It is generally seen that those patients subjected to adjuvant chemotherapy or radiotherapy have worse cosmetic results with breast reconstruction than those not subjected to it (Von Smitten and Sundell, 1992). Because radiotherapy can affect the overlying skin, making it inelastic, patients are not suitable for implant reconstruction if they have had radiotherapy. Radiotherapy to an implant or an expander is possible, however, after immediate breast reconstruction when healing has occurred. Those women who have flap surgery and require radiotherapy have good cosmetic results and the radiotherapy is well tolerated. If radiotherapy is required, therefore, it is sensible to avoid prosthetic reconstruction and opt for flap surgery.

Implant surgery:

- Length of operation: 1–2 hours.
- Hospital stay: 4–7 days.
- Convalescence/recovery time: 4–6 weeks.

Pre-operative marking up by the surgeon is essential. Breast width measurement is more important than volume measurement. Implants feel firmer than the natural breast, remain upright while the woman is lying down and feel a little cooler than the remaining breast. The implant usually has little movement. (See Figure 7.1.)

Autogenous Tissue Reconstruction

This type of breast reconstruction involves taking muscle and subcutaneous tissue, plus or minus skin, from a donor site and transferring it to the breast site. The donor site is either the tissue of the lower abdominal wall based on the rectus abdominus muscle or the back muscle (latissimus dorsi). Occasionally the gluteus maximus muscle can be used.

The pedicled latissimus dorsi flap (Figures 7.5, 7.6)

The latissimus dorsi muscle is a fan-shaped muscle that extends over the back from the lower six thoracic spines and thoracolumbar fascia to the humerus.

With this type of reconstruction, the latissimus dorsi muscle from the back with its overlying skin and blood supply is dissected and rotated under the arm and placed on the front of the chest wall, where the diseased breast has been removed. Depending on the size of the contralateral breast a woman usually requires an implant to go under the muscle and skin. The

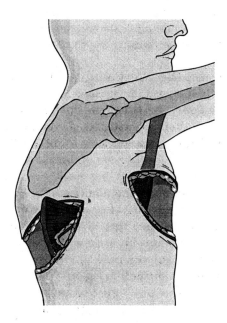

Figure 7.5: Latissimus dorsi flap reconstruction, side view.

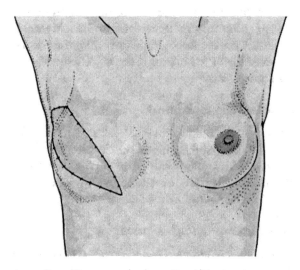

Figure 7.6: Latissimus dorsi flap reconstruction, front view.

woman has either a horizontal scar on her back or a more recent technique is a vertical scar hidden when the arm is placed by one's side. This type of reconstruction is recommended when a woman is larger breasted, where there is inadequate skin or muscle on the chest wall or damaged skin from radiotherapy, a failed attempt at tissue expansion or when the patient chooses it. It is not recommended for women who are very slim or who require their latissimus dorsi muscle, for example rock climbers or tennis players.

A latissimus dorsi skin flap can also be used to close a wound following mastectomy where there is insufficient skin, for example, following radical surgery for a large tumour. The latissimus dorsi muscle alone can be used when there is sufficient skin, but not enough volume, for example, after a wide local excision. This is known as a miniflap. Women with ductal carcinoma in situ and who are very keen on breast conservation, but would lose most of the breast tissue following a wide excision, benefit from a miniflap. Some surgeons perform the miniflap at a second operation when they are sure excision margins are clear and have been examined. Other surgeons perform this at the same time as removing the initial cancer. The latissimus dorsi muscle can also be used with a skin-sparing mastectomy where the skin and nipple are preserved and where the deficit needs filling with the muscle only and an implant.

The advantages of a latissiumus dorsi reconstruction include its safety, and that it gives a good contour, is reliable and dependable and gives a more natural-looking breast with some ptosis. It also has a good blood supply. Women often choose this reconstruction instead of a transverse rectus abdominis musculocutaneous flap (TRAM) reconstruction to prevent the potential problems of a longer operation and possibly a longer recovery.

The disadvantages include some shoulder impairment, scars either on the back or vertically on the side and the fact that women still require an implant in many cases. Potential complications with this type of breast reconstruction include: seroma formation on the back, infection, flap necrosis and capsular contracture, although contracture rates are lower when the latissimus dorsi muscle is used than when an implant is used alone (Vasconez et al., 1991).

- Length of operation: 3–5 hours.
- Hospital stay: 7–10 days.
- Convalescence/recovery time: 2–3 months.

The transverse rectus abdominis musculo cutaneous flap (TRAM)

The rectus abdominis muscle is a long flat muscle that runs from the fifth, sixth and seventh ribs to the pubis. The transverse rectus abdominis flap (TRAM) was developed in the early 1980s. Women who benefit from this type of surgery include larger breasted women with ptotic breasts. Women who choose this type of reconstruction are averse to the implant method of breast reconstruction and have enough abdominal tissue to remove. The TRAM reconstruction gives a more natural feel and look to the breast and women often think that because it is their own tissue and muscle it is more natural. Also, the skin from the abdomen provides a better colour and texture match than the latissimus dorsi flap. The TRAM flap can be performed either using a pedicle or as a free flap.

The pedicled TRAM flap

The pedicled TRAM flap is performed by removing an area of skin and fat from the abdomen with its blood supply, rotating the abdominal muscle and passing it through a subcutaneous tunnel onto the chest wall where it is constructed into a breast shape. Women often feel that the tram flap operation also gives them a tummy tuck by removing excess fat from their abdomen. Women who are heavy smokers, have diabetes, are generally unfit and have had an extensive abdominal operation in the past are not suitable candidates for this operation. It is a long operation to perform and thus is classed as major surgery (approximately 5–6 hours) and the blood supply is impaired if the woman is a heavy smoker, which compromises healing and the survival of the flap. Recovery from this operation is longer than from both the implant and the latissimus dorsi operation. Flap failure and donor site morbidity are higher with the TRAM method of reconstruction than the pedicled latissimus dorsi. Occasionally an implant is also required with a TRAM flap reconstruction. The disadvantages of this operation include a longer recovery, horizontal scars on the abdomen, abdominal muscle weakness, and therefore the potential for hernia formation and fat necrosis where ischaemia to the flap occurs, which can be very painful. Women who have had flap breast reconstruction sometimes have a normal or reduced sensation of the breast, especially if the skin envelope has been preserved. Flap surgery also tends to move with the patient on mobility and is generally softer than an implant. When a woman's weight changes, the TRAM flap can also change in size (Vasconez et al., 1991). (See Figures 7.7 and 7.8.)

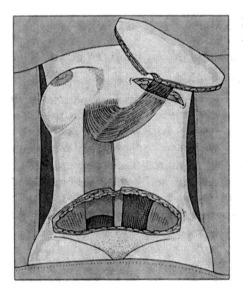

Figure 7.7: Transverse rectus abdominus musculo cutaneous (TRAM) flap.

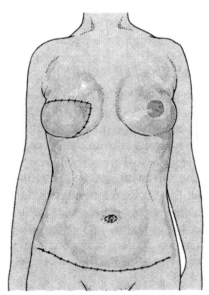

Figure 7.8: TRAM flap 2.

Free TRAM flap

This is tissue and muscle cut completely free from the abdomen with its own blood supply and moved to the breast area where it is reconnected to vessels in the axilla using microsurgical techniques. This technique can be used for unilateral or bilateral breast reconstruction. This method relies on the more robust deep inferior epigastric vessels and has less fat necrosis, and less risk of ischaemia and partial flap loss than the pedicled TRAM flap. It carries a larger volume of skin and fat than the conventional tram flap so it is most suitable for larger breasted women. Patients who are obese, smoke, have diabetes, peripheral vascular disease, autoimmune disease or cardiovascular disease are not suitable patients to undergo this procedure. Its downfall is the amount of theatre time required, its difficulty to perform and the possibility of total flap loss, which is in the region of 5–6 per cent (Arnez et al., 1991). Free flaps also avoid the bulge in the epigastrium from tunnelling of the pedicled flap. This technique is more difficult to perform and now less common. (See Figures 7.9, 7.10 and 7.11.)

TRAM reconstruction:

- Length of operation: approximately 4–7 hours.
- Hospital stay: 7–12 days.
- Convalescence / recovery time: 2–9 months.

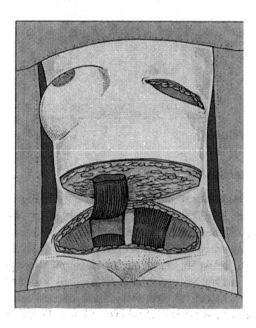

Figure 7.9: Free TRAM flap.

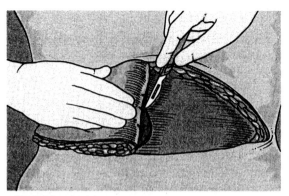

Figure 7.10: Free TRAM flap incision.

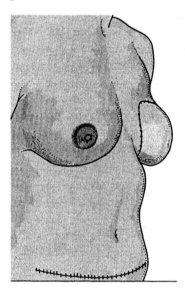

Figure 7.11: Free TRAM flap 2.

The DIEP flap (perforator flap)

This is the latest innovation; it is similar to the TRAM but uses the abdominal fat and tissue only. The deep inferior epigastric artery and veins are disconnected from their anatomical source and the vessels are then connected to the internal mammary artery. This technique involves microvascular surgery, which spares the muscle, resulting in minimal disruption to the rectus muscle. Hernias and bulges are therefore avoided and for the patient there is less pain and a reduced hospital stay. Also there is no need to close the abdomen with a tight synthetic mesh as with the TRAM flap. This is ideal for the young athletic patient for whom an intact abdominal wall is important, and also for those wanting bilateral breast reconstruction as preserving the rectus abdomini muscle significantly decreases donor site morbidity (Vasconez et al., 1991).

Inferior gluteus maximus musculocutaneous flap reconstruction

This is one of the most favourable free flaps because the patient has a breast reconstruction and a buttock reduction and lift. The main advantage of this flap is that an extremely large flap can be based on the vessel and muscle. The main disadvantage is the position of the patient on the operating table because the patient needs to be on her side when the flap is harvested. In addition the posterior cutaneous nerve of the thigh has to be sacrificed, which results in a small area of sensory loss on the posterior thigh. This technique is rarely performed by breast surgeons and is more popular with plastic surgeons because it involves microsurgery to restore the blood supply to the flap.

Although the incidence is low, complications from any type of breast reconstruction include seroma formation, infection, pain, flap loss and fat necrosis, capsular contracture with an implant, asymmetry, rupture and leaking, hypertrophic scars and a weakness at any of the donor sites. Many of the women undergoing breast reconstruction will need some form of extra minor surgery to rectify small surgical problems and obtain better symmetry (Vasconez et al., 1991).

Skin-sparing Mastectomy

Skin-sparing mastectomy was introduced in 1991 by Toth and Lappert. This technique removes the breast, nipple areola complex and the tumour. Local recurrence rates are not increased with this technique but complication rates can be higher. Its advantages include preserving the native skin and infra-mammary fold, lessening the chance of performing surgery on the contralateral breast and reduces the size of the mastectomy scar. The peri-areola incisions are also inconspicuous. An implant plus or minus a flap using the latissimus dorsi muscle is used to fill the deficit.

Peyser et al. (2000) reported that this technique is oncologically safe and involves minimal scars but they emphasize that it needs to be performed by surgeons trained in oncoplastic techniques.

Risk-reducing Mastectomies

It is easier to create symmetric breasts if both breasts need to be reconstructed. This type of surgery is ideal for implants or expanders because symmetry can be achieved. All of the breast tissue with skin and nipple is usually taken to ensure safe removal and reduce the risk of local recurrence. It cannot be guaranteed, however, that all of the breast tissue has been removed.

Subcutaneous Mastectomy

This is where all of the breast tissue is removed but the skin and nipple remain. Implants are then placed under the skin and not under the muscle. This is nowadays rarely carried out; the safety of the operation is questionable and the cosmetic results with implants are poor, because of contractures.

Nipple/Areola Reconstruction

Most operations for a mastectomy involve removing both the areola and nipple in order to successfully remove all the disease. A new nipple, however, can be created on the reconstructed breast giving some symmetry in an attempt to achieve a more natural look. This is usually performed at a later date following the breast reconstruction to allow the reconstruction to settle into its final shape and allow time for healing. Some women, however, do not want another operation and decide to wear a silicone stick-on nipple which can be custom made, to match the shape and colour of their existing nipple, or ready made. There are two method of nipple reconstruction: the skate flap and the C-V flap. With both methods a layer of skin and fat on the reconstructed breast is shifted to the centre of the future nipple areola area and formed into a nipple. The skin is used to create the nipple and the underlying fat is used to add bulk. With the skate flap much of the skin is taken from the site of the future areola to form the nipple. With the C-V flap, not as much local tissue is used so it may not produce as large or projecting a nipple as the skate flap. A new nipple can also be created by taking part of the nipple from the remaining natural breast. This is only performed, however, if the patient has large nipples and breast cancer has been ruled out. This gives the best match for size, colour and texture. Healing of the reconstructed nipple can take many months. There is usually no sensation in the reconstructed nipple and it does not function as a natural one.

Methods for re-creating the areola range from simple tattooing to the more complex use of grafts. The areola can be reconstructed using a graft of tissue from the upper inner thigh but this can result in a painful donor site and an extra scar. It can also be tattooed using a pigmented dye.

Although with any breast reconstruction the aim is to achieve as natural a look as possible for the woman, it does not look exactly the same as before. It may look bigger, smaller, flatter, firmer, higher or lower that the natural breast. The reconstructed breast can change shape over time especially after flap surgery where the muscle can atrophy and the breast can become smaller. Therefore surgery to the contralateral breast is often required. This can be carried out at the same time as the initial reconstruction but more often it is advised as a delayed procedure. Contralateral surgery can be in the form of a reduction mammoplasty, a mastopexy or an augmentation (Vasconez et al., 1991).

(a) Nipple reconstruction 1

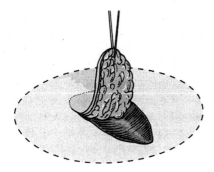

(b) Nipple reconstruction 2

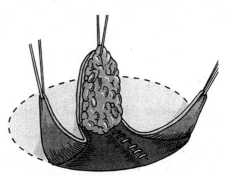

(c) Nipple reconstruction 3

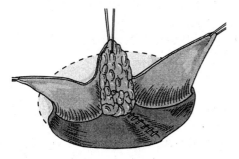

(d) Nipple reconstruction 4

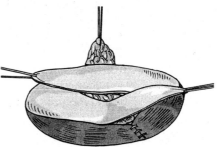

(e) Nipple reconstruction 5

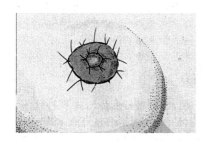

Figure 7.12: Nipple reconstruction.

Reduction Mammoplasty

When a woman's remaining breast is large she may wish to have it reduced to match the reconstructed breast. A reduction mammoplasty may also make it easier to match the breast reconstruction on the treated side. The incision used for a breast reconstruction resembles an upside-down T. If only a moderate amount of tissue needs removal, smaller, shorter scars can be achieved. The final result is a faint scar around the nipple, which is lifted and repositioned, a vertical scar down the middle of the breast and in some cases a small scar in the infra-mammary fold. For larger amounts of tissue to be removed the nipple will need to be used as a free graft and repositioned but the rate of nipple loss is higher with this surgery.

Mastopexy (Lift)

If the remaining breast is of a reasonable size but sags because of excess skin, a mastopexy may improve the situation. With this technique the surgeon moves the nipple areola upwards to a new position on the breast and removes the skin below the nipple and above the lower breast crease.

The incisions are similar to a breast reduction but may be shorter. When the breast does not sag too much an incision around the areola and down to the infra-mammary fold may be all that is necessary.

Breast Augmentation

If a woman's remaining breast is small and flattened an option after mastectomy and breast reconstruction is to consider having the existing breast enlarged. The reconstructed breast can then be created to resemble the larger breast especially if an expander has been used. The incision for augmentation is usually made under the breast and an implant is inserted behind the breast tissue or muscle.

Finally, women differ in their satisfaction with the breast reconstruction's end result and so expectations of this are especially important to identify. For this reason, all women considering undergoing breast reconstruction should receive appropriate in-depth counselling and should see the surgeon, the specialist nurse and possibly a patient volunteer. Photographs should be seen of realistic results and all information needs should be addressed.

Timing of Breast Reconstruction

Breast reconstruction can be carried out at the same time as a mastectomy (immediate breast reconstruction – IBR) or as a delayed procedure (delayed breast reconstruction – DBR). If it is to be carried out as a DBR it must be delayed for at least 3–6 months to allow adequate recovery. Evidence to date on the correct timing of breast reconstruction is inconclusive and inconsistent. One of the worries of surgeons in the past was that IBR may delay the administration of adjuvant therapies such as chemotherapy but this does not seem to be the case and it does not increase the time to treatments (Allweis et al., 2002).

This is supported by Malata et al. (2000) who found that IBR is safe, acceptable and there is no evidence that it has untoward oncological consequences.

Pre-1980, however, most breast reconstructions were carried out in a separate operation so that any treatment necessary could be completed and there would be greater healing of the mastectomy scar. For many surgeons delaying a breast reconstruction gave a woman time to grieve and to accept the loss (Winder and Winder, 1985).

Various arguments have been put forward supporting both immediate and delayed breast reconstruction. Generally, the main reason for offering women IBR is to spare them the psychological and psychosocial problems associated with breast loss (Maguire et al., 1978; Fallowfield et al., 1986) as well as being more cost effective. Furthermore IBR compared with DBR not only offers the benefits of being more cost effective but some women have a quicker recovery and there is less inconvenience for the patient, preventing the need for a separate admission (Bremner-Smith et al., 1996). Also, women who have had IBR have reported less distress at the time of the mastectomy and less of a fear about cancer (Rosenqvist et al., 1996). Other authors have also reported that post-operative psychological morbidity is lower in those who have IBR (Stevens et al., 1984; Singletary 1996), although the evidence is not compelling. Some authors, however, argue that IBR gives a lower score of satisfaction amongst patients (Wellisch et al., 1985). In addition, those women undergoing IBR have no experience of living without a breast for comparison.

Initially, the basic premise was that women need to have experience of a mastectomy in order to benefit from breast reconstruction, despite the fact that there is lack of sound research evidence to support any of the initial theories. It is also a general feeling that DBR may produce psychological trauma and morbidity (Scott et al., 2001) but again the evidence to support this is limited. Most of the studies on breast reconstruction are retrospective and assess decisions after they have been made, failing to portray actual feelings at the time. Furthermore many of the studies on breast reconstruction are not randomised controlled trials and do not compare like with like. Breast reconstruction can be a traumatic and upsetting experience for some women whether immediate or delayed (Ward, 1981; Fentiman, 1990) but have a positive and rewarding outcome for others.

Psychological Benefits of Breast Reconstruction

We restore, repair and make whole those parts, which nature has given but which fortune has taken away, not so much that they may delight the eye but that they may buoy up the spirit, and help the mind of the afflicted. (Tagliacozz, F, De Curtorum 1597 in Walsh Spencer, 1986, p. 131)

After a critical review of the literature, it is obvious that there is a lack of conclusive evidence on the psychological aspects of breast reconstruction (Harcourt, 2001). This is mainly due to the number of inadequate randomized controlled prospective studies. Most studies to date are retrospective.

According to the literature, the main reasons for undertaking breast reconstruction include practical reasons, for example ability to wear certain clothing and go swimming, improvement in confidence and self-esteem, taking the emphasis off the cancer and allowing women to be less sexually inhibited. Reasons against breast reconstruction include fear of scars, pain, not meeting expectations, not being essential for one's well-being and the possibility of an unclear future (Schain, 1991), and these facts remain consistent. It is also well documented that women undergoing breast-conserving surgery report significantly more positive body image than women who have mastectomy either with or without reconstruction (Mock, 1993). Furthermore, Al Ghazal et al. (2000) found that patients undergoing breast-conserving surgery had less psychological morbidity and greater satisfaction than patients undergoing mastectomy with reconstruction. However, other quality of life issues, for example, anxiety and depression, have been reported to be worse for women undergoing breast-conserving surgery or breast reconstruction (Nissen et al., 2001). The greatest mood disturbance and poorest well-being was actually reported in the mastectomy with reconstruction group (Nissen et al., 2001). In addition, Gilboa and co-workers in 1990 reported higher levels of anxiety and depression in the younger patient requiring adjuvant treatment despite having undergone breast reconstruction. Although some studies have reported psychological benefits and less psychological disturbance to patients undergoing breast reconstruction (Dean et al., 1983; Berry et al., 1998), results concentrate mainly on satisfaction rates and techniques. Many other authors have reported no significant difference between women who undergo breast reconstruction and those who do not in terms of body image, depression, anxiety, social support and self-esteem (Owens et al., 1988; Reaby and Hort, 1995; Holly and Kennedy, 1998).

Psychological assessment is also very difficult because of the complexity of the issues involved, as there is no gold standard assessment for body image, so researchers develop their own tools. Despite the inconclusive evidence, however, it is a general view that women who undergo breast reconstruction have good psychological functioning and adaptation (Anderson and Kaczmarek, 1996).

It is also a general belief that women who do not undergo breast reconstruction will not cope with their mastectomy. In 1991 McKenna et al. wrote:

> ... not electing for breast reconstruction may add to the cost of medical and psychiatric follow up. (p. 1182)

They thus suggest that breast reconstruction is essential for all women to prevent psychological problems. This reinforces the fact that many clinicians may not fully understand the patient and the complexity of the decision process. In 1983, Morris wrote:

> ... there is still much ignorance of what women feel and many assumptions are made on their behalf by clinicians treating them. (p. 1725)

Nursing Care

Pre-operative Care

This is the most important time for the patient and the nurse specialist to address all of the information needs and make an assessment of the patient. Women with breast cancer should have access to a specialist nurse in breast care who has received adequate training in the area and works as part of a multidisciplinary team. This is in line with both national and local guidelines. There is also no doubt that women facing decisions about their treatment for breast cancer need support and this has been widely acknowledged (Fallowfield et al., 1994). Furthermore there is now strong evidence that the clinical nurse specialist has a significant impact on psychological outcome (McCardle et al., 1996). It is also felt that breast care nurse specialists should extend their support to include care of the woman undergoing breast reconstruction (Harcourt, 2001).

The decisions women and their partners have to make often run far beyond the type of surgery they want to undergo at initial diagnosis. They have to make decisions on issues which include surgery and adjuvant treatment, e.g. chemotherapy, radiotherapy, hormone therapy, sentinel node biopsy, clinical trials and breast reconstruction. Nurses caring for women with breast cancer include ward nurses, clinic nurses, district nurses and practice nurses and so a sound knowledge of breast care is also imperative for all the above to ensure continuity for the patient.

The decision regarding breast reconstruction is an extremely difficult one to make for some women, especially when a woman has just been diagnosed, is vulnerable and is not taking in all the information the professionals are imparting. Clifford (1979) found that a quarter of patients used denial or avoidance when working through the decision process of breast reconstruction. Excellent communications skills as well as a sound knowledge in breast reconstruction are paramount when caring for such women and their families. Women considering breast reconstruction may not always be those who have just been given the initial diagnosis of breast cancer. They may be women who have just been told that the conservative treatment they have undergone has been unsuccessful. They may also be women who have developed a recurrence or been referred from another hospital. The psychology therefore for these groups of women is extremely diverse and individual assessment is critical.

When a woman is diagnosed with breast cancer this is not always the best time to discuss the surgical options, especially in a busy clinic. Most clinical nurse specialists make appointments to see the woman and her family either in their home, which ensures privacy, or in a separate private counselling room. All nurses working with the patient can assess the individual's meaning of the diagnosis of breast cancer. The anxiety levels, fears and feelings about having a mastectomy with or without breast reconstruction can also be determined. Basic communication skills of listening, gentle probing and reflection can assess what the most important issues are for the woman. The clinical nurse specialist is in an ideal position to build a good rapport with the patient and family owing to her autonomy, availability, experience, advanced clinical decision making and expertise. A woman's individual femininity, sexuality and body image are especially important to ascertain because these issues can ultimately affect the decision she finally makes on breast reconstruction. However, the nurse specialist can only identify these issues when a sound relationship has been established with trust and when a woman feels there is confidentiality. Nurses often feel inadequate when faced with issues of sexuality and feel they do not possess the skills to assess these sensitive issues but much can be assessed by what the patient initially says and her actions, without any strong enquiry from the nurse. Often women think they want breast reconstruction but after talking to the specialist nurse and surgeon, seeing relevant photographs and speaking to other women, they decide against it. Body image and sexuality are important issues in the decision to have breast reconstruction but are not the only factors that influence a woman. Other issues surrounding the decision process include: the support network within the family, occupation and financial issues, dependants, amount of information available, final results and the likely adjuvant treatment required. There is, however, little research evidence on the factors that enable women to decide on breast reconstruction and their coping abilities around this decision period (Harcourt, 2001).

The surgeon would have already physically assessed the patient's suitability for breast reconstruction before it is offered. In order to make such a huge decision a woman needs adequate information, given clearly and in stages, both verbally and written by the nurse specialist. She also needs time to decide. Clifford (1979) reported that several women felt that not enough time had been given for them to decide. Often, women benefit from talking to someone who has undergone the procedure, and seeing photographic results to consider the pros and cons of the procedures involved. Some women are well informed about breast reconstruction, others know very little. The woman who does not want to discuss breast reconstruction or wants minimal input from any nurse including the clinical nurse specialist has to be respected; the nurse can only offer her support and a contact number should the woman change her mind.

Once the surgeon and the patient have discussed briefly the breast reconstruction options there is usually one option that appeals to a woman. For example the TRAM reconstruction is popular because it usually does not involve an implant and gives a 'tummy tuck' at the same time. However, some women, because of their shape, size, health status and previous circumstances, e.g. radiotherapy, may only be suitable for one option. This makes it easier for the nurse specialist to discuss with the patient. When a woman has the option of all three methods of breast reconstruction and is unsure, she will need more information, more time and support to enable her to decide on the right option.

Some women have unrealistic expectations of the final result and the preoperative time is very important for discussing all the issues. It has been found that specific pre-operative counselling for breast reconstruction does not increase the likelihood that a woman will choose breast reconstruction; it has more to do with a woman's own desires than access to education (Finlayson et al., 2001). Nevertheless, quality information, time to make an informed decision and careful patient selection are paramount. Pre-operative counselling not only enables the woman to consider all the issues but allows the nurse specialist to make a thorough psychological assessment of the patient.

Continuous education and support are very important for women who accept or refuse breast reconstruction. Those who refuse may want to reconsider, change their mind, or have a delayed breast reconstruction.

If surgery needs to be performed on the contralateral breast, photographs can also be seen of this surgery. Again a volunteer can be provided if the woman so wishes and the procedure needs to be fully discussed. In addition to the education and information given by the nurse specialist and nurses caring for the woman, information booklets provided locally or by cancer organizations such as Breast Cancer Care and CancerBacup can be given. For many women, the role of the nurse specialist extends beyond the initial pre-operative assessment to full recovery. Although policies vary between regions, a contact number is usually given even if the clinical nurse specialist cannot visit in the community. Women who refuse breast reconstruction need to feel just as supported. The relationship with the primary healthcare team is also very important. Support may be given from the district nurses, GP and possibly practice nurses.

When the patient is admitted to the hospital the ward nurses care for her, so it is imperative that good communication exists between the nurse specialist and the ward team, ensuring continuity of care. Pre-operative marking up is essential, especially for nipple reconstruction, and it is a good idea for patients to wear a prosthetic nipple a few weeks prior to surgery to enable accurate placement of the new nipple. On admission the patient will have an anaesthetic assessment and a general history will be taken.

Post-operatively

Following surgery the ward nurses take the usual observations for blood pressure, temperature, pulse, pain and any post-operative complications, for example bleeding. The breast reconstruction should also be monitored – especially 'flap' surgery – for colour, temperature and swelling: if the flap is not a healthy pink colour but dark and cold to the touch this needs to be reported as it indicates venous congestion. Blanching, which is touching the flap to ensure venous return, can be performed by the nurse. These observations are usually carried out half-hourly until stable. Most women have PCA in place (patient controlled analgesia) to stabilize their own pain, especially women undergoing TRAM reconstruction, which can be very uncomfortable. Pain management is extremely important. Women vary in their recovery and progress. An intravenous infusion is also in place until the woman is eating and drinking, and there are always drains in place that require either changing daily or careful output recording. Removal of drains will depend on the hospital policy and particular surgeon. The drains should be observed for excess blood volume, indicating bleeding, and also for patency to ensure the drain is draining freely. Drains may reduce the risk of infection and haematoma, although there is no evidence to support this.

No tight dressings or pressure of any kind should be put on the wounds following surgery as they may interfere with the circulation, especially in the case of flap surgery. For those women with implant surgery, the chest wall may already feel very tight. Women need to be informed that post-surgery they will feel a tightness across their chest where the implant has been placed under the muscle and that when they relax and become more mobile the tightness will improve. The wounds need to be observed for bleeding or swelling, which may indicate a haematoma.

As the patient recovers and the hospital stay lengthens, the woman becomes more mobile, the drains are removed, the dressings are changed according to the surgeon's preference and arm exercises are increased. The physiotherapist normally visits the woman, as well as the specialist nurse and ward nurses, and arm exercises are encouraged and demonstrated as soon as possible. Women need reassurance that they will not damage anything by moving their arm as soon as possible and that the arm can be particularly painful after axillary surgery. Leaflets on arm exercises can also be given. In addition, the arm can be particularly painful after axillary surgery. The wounds must also be observed for signs of infection and tissue necrosis. Any signs of redness, heat, discharge or a rise in temperature need reporting. Infection must be addressed immediately as it may compromise the success of the breast reconstruction. Antibiotics are commenced if infection occurs but will also be given in theatre prophylactically. The chances of an implant needing removal after surgery as a result of infection are low, as is the need for more surgery following flap breast reconstruction because of necrosis. The clinical nurse specialist will usually visit the patient on the ward, check wounds and support the patient psychologically.

Hospital stay varies for each woman and for each breast reconstruction technique and particular hospital. It is now commonplace to discharge women home with the drain in place so this could be as early as 4–5 days post-operatively. Seroma formation after removal of drains, whether in hospital or at home, is a possibility and is common. It occurs in 10 to 52 per cent of patients (Tadych and Donegan, 1987). The patient is made aware of this and told that any signs of swelling in the wound need to be reported, and reassurance needs to be given that it can easily be aspirated. District nurses are also involved with the patient on discharge, which means patients have the primary healthcare team, the ward and the breast team as sources of contact. Some clinical nurse specialists visit the patient at home post-surgery and can assess for any physical or psychological problems and refer to the appropriate person. It must be remembered that women are not only coming to terms with their new body image and reconstruction but may also have worries concerning the cancer, survival and adjuvant therapy.

Women usually return to the hospital a few weeks following surgery for their results and to check their wounds. When healing has taken place the breast reconstruction can change shape and look very different from the initial post-operative period when swelling and bruising has disappeared.

Any signs of tissue necrosis (dark hard areas) need to be reported early and therefore the primary care team are invaluable following discharge. Any discoloration of skin, discharge, protrusion of an implant from a mastectomy wound, or any signs that a wound is not healing should be reported. An earlier outpatient appointment may be necessary. The clinical nurse specialist usually makes contact post-surgery and becomes aware of any complications. Advice on bras is given by the nurse specialist and also the ward nurses. Initially a soft bra is advised and then a more supportive bra when the wounds have healed. Wearing a bra is very individual and there is no evidence that wearing one immediately affects the breast reconstruction. It is, however, more comfortable for the larger breasted patient. Patients who want to wear underwired bras are able to do so once healing has taken place. Information, support and psychological care are usually continued after discharge until the patient and nurse feel these can be given less frequently. The patient should always have a contact number. For those patients assessed by the clinical nurse specialist to be in need of more expert intervention, referrals to counsellors, psychologists or psychiatrists can be made.

Summary

Breast reconstruction is not essential for everyone in order to improve psychological well-being, but access to breast reconstruction should be available to all women. Although there have been major improvements in surgical techniques and availability, breast reconstruction is not accepted by the majority of women facing breast surgery. Generally, those who do accept it are younger patients, whose appearance is a high priority. Satisfaction rates are generally very high. Those not suitable seem to select themselves out after adequate counselling by the clinical nurse specialist and surgeon.

To date there is clearly little conclusive research evidence surrounding the psychological benefits of breast reconstruction and in particular little is known of the decision process, enabling or disabling factors influencing women at the time (Harcourt, 2001). This in itself presents the clinical nurse specialist and other nurses involved with such patients with a major nursing challenge because they are at the forefront of care. To date, the key psychological influences include body image, personality, sexuality, cancer treatments, fear, expectations, scars and the amount and quality of available information.

Although body image and sexuality are two recurring factors influencing the decision on breast reconstruction, they are not the only ones. Some women with a high body image, for example, refuse breast reconstruction because of many of the other issues involved.

The clinical nurse specialist in breast care has a key role to play caring not only for the woman with breast cancer but also those with breast cancer who are considering breast reconstruction. Her advanced nursing skills and in-depth knowledge, as well as the close relationship and rapport built with the patient, equip her with the necessary resources to do this.

In conclusion, patients considering breast reconstruction need and want information, both written and verbal. This information needs to be given in stages and it has been suggested that a video would also be helpful. Too much information given too soon is not processed and patients may require continuous support in order to make a final decision. A few consultations may be necessary. Patients value the input of the clinical nurse specialist, who is in an ideal position to make physical and psychological assessments because of her understanding of the whole cancer process for the patient. This can then be communicated to the multidisciplinary Breast Team thereby ensuring individualized intervention and careful patient selection.

References

Al Ghazal SK, Fallowfield L, Blamey RW (2000) Comparison of psychological aspects and patient satisfaction following breast conserving surgery, simple mastectomy and breast reconstruction. European Journal of Cancer. 15(36): 1938-43.

Allweis TM, Boisvert ME, Otero SE, Perry DJ, Dubin NH, Priebat DA (2002) Immediate reconstruction after mastectomy for breast cancer does not prolong the time to starting adjuvant chemotherapy. American Journal of Surgery 183(3): 218-21.

Anderson R, Kaczmarek B (1996) Psychological well-being of the breast reconstruction patient: a pilot study. Plastic Surgical Nursing 16: 185-8.

Arnez ZM, Bajec J, Bardsley AF, Scamp T, Webster MH (1991) Experience with 50 TRAM flap breast reconstructions. Plastic Reconstruction Surgery 87: 470–8.

Barreau-Pouhaer L, Le MG, Rietjens M, Arrlagada R, Contesso G, Martins R (1992) Risk factors for failure of immediate breast reconstruction with prosthesis after mastectomy for breast cancer. Cancer 70 1145–51.

Beasley ME, Ballard AR (1990) Immediate breast reconstruction: a comparison of techniques utilizing the pedicled TRAM and tissue expanders. Paper presented at the Annual Meeting of the American Association of Plastic Surgeons, Hot Springs, VA, 7 May.

Berry MG, Al-Mufti RA, Jenkinson AD, Denton S, Sullivan M, Vaus A, Carpenter R (1998) An audit of outcome including patient satisfaction with immediate breast reconstruction performed by breast surgeons. Annals of the Royal College of Surgeons of England 80: 173.

Bostwick III J (1990) Plastic and Reconstructive Breast Surgery, Vol. II. St Louis, MO: Quality Medical Publishing.

Bremner-Smith A, Straker V, Abel A, Rainsbury R (1996) Choices and experiences of women offered breast reconstruction. Paper presented at British Association of Surgical Oncologists, Winter Meeting, Royal College of Surgeons, London.

Callaghan CJ, Couto E, Kerin MJ, Rainsbury RM, George WD, Purushotham AD (2002) Breast reconstruction in the UK and Ireland. British Journal of Surgery 89: 335–40.

Clifford E (1979) The reconstruction experience: the search for restitution. In Georgiade NG (Ed) Breast Reconstruction following Mastectomy. St Louis, MO: Mosby, pp. 22–34.

Cotton T, Locker A, Jackson L et al. (1991) A prospective study of patient choice in treatment for primary breast cancer. European Journal of Surgical Oncology 17: 115–17.

Dean A, Chelty N, Forrest APM (1983) Effects of immediate breast reconstruction on psychological morbidity after mastectomy. Lancet: 459–62.

Department of Health (1996) Hospital Episode Statistics. London: Department of Health.

Department of Health (1999) Withdrawal of oil based breast implants. Department of Health Website [http://www.doh.gov.uk/cmo99_01.htm].

Dickson MG, Sharpe DT, Dickson WA, Wilde GP, Brennan TG, Roberts AH (1987) Breast reconstruction by tissue expansion. Annals of the Royal College of Surgeons of England 69: 19–21.

Fallowfield LJ, Baum M, Maguire P (1986) Effects of breast conservation on psychological morbidity associated with diagnosis and treatment of early breast cancer. British Medical Journal 193: 1331–3.

Fallowfield LJ, Hall A, Maguire P, Baum M, A'Hern RP (1994) A question of choice: results of a prospective 3 year follow up study of women with breast cancer. The Breast 3: 202–8.

Faulder C (1982) Breast Cancer: A Guide to its Early Detection and Treatment. London: Pan Books.

Fentiman IS (1990) Detection and Treatment of Early Breast Cancer. London: Martin Dunitz.

Finlayson CA, Macdermott TA, Jyoti Arya MD (2001) Can specific pre-operative counselling increase the likelihood a woman will choose post mastectomy breast reconstruction. American Journal of Surgery 182: 649–53.

Fisher B, Redmond C, Poisson R et al. (1989) Eight year results of a randomized controlled study comparing total radical mastectomy and lumpectomy with or without radiation in the treatment of breast cancer. New England Journal of Medicine 320: 822–8.

Gilboa D, Borenstein A, Floro S (1990) Emotional and psychological adjustment of women to breast reconstruction and detection of sub-groups at risk for psychological morbidity. Annals of Plastic Surgery 25: 397–401.

Goldberg IA, Scott RN, Davidson PM, Murray GD, Stallard S, George WD, Maguire GP (1992) Psychological morbidity in the first year after breast surgery. European Journal of Surgical Oncology 18: 327-31.

Handel N, Silverstein MJ, Waisman E, Waisman JR (1990) Reasons why mastectomy patients do not have breast reconstruction. Plastic & Reconstructive Surgery 86(6): 1118-25.

Harcourt D (2001) Psychological aspects of breast reconstruction: a review of the literature. Journal of Advanced Nursing 4(35): 477-87.

Holly P, Kennedy P (1998) The psychological benefits of immediate breast reconstruction in women who have undergone surgery for breast cancer. Proceedings of the British Psychological Society 6: 32.

Kagawa-Singer M, Wellisch DK, Durvasula R (1997) Impact of breast cancer on Asian American and Anglo American Women. Culture, Medicine and Psychiatry 21(4): 449-80.

Kasper AS (1995) The social construction of breast loss and reconstruction. Women's Health 1(3): 197-219.

Kissane DW, Clarke DM, Ikin J, Bloch S, Smith CG, Vitetta L, McKenzie DP (1998) Psychological morbidity and quality of life in Australian women with early stage breast cancer: a cross sectional survey. Medical Journal of Australia 169(4): 192-6.

Krueger EA, Wilkins EG, Strawderman M, Cederna P, Goldfarb S, Vicini FA, Pierce LJ (2001) Complications and patient satisfaction following expander/implant breast reconstruction with and without radiotherapy. International Journal of Radiation Oncology Biological Physics 1/49 (3): 713-21.

Maguire GP, Lee EG, Bevington DT (1978) Psychiatric problems in the first year after mastectomy. British Medical Journal 282: 963-5.

Malata CM, McIntosh SA, Purushotham AD (2000) Immediate breast reconstruction after mastectomy for cancer. British Journal of Surgery 11(8): 1455-72.

McCardle J, George W, McCardle C, Smith D, Moody A, Hughson A, Murray G (1996) Psychological support for patients undergoing breast cancer surgery: a randomised study. British Medical Journal 312: 813-17.

McKenna R, Grene T, Hang-Fu L, Hayes D, Scanlon E, Schweitzer R, Strax P, Winchester D, Wood W (1991) Implications for clinical management in patients with breast cancer. Cancer 68 (Suppl.): 1182-3.

Mock V (1993) Body image in women treated for breast cancer. Nursing Research 42(3): 153-7.

Morris T (1983) Psychosocial aspects of breast cancer: a review. European Journal of Cancer and Clinical Oncology 19: 1725-33.

Morrow M, Bucci C, Rademaker A (1998) Medical contraindications are not a major factor in the utilization of breast conserving therapy. Journal of the American College of Surgeons 186(3) 269-73.

Nissen MJ, Swenson KK, Ritz LJ, Farrell JB, Sladek ML, Lally RM (2001) Quality of life after breast carcinoma surgery: a comparison of 3 surgical procedures. Cancer 91(7): 1238-46.

Owens RG, Ashcroft JJ, Slade PD, Leinster SJ (1988) Psychological effects of the offer of breast reconstruction following mastectomy. In Watson M (Ed) Psychosocial Oncology. Oxford: Pergamon.

Peyser PM, Abel JA, Straker VF, Hall VL, Rainsbury RM (2000) Ultra conservative skin sparing key-hole mastectomy and immediate breast and areola reconstruction. Annals Royal College of Surgeons of England 82: 227-35.

Pierce P (1993) Deciding on breast cancer treatment: a description of decision-making behaviour. Nursing Research 42: 22-7.

Reaby LL, Hort LK (1995) Post mastectomy attitudes in women who wear external breast prosthesis compared to those who have undergone breast reconstruction. Journal of Behavioural Medicine 18: 55-67.

Rosenqvist S, Sandelin K, Wickman M (1996) Patients' psychological and cosmetic experience after immediate breast reconstruction. European Journal of Surgical Oncology 22: 262-6.

Rowland J, Dioso J, Holland J C, Chaglassian T, Kinne D (1995) Breast reconstruction after mastectomy. Who accepts it, who refuses! Plastic and Reconstructive Surgery 95(5): 812-22.

Schain WS, Wellisch DK, Pasnaw RO, Landsverk J (1985) The sooner the better: a study of psychological factors in women undergoing immediate versus delayed breast reconstruction. American Journal of Psychiatry 142: 40-7.

Schain WS (1991) Breast reconstruction: update of psycho-social pragmatic concerns. Cancer Supplement 68(5): 1170-5.

Schover LR (1991) The impact of breast cancer on sexuality. Body image and intimate relationships. Cancer Journal for Clinicians 41(2): 112-20.

Scott L, Spear MD, Spittler CJ (2001) Breast reconstruction with implants and expanders. Plastic and Reconstructive Surgery 107: 177-87.

Singletary SE (1996) Skin sparing mastectomy with immediate breast reconstruction: the MD Anderson Cancer Centre experience. Annals of Surgical Oncology 3: 411-16.

Stevens LA, McGrawth M, Druss RG, Kister SJ, Gump FE, Forde K (1984) The psychological impact of immediate breast reconstruction for women with early breast cancer. Plastic and Reconstructive Surgery 73: 619-28.

Tadych K, Donegan WL (1987) Post mastectomy seroma and wound drainage. Surgical, Gynaecology & Obstetrics 165: 483-7.

Vasconez LO, Lejour M, Gamboa-Bobadilla M (1991) Atlas of Breast Reconstruction. New York: Gower Medical Publishing.

Veronesi V, Saccozzi R, Vecchio M (1981) Comparing radical mastectomy with quadrantectomy, axillary dissection and radiotherapy in patients with small cancers of the breast. New England Journal of Medicine 305: 6-11.

Von Smitten K, Sundell B (1992) The impact of adjuvant radiotherapy and cytotoxic chemotherapy on the outcome of immediate breast construction by tissue expansion after mastectomy for breast cancer. European Journal of Surgical of Surgical Oncology 18: 119-23.

Walsh Spencer K (1986) The significance of the breast to the individual and society. Plastic Surgical Nursing 16(3): 131-2.

Ward CM (1981) Breast Reconstruction after cancer. Aesthetic triumph or surgical disaster? British Journal of Plastic Surgery 34: 124-7.

Watson JD, Sainsbury DRD, Dixon JM (1995) ABC of breast disease: Breast reconstruction after surgery. British Medical Journal 6310: 117.

Wellisch DK, Shain WS, Noone RB, Little JW (1985) Psychosocial correlates of immediate versus delayed reconstruction of the breast. Plastic and Reconstructive Surgery 76: 713-18.

Winder AE, Winder BD (1985) Patients counselling: clarifying a woman's choice for breast reconstruction. Patient Education and Counselling 7: 65-75.

Young-McCaughan S (1996) Sexual functioning in women with breast cancer after treatment with adjuvant therapy. Cancer Nursing 19(4): 308-19.

CHAPTER 8

Chemotherapy as a Treatment for Breast Cancer

JOAN MCCOY

Introduction

The term chemotherapy was first coined to describe the use of chemicals or drugs to treat microbial and later neoplastic diseases. After the first promising results of cytotoxic treatment during studies in the 1940s, there was a tremendous surge of activity to discover new anti-cancer agents in the hope of finding the ideal drug that would eradicate the tumour whilst having no harmful effects on normal tissue. More than 50 years later this hope is yet to be realized but the search for new cytotoxics has yielded many hundreds of compounds with possible therapeutic applications, though only 40 or so are in common use.

Chemotherapy in breast cancer has become firmly established as one of the major therapeutic modalities. Although introduced much more recently than other treatments, chemotherapy has assumed increasing importance.

This chapter will explain how chemotherapy works, how it is used and the side effects of treatment with some basic detail on side effect management.

In recent years we have seen the development of new approaches in treating breast cancer. The use of the new monoclonal antibody Herceptin® is explained, including administration and side effects.

How Chemotherapy Works

Cytotoxic drugs are defined as 'cell killing drugs' and they act against cancer cells in two main ways:

1. to kill dividing cancer cells;
2. to interfere with cell reproduction.

In this way such drugs eradicate or control cancer cell growth.

Chemotherapy cannot, however, distinguish between normal and malignant cells. This means that when a cytotoxic drug is introduced into the body it will attack not only dividing cancer cells but also normal cells which are proliferating as part of the normal physiological processes of repair and replacement, e.g. bone marrow, hair, gastrointestinal tract, skin, etc. It is this that leads to the well-known side effects of these drugs including neutropenia, nausea and vomiting, stomatitis and alopecia. These side effects will be discussed in more detail later in this chapter.

A knowledge of the way in which normal cells and tumours grow is important in understanding the way in which cancer chemotherapy is used.

The Cell Cycle

M: mitosis;
G_0: resting phase;
G_1: early growth phase;
S: DNA synthesis;
G_2: later growth phase.

After cell division, each cell enters a growth phase, G_1, which lasts for a variable length of time in different tissues. Cells that are not dividing are said to be in the G_0 phase. After G_1 the cells move into the phase of DNA

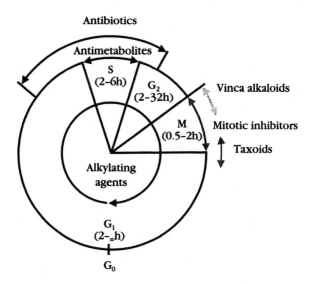

Figure 8.1: Cell Cycle Diagram and sites of action of cytotoxic agents.

synthesis, the S phase, in which the amount of chromosomal material is doubled. The cell then passes through a premitotic phase, G_2, and then into mitosis, M, in which the pairs of chromosomes separate and the cell divides.

The rate of cell division in human tumours and the speed at which their size increases vary considerably from one disease to another.

Classification of Cytotoxic Drugs

Cytotoxic drugs are divided into:

- Cell cycle phase specific drugs. Only a limited number of cells will be sensitive to these drugs; they are more powerful in specific phases of the cell cycle, e.g. vinblastine is specific to the M phase.
- Cell cycle phase non-specific drugs. These drugs are toxic to cells in the cycle, regardless of the phase, e.g. cyclophosphamide.
- Cell cycle non-specific drugs. These drugs act on the cell in or out of the cycle, e.g. BCNU.

Cytotoxic drugs are classified into six biochemical groups:

1. Alkylating agents: Alkylating agents prevent certain enzymes from carrying out their biological role within the cell, preventing formation of new DNA and inhibiting mitosis. They also form breakages and cross-links with DNA chains. Most are cell cycle non-specific, destroying resting and dividing cells.

Example: cyclophosphamide.

2. Anti-metabolites: The chemical structure of these drugs is similar to some essential metabolites required for synthesis of nucleic acid and protein. These drugs are taken in place of essential components and cause breakdown of synthesis and thus prevent cell division. They are most active in the S phase and are therefore cell cycle phase specific.

Examples: methotrexate, 5-fluorouracil.

3. Vinca alkaloids: These drugs are derived from the periwinkle plant. They prevent spindle formation and mitosis at metaphase by binding tubulin, which is an intracellular protein required to achieve mitosis.

Examples: vinblastine, vinorelbine.

4. Antimitotic antibiotics: These drugs bind directly to the DNA and change its make-up therefore preventing normal duplication. There are two groups:
   - Anthracyclines, e.g. doxorubicin and epirubicin;
   - non-anthracycline antibiotics, e.g. mitomycin C.
5. Taxanes: These are derived from yew trees and work by inhibiting mitosis.

Examples: Taxotere, Taxol.

6. Miscellaneous compounds: The action of these drugs is not fully understood and does not conform to other groups.

This group includes: cisplatin, carboplatin, etoposide and dacarbazine.

Combination Chemotherapy

Many cancers are treated with a combination of several drugs. The principles of this are:

- A combination of drugs, with different mechanisms of action, reduces the risk of developing drug resistance. They may be synergistic, interacting with each other to produce increased activity, which is greater than the effect achieved by giving the same drugs separately.
- A combination of drugs with different toxicity can be given to a maximum tolerated dose without causing unacceptable or irreversible toxicity.

The principles for choice of drugs in combination chemotherapy include:

- Drugs should be proven to have value in the treatment of the disease.
- Drugs should have different modes of cytotoxic action.
- The dose-limiting toxicity of drugs should be different, so additive toxicity does not limit dose or intensity of treatment.

Scheduling of Chemotherapy Treatments

The interval between treatments is very important. Too short an interval and normal cells do not have sufficient time to recover and repair. Too long an interval and cancer cells have more time to replicate and the tumour may get larger.

Most chemotherapy treatments for breast cancer are delivered every 21 to 28 days for 6–8 cycles.

A given dose of chemotherapy kills a proportion of cells, not a given number. Because only a proportion of the cells die with a given treatment, repeated doses of chemotherapy must be used to continue to reduce the number of cells.

In an ideal system, each time the dose is repeated the same proportion of cells, not the same absolute number, is killed. The 'log kill graph' in Figure 8.2 demonstrates this diagrammatically.

Between doses, cell regrowth occurs. When therapy is successful, cell killing is greater than cell regrowth. Drugs should therefore be scheduled in such a way as to produce maximum killing. This will depend on the rate of recovery of the normal tissues that have been most damaged by the drug. These tissues are usually the gut and bone marrow, which regenerate quickly in comparison with most cancer tissue. For this reason pulsed intermittent therapy, with time for normal tissues to recover, is the usual method of drug administration.

It is also important to note that in some instances breast cancer cells can be completely resistant to the cell-killing effects of cytotoxic drugs.

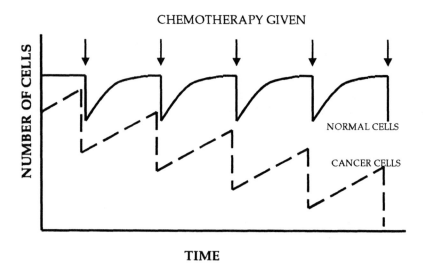

Figure 8.2: 'Log kill graph' – demonstrating the effect of chemotherapy on normal and malignant cells in a tumour which is responding to treatment.

Role of Cytotoxic Chemotherapy in Breast Cancer

Chemotherapy has an important part to play in the treatment of breast cancer. The treatment aims to cure some women but for others who are not going to be cured it serves to prolong life and affect or palliate symptoms. Current chemotherapy approaches include:

1. Neoadjuvant chemotherapy. Chemotherapy may be used as first-line treatment for large breast tumours. The aim of this approach is to shrink the tumour prior to surgery. This may avoid mastectomy and often renders inoperable breast tumours operable (Mansi et al., 1989). This method of treatment has been shown to prevent up to 90% of women undergoing mastectomy (Bonadonna et al., 1990).
2. Adjuvant chemotherapy. This approach involves the administration of chemotherapy following local treatment for the tumour by surgery or radiotherapy. The aim of adjuvant chemotherapy is to reduce the risk of metastatic disease and improve disease-free survival. It is normally used for women who have poor prognostic indicators such as lymph node metastases. However, there has been an increasing trend to give chemotherapy to almost all young patients with operable breast cancers regardless of lymph node status as there is increasing evidence of real benefit in disease-free survival.
3. High-dose chemotherapy. This approach involves the delivery of high doses of chemotherapy in an attempt to eradicate the cancer. However, to date, the results of clinical trials using high-dose chemotherapy regimens have not been encouraging. Several international studies looking at high-dose treatment for metastatic disease and in the adjuvant setting have shown that there is no appreciable survival benefit over conventional treatment (Berger, 1999).
4. Palliative chemotherapy. Palliative chemotherapy sees its place in the management of symptoms associated with advanced metastatic disease, for example, liver pain in patients with hepatic metastases, or dyspnoea in patients with pulmonary metastases. The overall aim of treatment is to improve quality of life. The benefits must always outweigh the side effects. It is important that patients fully understand the treatment intention in these circumstances. Nurses fulfil an important role in meeting information needs and ensure that patients have realistic expectations.

Drug Administration

Dose Calculation

The dose of drug to be administered is generally based on the individual's body surface area (BSA), usually expressed in milligrams per square metre. The patient's body surface area is determined by a height and weight nomogram.

Chemotherapy agents for breast cancer are most commonly administered via the intravenous route. This is the most reliable method of drug delivery. It is important to note that patients who have undergone breast surgery should always have the intravenous drugs administered through the veins on the contralateral arm.

It is not uncommon for patients to be prescribed oral chemotherapy. Currently the most commonly used oral cytotoxic drug for the treatment of breast cancer is cyclophosphamide.

Cytotoxic drugs commonly used to treat breast cancer

Currently the drugs commonly used to treat breast cancer include:

- doxorubicin;
- epirubicin;
- cyclophosphamide;
- methotrexate;
- 5-fluorouracil (5-FU);
- mitomycin C;
- mitozantrone;
- docetaxel (Taxotere);
- vinorelbine;
- paclitaxel (Taxol).

These drugs can be used as single agents but are more commonly used in combination.

Examples of some widely used combination regimens include:

CMF = cyclophosphamide, methotrexate, 5-FU;
AC = doxorubicin, cyclophosphamide;
FEC = 5-FU, epirubicin, cyclophosphamide.

These chemotherapy regimens may be used in the neoadjuvant, adjuvant and palliative settings.

Taxotere is commonly used as a monotherapy in patients with locally advanced metastatic breast cancer. Clinical trials suggest that half of all patients whose disease is resistant to anthracyclines may achieve either a complete or partial remission when administered Taxotere. Its place in the adjuvant setting is still to be fully elucidated.

Professional Issues

The delivery of chemotherapy, as well as the education of the patient and family, is primarily the responsibility of the registered nurse. Only specially trained nurses working as part of a multidisciplinary oncology team should administer chemotherapy (Calman and Hine, 1995).

Each Hospital Trust involved in the delivery of chemotherapy should have a comprehensive policy detailing all the necessary precautions for the safe handling and administration of cytotoxic drugs.

The 'Manual of National Cancer Standards' (Department of Health, 2001) details the minimum standards a hospital must meet in order to be recognized as delivering the minimum standards of safe practice.

Common Side effects of Breast Cancer Chemotherapy (Figure 8.3)

The common side effects of anti-cancer cytotoxic agents used to treat breast cancer include the following.

Bone Marrow Depression (Myelosuppression)

Myelosuppression is not only the most common dose-limiting side effect of chemotherapy but also potentially the most life threatening (Maxwell and Maher, 1992). All haematopoitic cells divide rapidly and are therefore vulnerable to chemotherapy.

Neutropenia (drop in white blood cells) typically develops 8–12 days post-chemotherapy, with full recovery 21–28 days post-treatment. Occasionally the white blood count can drop to a level where the patient cannot fight infection normally.

Most patients receiving chemotherapy for breast cancer will receive this as an outpatient and will only need admission to hospital if they become neutropenic and febrile.

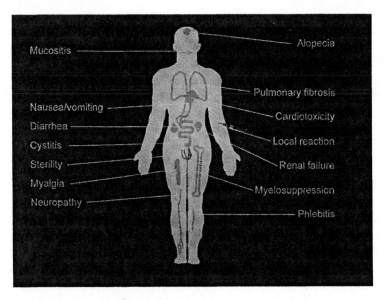

Figure 8.3: Side effects of chemotherapy

If admitted to hospital, the patient will need to be nursed in protective isolation in line with local infection control policy and procedure and be assessed for the source of infection. They will almost certainly require intravenous antibiotic therapy and will need close observation of vital signs, observing for septic shock, signs of which include high temperature with low blood pressure. This should be reported to a member of the medical team urgently as septic shock leads to fatality if not treated immediately.

Patients should be given only food that is hot and freshly cooked to minimize the risk of infection by pathogens carried in food. They should be advised to avoid uncooked and unpasteurized foods including shellfish, salads and soft cheeses. Fruits with thick skins, which can be peeled, are safe to eat including bananas and oranges. This advice is also applicable to patients who are at home and have a low white blood count, and it is also important to remind patients that food from the local 'take away' should also be avoided!

Neutropenic patients who are at home should be advised to monitor themselves for fever, sore throat, dysuria or productive cough. If a patient has any sign of infection she/he should be advised to contact the hospital chemotherapy unit immediately.

In some cases it may be necessary for the patient to be prescribed a granulocyte colony stimulating factor (GCSF) to promote the production of neutrophils by the bone marrow. This is used to prevent or recover low blood counts and may contribute to the reduction of febrile episodes during neutropenia.

It can be administered either by the patient her/himself at home or the district nurse may need to get involved. It would be the nurse's role to teach the patient self-administration of the subcutaneous injection.

Chemotherapy units will have comprehensive guidance available for the care of a myelosuppressed patient. It is advisable that such patients should be cared for on wards where the nursing staff have experience of managing post-chemotherapy complications.

Alopecia

Alopecia is the most noticeable and often the most distressing side effect. Although not a life-threatening event, loss of hair has a profound social and psychological impact on individuals and their acceptance of treatment. Some may even refuse potentially curative treatment for fear of this effect (Freedman, 1994).

Cancer chemotherapy agents affect actively growing hairs. As actively growing hair is the most rapidly proliferating cell population in the human body, alopecia is a common toxic manifestation of these drugs. The extent of hair loss ranges from thinning of scalp hair to total body hair loss. With an average of 85 per cent of scalp hair follicles in the active growing phase at any one time, the most common location for hair loss is the scalp.

Unlike natural hair loss, chemotherapy-induced alopecia occurs rapidly and usually starts two to three weeks following a dose of chemotherapy. It is most apparent after one to two months. Hair loss is diffuse and usually asymptomatic; however, some patients have described scalp discomfort one to two days prior to and during hair shedding.

Alopecia is temporary and reversible. After discontinuation of the drugs, regrowth is visible within six to eight weeks. As hair grows back, alterations in hair pigment (lighter or darker), texture (finer or coarser) and hair type (straight or curly) may be evident.

Prevention of alopecia

Since the 1960s considerable efforts have been directed at reducing the incidence and severity of alopecia using scalp hypothermia or scalp cooling (Dean et al., 1983). The rationale is that it causes vasoconstriction of the superficial scalp veins, temporarily preventing drug uptake, and it also reduces cellular uptake of drugs that are temperature dependent such as doxorubicin. There are several types of scalp-cooling systems available in the United Kingdom (e.g. Penguin, Paxman), all working on the above basic principles but employed slightly differently. Therefore, I shall not endeavour to discuss the specifics of the procedure.

Hair contributes greatly to body image, consequently the loss of hair can have a devastating emotional impact on a patient. In the absence or failure of hair-preserving techniques, more emphasis needs to be placed on the psychological support of the patient and on creative measures to preserve self-image. Advice on the use of scarves and hats may also help patients to cope with hair loss, and an information booklet is available from the cancer charity BACUP entitled 'Coping with Hair Loss'. These are available free of charge to patients and their relatives.

One UK charity, 'Look Good... Feel Better', offers free consultation to patients on applying make-up and skin care for patients with cancer. This service aims to improve self-esteem and confidence for women with cancer.

It is often helpful for patients to prepare for probable alopecia by obtaining a wig before it becomes absolutely necessary. This will reduce the anxiety associated with uncertain timing of hair loss and makes it easier for a hairstylist to match colour and style

Nausea and Vomiting

Nausea and vomiting associated with cancer chemotherapy can be classified as anticipatory, acute and delayed.

Anticipatory nausea and vomiting occurs in approximately 25 per cent of patients (Aappro, 1991) before chemotherapy is administered. It is difficult to control and is associated with worsening acute nausea and vomiting (Goodman, 1997). Triggers for anticipatory nausea and vomiting include previous unsuccessful control of emesis, smells, sight of chemotherapy nurse, hospitals, etc.

The administration of lorazepam prior to treatment has been found to relieve anticipatory effects (Malik et al., 1995).

Acute nausea and vomiting occurs from a few minutes to one to two hours after treatment, usually resolving within 24 hours. This is generally associated with the emetogenicity of the drugs administered and can be counteracted with the administration of appropriate anti-emetics prior to administration.

Delayed nausea and vomiting persists or develops 24 hours after chemotherapy administration. Oral granisetron or ondansetron (5HT3 antagonists) have been found to control delayed nausea and vomiting for up to 72 hours post-chemotherapy.

Management of nausea and vomiting

Management should begin by obtaining an in-depth emetic history and developing a prevention action plan with anti-emetics. Characteristics that affect the occurrence of nausea and vomiting include susceptibility to motion sickness, poor previous emetic control and being young. Individuals with a heavy alcohol intake seem to have a decreased occurrence of nausea and vomiting (Aapro, 1991; Goodman, 1997).

Anti-emetics interrupt the stimulation of the vomiting centre in the brain. The choice of anti-emetic drugs should be made according to the emetic potential of the chemotherapy drugs. Anti-emetic protocols direct the healthcare professional to prescribe the most effective anti-nausea drugs. Each chemotherapy unit will have a detailed anti-emetic protocol. Anti-emetic drugs commonly used with chemotherapy include:

- granisetron;
- domperidone;
- ondansetron;
- cyclizine;
- dexamethasone;
- metoclopramide.

As part of patient education it is important to inform patients about the potential side effects of anti-emetic therapy; for example, dexamethasone (steroid) can cause hyperactivity, sleeplessness and weight gain; granisetron/ondansetron can cause constipation and headaches.

Skin and Nails

Several chemotherapy drugs are associated with altered skin pigmentation. This is a purely cosmetic reaction and the aetiology is poorly understood. It is unclear why some drugs are associated with widespread pigmentation and others are confined to darkening specific areas, e.g. nails and tongue. Hyperpigmentation occurs more commonly in dark-skinned individuals.

Hyperpigmentation associated with cyclophosphamide can be diffuse or confined to the palms, soles, nails or gums. With 5-FU hyperpigmentation occurs most readily in sun-exposed areas. Patients may also experience hyperpigmented streaks overlying veins that have been used repeatedly for infusions of 5-FU. This generally occurs without any clinical evidence of cutaneous inflammation or phlebitis.

Cyclophosphamide, doxorubicin and 5-FU have been associated with hyperpigmentation of the oral mucosa and tongue, especially in Afro-Caribbean patients. Doxorubicin and 5-FU may also cause skin darkening over the knuckles.

Hyperpigmentation subsides once treatment is finished.

Changes in toe- and fingernails are commonly seen in patients receiving chemotherapy. Pigmentation is seen most commonly and occurs more regularly and intensely in Afro-Caribbeans than in Caucasians. The pigment is deposited at the base of the nail causing dark lines, corresponding with the times the drug was administered. This reaction occurs most commonly with cyclophosphamide, doxorubicin and docetaxel.

Beau's lines (transverse white lines or grooves in the nail) indicate a reduction or cessation in nail growth in response to cytotoxic chemotherapy.

After treatment the nails will resume a normal growth pattern and the evidence of any damage will grow out.

It is invaluable that nurses are aware of these effects, which are all too often overlooked. Although these effects do not make the patient unwell, the period when they occur can be very frightening. The alteration in skin and nail pigmentation will add to patients' altering self-image. Nail varnish can be used to disguise pigmented nails and patients may find value in seeking make-up and skin care advice from the charity 'Look Good... Feel Better'.

Weight Gain

Weight gain is a troublesome side effect of chemotherapy, and is due to increased calorie intake (Grindel et al., 1989). Significant correlations exist between weight gain and subjective feelings of unhappiness and worry. Factors contributing to weight gain include use of steroids, taste changes, increased appetite, depression, mild nausea that is relieved by eating and psychological distress (Knobf et al., 1983; Knobf, 1986; Grindel et al., 1989).

It is not unusual for some women to gain as much as 6 kilograms (1 stone) in weight.

The potential problem of significant weight gain should be discussed with patients prior to commencing treatment, as most patients assume that they will lose weight during treatment. Weight gain can add to poor self-image and self-esteem.

Fatigue

Fatigue is a common subjective complaint associated with adjuvant therapy, and symptoms such as total body tiredness, forgetfulness and wanting to rest increase over time throughout therapy (Knobf et al., 1983).

Patients should be advised to take regular breaks throughout the day as necessary.

Stomatitis

The oral mucosa, which has a rapid proliferation rate, is a prime target for complications secondary to cancer chemotherapy. In breast cancer treatment, the drugs that are most likely to cause stomatitis are doxorubicin, epirubicin and methotrexate.

Oral complications resulting from treatment can be acute or chronic.

Acute:

- mucosal inflammation;
- ulceration;
- infections including herpes simplex and candida.

Chronic:

- taste alteration;
- xerostomia (salivary gland dysfunction causing a dry mouth).

Treatment of drug-induced stomatitis is essentially palliative, involving topical anaesthetics (e.g. Difflam or cocaine mouthwash for severe stomatitis), analgesics, coating agents (e.g. Gelclair) and cleansing mouthwashes (e.g. Corsodyl).

Infections need to be treated with the appropriate agents: e.g. candida should be treated with anti-fungal preparations, which include topical treatment with mouthwash/lozenges or systemic treatment with fluconazole.

Herpes simplex can be treated topically with acyclovir cream or systemically with intravenous or oral preparations of acyclovir. This will be dependent on the severity of the infection and whether the patient is neutropenic or not.

All the above preparations will need to be prescribed by a doctor.

It is the nurse's role to provide education on good oral hygiene. There is evidence to suggest that the performance of good oral care may be of greater significant benefit in reducing the effects of chemotherapy than the actual agents used.

The patient should be advised to clean her/his teeth twice per day with a soft toothbrush, and the brush rinsed well after use. A chlorhexidine (0.2%) based mouthwash, e.g. Corsodyl, should be used after brushing in an aim to prevent stomatitis. This can be used in conjunction with an anti-fungal mouthwash such as nystatin. If the patient has a dental plate or full dentures these should also be rinsed in the chlorhexidine solution before replacing.

In an attempt to relieve xerostomia, patients can be advised to chew sugarless gum, suck a hard sour sweet or use regular mouth rinses with iced water to promote saliva production. It may be necessary to employ a saliva substitute. Patients should be advised that irritants such as tobacco, alcohol and caffeine should be avoided as they dry and irritate the mucous membranes.

Chemotherapy drugs cause direct injury to taste cells composing the taste buds, resulting in taste changes that vary widely. Common changes include an increased threshold for sweet taste, a decreased threshold for bitter taste and complaints of a metallic taste. Some agents, such as cyclophosphamide, can be tasted while being injected.

Unless patients are specifically questioned, taste alterations are seldom reported.

Fertility

Infertility and sterility after chemotherapy have been noted since the early 1970s, with reports of amenorrhoea after single-agent or combination therapy. The likelihood that chemotherapy will affect a patient's fertility depends on gender, age and the specific drugs (Lamb, 1995).

Many pre-menopausal women who receive chemotherapy for breast cancer will experience ovary failure and early menopause. In contrast with males, the age of women is an important predictor of treatment-induced sterility. The probability of premature menopause occurring and being permanent increases for women as they near the age of 40 years (Chapman, 1982).

For most, menses (periods) cease during therapy or become erratic over two to three years and amenorrhoea occurs. Levels of follicle stimulating hormone (FSH) increase gradually and remain elevated for two to five years. FSH levels > 30 ng/l are generally considered diagnostic for ovarian failure.

Estradiol and testosterone levels decrease by 60 per cent, which may account for the reports of lessened sexual desire and arousability (Goodman, 1996).

Pre-menopausal women who receive chemotherapy should be clearly informed of their risk for temporary or permanent ovarian failure. Menopausal symptoms that commonly occur include hot flushes, night sweats, vaginal dryness and irregular menses. Patients will need support and advice on how to manage these symptoms.

Contraception

Although many patients experience reproductive dysfunction during chemotherapy, information should still be given concerning contraception. A woman may still be fertile during treatment even if her menstrual cycle is irregular. The combined oral contraceptive pill is not currently recommended in patients with breast cancer so alternatives will need to be explored with the patient and her partner.

Patients who survive cancer and are considering starting a family are generally advised to wait at least two years from the completion of therapy. The main reason for waiting is that most recurrences of cancer occur within two years (Shrover, 1991).

In general most chemotherapy drugs are excreted from the body within 72 hours of administration. Patients need to be advised to use condoms and to avoid oral sex during this period because vaginal secretions may contain chemotherapy metabolites.

Accurate information can make a significant difference in the patient's ability to deal with sexual concerns regarding chemotherapy.

New Developments in Breast Cancer Management

Herceptin®: a Monoclonal Antibody

Herceptin is a monoclonal antibody that binds to the HER-2 (Human Epidermal growth factor Receptor 2) cell surface receptor, which is over-expressed in some breast cancer patients. It is used to treat patients with metastatic disease whose tumours over-express HER-2. Herceptin is the only licensed monoclonal antibody for the treatment of breast cancer.

HER-2 is a protein product of a specific gene with cancer-causing potential. Under normal conditions, two copies of the HER-2 gene in a cell produce small amounts of a protein product on a cell surface called the HER-2 growth factor cell surface receptor, which appears to play a role in transmitting growth signals and controlling normal cell growth and division.

Researchers have discovered that sometimes the HER-2 gene is amplified, resulting in multiple copies in a single cell. It is not yet known what factors trigger this genetic event. This in turn triggers HER-2 over-expression. The overproduction of HER-2 receptors seems to stimulate some cells to divide, multiply and grow at a faster rate than normal cells, thus contributing to the occurrence and progression of cancer. Slamon et al. (1989) demonstrated that HER-2 is amplified or over-expressed in as many as 20–30 per cent of breast cancer patients.

The significance of over-expression of HER-2 in breast tissue is that these patients are at greater risk of aggressive disease. These markers are directly related to a poor overall prognosis, with faster relapse and shorter survival time at all stages of breast cancer development (Slamon et al., 1989). When compared with women whose tumours do not over-express HER-2, these women's cancer may spread to other parts of the body at a faster rate, progress more rapidly after standard treatment including chemotherapy, and affect long-term survival.

Herceptin works by binding to the HER-2 cell surface receptors, thus blocking their action. Unlike cytotoxic chemotherapy Herceptin does not have a significant effect on normal healthy cells. The presence of Herceptin stimulates the body's own natural defences (killer cells and macrophages) to help destroy the tumour cells.

Herceptin is administered as a weekly short intravenous infusion; the first dose is administered over 90 minutes and subsequent doses are administered over 30 minutes. Any adverse reactions are generally manageable. Patients can receive this treatment in the outpatient setting, thus minimizing disruption to their lifestyle (Cobleigh et al., 1999).

The major difference between chemotherapy and Herceptin is the side effect profile. Herceptin does have side effects, including transient infusion-associated fevers, chills and pain. These are experienced with the initial infusion in around 40 per cent of patients (Baselga et al., 1996; Cobleigh et al., 1999) but do not usually occur during subsequent infusions.

Although these adverse effects can be managed effectively, the experience can be very frightening for the patient and the nurse. It is therefore imperative that oncology nurses caring for patients receiving Herceptin are confident in the management of adverse effects and that emergency drugs and equipment are readily available for the treatment of anaphylaxis. Close observation of the patient is essential during the infusion. Adverse effects can be managed using an analgesic/antipyretic such as parac-etamol or an antihistamine such as Piriton.

The adverse effects are caused by the body's natural response to a foreign agent but are usually mild because Herceptin is a humanized antibody.

Because Herceptin is a protein produced by living cells, the body accepts the agent more readily and usually adapts to it after the first infusion.

The most concerning adverse side effect reported with Herceptin is cardiac dysfunction (Stebbing et al., 2000). Cardiac dysfunction has been reported in approximately 5 per cent of patients treated with Herceptin alone (Cobleigh et al., 1999), and 13 per cent of patients receiving Herceptin in combination with chemotherapy (Slamon et al., 1989). However, later studies suggest that it is a much greater problem, with a 28 per cent incidence when administered with concomitant anthracycline chemotherapy. As a result of these findings it is recommended that, when Herceptin is to be administered with chemotherapy, it is given with taxanes as opposed to anthracyclines (e.g. doxorubicin, epirubicin). Taxanes have a lower risk of associated cardiotoxicity.

As a new development in breast cancer treatment HER-2 testing and the use of Herceptin signify innovative and promising advances in the treatment of metastatic breast cancer.

Conclusion

There are currently national comprehensive guidelines for the treatment and management of breast cancer but it remains important that a patient's treatment should, as far as possible, be tailored to the individual. The current emphasis is on multidisciplinary decision making and treatment planning involving breast care nurses, surgeons, oncologists, histopathologists and oncology nurses, to name but a few. This is breaking down historical barriers and is a positive step towards the delivery of seamless care.

Most, if not all, of these treatments are medically prescribed, but we should never underestimate the benefit of nursing in caring for these patients. There is a great deal of scope for nursing creativity in supporting patients throughout their cancer treatment experiences.

References

Aapro MS (1991). Controlling emesis related to cancer therapy. European Journal of Cancer 27: 356–61.

Baselga J, Tripathy D, Mendelsohn J et al. (1996) Phase II study of weekly intravenous recombinant humanised anti-p185 HER-2 monoclonal antibody in patients with HER-2/neu-overexpressing metastatic breast cancer. Journal of Clinical Oncology 14(3): 737-44.

Berger A (1999) High dose chemotherapy offers little benefit in breast cancer, new article. British Medical Journal 318: 1440.

Bonadonna G, Veronesi U, Brambilla C, Ferrari L, Luini A, Greco M et al. (1990) Primary chemotherapy to avoid mastectomy in tumours with diameters of three centimeters or more. National Cancer Institute 82: 1539–45.

Calman K, Hine D (1995) A Policy for Commissioning Cancer Services. A Report by the Expert Advisory Group on Cancer to the Chief Medical officers of England & Wales. London: Department of Health.

Cobleigh M, Vogel C, Tripathy D, Robert N, Scholl S, Fehrenbacher L et al. (1999) Multinational study of the efficacy and safety of humanized anti-HER-2 monoclonal antibody in women who have HER-2 overexpressing metastatic breast cancer that has progressed after chemotherapy for metastatic disease. Journal of Clinical Oncology. 17(9): 2639–48.

Chapman RM (1982) Effect of cytotoxic therapy on sexuality and gonadal function. Seminars in Oncology 9: 84–94.

Dean JC, Griffiths KS, Cetas TC et al. (1983) Scalp hypothermia: a comparison of ice packs and the Kold Kap in the prevention of doxorubicin induced alopecia.   Journal   of Clinical Oncology 1: 33–7.

Department of Health (2001) Manual of National Cancer Standards. London: Department of Health. Maxwell MB, Maher KE (1992) Chemotherapy induced myelosuppression. Seminars in Oncology Nursing 8: 113–23.

Freedman TG (1994) Social and cultural dimensions of hair loss in women treated for breast cancer. Cancer Nursing 17: 334–41.

Goodman M (1996) Menopausal symptoms. In Groenwald SL, Frogge MH, Goodman M, Yarbro CH (Eds) Cancer Symptom Management. Boston, MA: Jones & Bartlett, pp. 77–93.

Goodman M (1997) Risk factors and antiemetic management of chemotherapy induced nausea and vomiting. Oncology Nursing Forum 124(7, Suppl.): 20–32.

Grindel CG, Cahill CA, Walker A. (1989) Food intake of women with breast cancer during the first six months of chemotherapy. Oncology Nursing Forum 16: 401–7.

Knobf M, Mullen J, Xistris D et al. (1983) Weight gain in women with breast cancer receiving adjuvant chemotherapy. Oncology Nursing Forum 10: 28–33.

Knobf MT (1986). Physical and psychological distress associated with adjuvant chemotherapy in women with breast cancer. Journal of Clinical Oncology 4: 678–84.

Lamb MA (1995). Effects of cancer on the sexuality and fertility of women. Seminars in Oncology Nursing 11(2): 120–7.

Malik IA, Khan WA, Qazilbash M. (1995) Clinical efficacy of oral lorazepam in prophylaxis of anticipatory, acute and delayed nausea induced by high doses of cisplatin. American Journal of Clinical Oncology 18: 170–5.

Mansi JL, Smith IE, Walsh G, A'Hern RP, Harmer CL, Sinnett HD, Trott PA, Fisher C, McKinna JA (1989) Primary medical therapy for operable breast cancer. European Journal of Cancer & Clinical Oncology 25(11): 1623–7.

Maxwell MB, Maher KE (1992) Chemotherapy induced myelosuppression. Seminars in Oncology Nursing 8: 113–23.

Shrover L (1991) Sexuality and Fertility after Cancer. New York: Wiley.

Slamon D, Godolphin W, Jones LA, Holt JA, Wong SG, Keith DE, Levin WJ, Stuart SG, Udove J, Ullrich A (1989) Studies of the HER-2/neu proto-oncogene in human breast cancer. Science 244: 707–12.

Stebbing J, Copson E, O'Reilly S (2000) Herceptin (trastuzumab) in advanced breast cancer. Cancer Treatment Reviews 26(4): 287–90.

Support Organizations

Look Good ... Feel Better
Albany House
Claremont Lane
Esher, Surrey KT10 9DA, UK
http://www.lookgoodfeelbetter.co.uk

Cancer BACUP
3 Bath House
Rivington Street
London EC2A 3DR,UK
http://www.cancerbacup.org.uk

CHAPTER 9

Radiotherapy as a Treatment for Breast Cancer

KAREN BURNET

Introduction

Comprehensive treatment for breast cancer can include surgery, hormone therapy, chemotherapy and radiotherapy. This chapter will concentrate on the treatment modality of radiotherapy with particular reference to what radiotherapy is, when it is used and how it can affect the patient. Nursing care for the patient undergoing radiotherapy involves many skills from a basic knowledge of radiation physics to understanding what physical effects radiation can have on the patient. The inclusion of radiotherapy in a patient's treatment programme needs careful explanation and preparation to make the unknown and often misunderstood less of an ordeal to that patient. This chapter aims to separate the facts from the fiction about radiotherapy for those who care for patients undergoing this treatment.

What is Radiotherapy?

Radiotherapy is the use of radiation to damage tumour cells. Radiation interacts with the DNA (deoxyribonucleic acid) within the nucleus of the tumour cells. The important cell-killing effect of radiotherapy on DNA is the double-strand break, that is a complete break in the DNA molecule. Although cells can repair some of these breaks, residual breaks lead to cell death, the desired effect against the tumour.

  X-rays were first discovered by Röntgen in 1895. He produced these rays by heating an electrode in a sealed airless tube and applying a voltage across it, which accelerated the electrons towards a target plate. Striking the target, the electrons changed their kinetic (movement) energy into X-rays. The term 'X' was used because at the time the nature of these rays was not understood. Röntgen quickly recognized the potential for medical diagnosis, and an early X-ray exists of his wife's hand, showing how well bones could be visualized with this radiation. The first treatment of a cancer using X-rays took place the next year, 1896.

Also in 1896 Becquerel described radioactivity, and his name is given to the modern SI (Système International) unit of its measurement (Bq). Shortly after, the Curies extracted radium from pitchblende, a radioactive substance of uranium oxides, contributing further to the understanding of radiation. Their name was given to the first unit of radioactivity (Ci).

X-rays (produced by electrons hitting a target) and gamma (γ) rays (produced by the decay of the nucleus of a radioactive atom) are identical forms of electromagnetic radiation. Of all the electromagnetic wave spectrum, which includes light waves, infrared and radio waves, only X-rays and gamma rays have the right amount of energy to produce the ionization of atoms that takes place when radiation passes through living tissue. These are the main sources of therapeutic radiation used today.

In the past, patients with breast cancer requiring radiotherapy were treated using ^{60}Cobalt machines. ^{60}Cobalt decays at a steady rate, with a half-life of five years, emitting gamma rays with high energy. The production of gamma rays is not changed by any external factors such as temperature or pressure and this, combined with its predictable rate of decay, makes it a reliable source of therapeutic radiation. The ^{60}Cobalt machine works by opening a shutter to expose the radioactive source every time the patient is treated but keeps the source shielded at all other times. Today these machines have mostly been replaced by the superior linear accelerators, or 'Linacs', which produce X-rays. Linacs are capable of accelerating electrons almost to the speed of light before they hit a target to produce X-rays. Some Linacs are equipped to allow use of the electron beam (beta particle radiation) itself to treat the patient. Linacs are able to produce a more defined beam than ^{60}Cobalt machines and can achieve greater-depth doses through tissue.

Radiation dose is measured as the amount of energy that is absorbed by tissue and is measured in the SI unit termed the gray, usually abbreviated to Gy. One gray is equal to one joule of energy absorbed per kilogram of tissue treated. Sometimes doses are expressed in centigray (cGy), 100th of a gray.

The penetrating power of high-energy X-rays and gamma rays means that some normal tissues will be irradiated as well as the tumour. With electrons, the radiation stops after a short distance in tissue, the depth of penetration depending on the energy of the beam. This is useful for giving a 'boost' of radiation to the site of the tumour (tumour bed) but using the decay phenomena to reduce the dose to the deeper structures of the chest wall, that is, ribs, lung and heart. When treating breast cancer a boost of radiation to the tumour bed has clearly been proved to reduce the rate of local recurrence (Bartelink et al., 2001).

How Does Radiotherapy Kill Cancer Cells?

Radiation kills cancer cells by:

- a direct hit, when the radiation damages DNA directly; or by
- an indirect hit, when the radiation produces free radicals in water adjacent to the DNA, which then damage the DNA.

This DNA damage leads to breaks in chromosomes, the collection of genes responsible for the particular characteristics of that cell. If a cell is unable to repair these breaks it will die when it tries to divide. Figure 9.1 gives a pictorial representation of what happens when a cell divides.

The damaging effects of radiation are less marked in cells that are hypoxic (have a limited oxygen supply), which could be relevant when treating large, inoperable breast cancers that are not well vascularized and are therefore not well oxygenated. There are also differences in sensitivity in different phases of the cell cycle but it is difficult to exploit this clinically (Hall and Cox, 1994).

Cell death is proportional to the amount of radiation given: the more radiation given the greater the number of cells killed. Unfortunately, the surrounding normal tissues also receive a dose of radiation. If very high doses of radiation are used, normal tissues may be permanently damaged, which could be very dangerous to the patient (Souhami and Tobias, 1995). The limiting of normal tissue damage is achieved by the biological strategy of dividing the course up into a number of treatments, called 'fractions', and by the physical strategy of careful planning to limit the amount of normal tissue

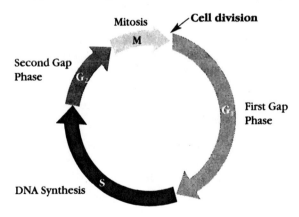

Note: With thanks to Dr Norman Kirkby, Department of Chemical and Process Engineering, University of Surrey.

Figure 9.1: The cell cycle.

treated. The challenge for the radiotherapist is to give enough radiotherapy to achieve optimal local control and survival of the patient, while avoiding normal tissue damage and ensuring a good cosmetic outcome.

When is Radiotherapy Used for the Treatment of Breast Cancer?

Breast irradiation is a major part of the radiotherapy workload in the UK using about 30 per cent of all radiotherapy resources. Radiotherapy has a role in the treatment of breast cancer in several clinical settings.

As a Treatment for Early Breast Cancer

Surgery for the treatment of breast cancer has become less radical over the last 30 years with the introduction of wide local excision of the tumour (see Chapter 5) and the use of primary chemotherapy to reduce the size of the tumour (see Chapter 8). If wide local excision has been used, radiotherapy is given to complete the treatment of the breast, as an added insurance against local recurrence. The breast surgeon will try to remove the entire breast tumour but there is always the risk that at a microscopic level some cancer cells will have been left behind, or that a separate focus of cancer has been missed. It has been shown that mastectomy can safely be replaced by wide local excision and radiotherapy (Fisher et al., 1995). There is also evidence that radiotherapy may contribute to the systemic control of the disease by improving overall survival of the patient as well as preventing local relapse in the treated breast (Overgaard et al., 1997).

Radiotherapy may be given after a mastectomy if the tumour was close to the chest wall or was large in volume. Patients who have a high number of lymph nodes involved with tumour, or who have received primary chemotherapy to shrink the breast tumour or in whom the tumour cannot be completely surgically excised will also be offered radiotherapy.

As a Treatment for a Locally Advanced Breast Cancer

Patients who present with a large, inoperable tumour may receive radiotherapy as a primary treatment to shrink the tumour. The response of the tumour to radiotherapy will be carefully assessed and the plan of treatment may change if the tumour shrinks enough to make surgery possible.

As a Treatment for Metastatic Breast Cancer

Radiotherapy has a very large part to play in the palliation and control of metastatic breast cancer and is generally well tolerated. When used on its own or in conjunction with other treatment modalities radiotherapy can do much to enhance the quality of life of the patient. Radiotherapy given for the treatment of metastatic disease is described in greater detail later in this chapter.

How is Radiotherapy Given to the Patient with Breast Cancer?

External Beam Radiotherapy (or Teletherapy)

External beam radiotherapy is given using a Linac or ^{60}Cobalt machine. The treatment is given in divided doses, known as fractions, on a daily or every other day basis to the breast, chest wall and sometimes to associated lymph nodes. It is recommended that treatment begin about a month after chemotherapy has finished or a month to six weeks after the surgery if no chemotherapy is given.

Brachytherapy

Although most patients in the UK receive breast radiotherapy from a Linac or ^{60}Cobalt machine, radiation can be delivered by a radioactive implant. This is called brachytherapy. Brachytherapy has its place, particularly for local recurrence of breast cancer where external beam radiotherapy has already been given and sometimes, particularly in Europe, to deliver the boost dose of radiation to the tumour bed (Sainsbury et al., 2000). This is discussed in greater detail later in this chapter.

Hyperthermia

Some radiotherapy centres have offered the use of hyperthermia (heat treatment) as an additional treatment, particularly when treating a local recurrence of breast cancer. The theoretical basis for this is that hyperthermia kills tumour cells, particularly hypoxic cells where radiotherapy is less effective. It may also affect particularly any cells that are in S phase, when they are the least radiosensitive. External beam radiotherapy is used concurrently and the treatments are thought to work synergistically. Heating the tissue to be treated can be achieved in several ways but in this situation is usually done with microwaves. Side effects include discomfort or pain during the procedure, and local skin reaction, pain, fever and, rarely, cardiac arrythmias. Only a few centres offer this treatment in the UK and it remains a partly experimental treatment.

Planning Radiotherapy

The patient's initial visit to the radiotherapy department will involve an accurate plan being made of where the radiotherapy will be given. This is called simulation. The first step is to position the patient in a way that is comfortable and also reproducible. The patient's arm is usually moved up (abducted) so it is clear of the breast area. In most centres, the patient is asked to hold on to a fixed point, often attached to the treatment couch, sometimes a pole, to keep her arm in the same position from day to day. The radiotherapy plan is based on pictures taken from an X-ray machine linked to an image intensifier called a 'simulator', and an outline of the shape of the patient's chest. Sometimes a limited CT scan is taken using the simulator to add information, such as the thickness of the chest wall and the position of underlying lung and heart.

The simulator reproduces the movement of the actual treatment machines so that angles and distances between the patient and Linac radiotherapy machine can be calculated. Marks are made on the woman's skin that will later be used to ensure that the treatment beam is accurately directed at the precise area required, avoiding as much as possible the delicate structures of the lung, the left anterior ascending coronary artery and the heart. These lines are made with a semi-permanent pen. Additional permanent 'tattoos' are also made, from a small drop of Indian ink introduced under the skin with a small-bore needle. These tattoos provide a permanent record of the location of the radiotherapy on the patient. The procedure is quick and painless but the need for these marks introduces yet another assault on the patient's body image that can be very difficult. The need for these tattoos needs to be explained to the patient with care and sensitivity ahead of the simulator appointment so that she is prepared.

During planning, which for complex treatments can take up to an hour, the patient will be asked to keep quite still, with her arm up. A good range of arm movement is essential after axillary surgery and if this has not been achieved the patient should be referred back to the physiotherapist for more individualized arm exercises. She will remain supine during her treatment. Clear communication is of paramount importance as this will usually be the first time a patient is introduced to the radiotherapy department. Being surrounded by large and complicated machinery can be very daunting, and then having to keep still for such a long period of time can make some patients very anxious.

Rarely, partial volumes of the breast may be treated if the patient had a very low-grade invasive breast cancer or DCIS. If the patient has undergone a wide local excision of her tumour, the whole breast will be treated, and sometimes a 'boost' of radiation to the tumour bed is given (Sainsbury et al., 2000). The location of the boost is defined by using the surgical scar as a guide. For patients who need radiotherapy to the chest wall following a mastectomy the chest wall is the target, and a boost is not usually required. Some primary breast tumours that have not been removed are visible to the naked eye or their dimensions can be defined with mammogram, ultrasound and occasionally MRI. If the patient has received primary chemotherapy a titanium clip is sometimes inserted into the breast at the time of the diagnostic biopsy to locate the tumour site for the radiotherapist. Depending on the surgical clearance of the axilla and the lymph node involvement the axillary lymph nodes and supraclavicular nodes may also be treated. There has been some discussion about the treatment of the axilla with radiotherapy because of the rare but serious complication of brachial nerve damage or plexopathy (Bates and Evans, 1995; Royal College of Radiologists, 1995) and an increased risk of lymphoedema. There is no consensus as to whether the axilla should be routinely treated or not although standardization of which areas of the breast and loco-regional nodes are to be irradiated is under consideration. Results of research looking at these issues are awaited to see if treating these areas is worthwhile (Dobbs, 2002).

For each patient the volume of tissue to be irradiated is assessed by the radiotherapist and the therapy radiographer. For treatment to the breast it is usual to use two directions of radiation beam or fields, striking the breast tangentially from opposite directions so that the beams intersect within the breast. This gives the most radiation to the tumour or the tumour bed while sparing the skin and normal tissues as much as possible. Since the chest wall is curved and radiation travels in straight lines, it is inevitable that the ribs and a small amount of the lung are treated. When treating the left side, where the heart lies just below the chest wall, it is especially important to minimize any radiation dose to the heart. If the woman has undergone a wide local excision a boost of radiotherapy may be given to the site of the tumour or the tumour bed after the whole breast has been treated. Treating the tumour bed will usually be by a single small electron beam, which can be produced from most Linacs. The radiation physics department will be involved with all treatment plans. Figure 9.2 shows a breast treatment plan. Note the different isodoses or concentrations of radiation throughout the breast shown by the separate contours. This plan shows how well the normal tissues can be spared by accurate and careful planning.

Delivering Radiotherapy Treatment

Once simulated to the satisfaction of the radiotherapist the patient is expected to adopt the exact position each time she is treated. Laser beams projected from the walls of the Linac room onto the patient are lined up on the tattoos and semi-permanent ink marks to ensure that the positioning is accurate daily throughout the weeks of treatment.

After the machine is positioned, each time the patient is treated she is left alone in the treatment room. The radiographers do watch the patient on

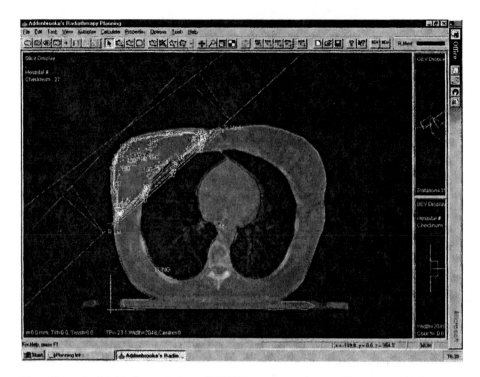

Note: Printed with kind permission of Nikki Twyman, Radiation Physicist, Addenbrooke's NHS Trust.

Figure 9.2: A breast treatment plan.

CCTV but the patient cannot see them. This can be quite frightening for some patients who have been diagnosed with a serious condition and then find themselves isolated whilst they receive the radiotherapy, yet another unknown experience. Sometimes music is left on in the treatment room making the solitude easier and the radiographers who operate the machinery have an audio link with the patient. Clear explanation of the procedure and the approximate time the patient is left alone can help to relieve her anxiety. For a two-field treatment to the breast alone, the whole treatment lasts only about 10 minutes, including setting up the patient, so the patient is alone in the room for only a minute or two at a time.

Radiotherapy Dose

Across the UK there is some variation between radiotherapists about the dose and number of fractions of radiotherapy that should be given to the patient (Yarnold et al., 1995). Generally, treatment fractions are given at a 2.0

gray per day in 25 fractions, over five weeks, or as 2.67 gray per day in 15 fractions over three weeks. A national trial has recently finished which aimed to discover the optimal treatment regime. Called START, the trial randomized women requiring radiotherapy between regimes of differing dose and fractions (START, 1998). The data are currently being analysed and the principle investigators are yet to report their findings but it is hoped that the information gained from this trial will be a useful guide to radiotherapists.

General Nursing Care for a Patient Undergoing Radiotherapy

Patients who need radiotherapy as part of their treatment for breast cancer can have significant concerns about this treatment. They may worry about being badly burned or being very unwell, thinking that the radiation is a systemic and not a local treatment. Some patients confuse the side effects of chemotherapy with radiotherapy and believe that they will lose their hair and be nauseated.

Most people never see a radiotherapy machine until they are being treated so any nursing care should be directed at helping patients to understand the unknown and supporting them through their treatment. Sometimes, for patients, attendance at a radiotherapy unit can mark the end of the fairly intensive support they will have received during chemotherapy and they should be encouraged to call their breast care nurse or treatment radiographer if they are feeling isolated. For many patients who have had adjuvant chemotherapy, radiotherapy is not as difficult but they find that they are still recovering from the physical side effects of their chemotherapy. In reality, radiotherapy is painless and quick once the planning has taken place, and for most women the only side effects they experience are fatigue and some skin sensitivity. Other side effects do occur but these are rare and the severity of such effects depends on the dose of radiation, the individual's sensitivity and the treatment site. If the patient knows what sort of side effects to expect, and that there are measures to alleviate them, she is usually able to cope much better (Ream and Richardson, 1996). Having to attend for daily or every other day radiotherapy may cause some problems for a mother, for the elderly or for someone who has a particularly demanding job. Although most radiotherapy centres are working to full capacity, it is often possible for a patient's treatment to be scheduled for early in the morning or later in the day to help her organize her life better and this should be discussed with the treatment radiographers. Each patient needs to be assessed and cared for as an individual. Patients are seen regularly throughout their treatment by the clinician and the radiographers, so this can be an opportunity to evaluate how things are going as well as assessing the physical effects of the radiotherapy. Most patients find that radiotherapy is not as bad as they were expecting, and meeting other patients who are going through the same treatment can help the individual cope with her fears and anxieties better.

All patients who receive radiotherapy will be given advice about skin care during their treatment. Patients should be encouraged to use aqueous cream or E45 cream to moisturize the area when radiotherapy commences to delay the onset of skin erythema. They should be encouraged to wash or shower their skin during the treatment period, using tepid water and mild soap, rinsing thoroughly and patting the area with a soft, clean towel. Patients should wear loose-fitting, cotton clothing next to the treated area and this clothing should be washed using a mild detergent. Bras should be soft but supportive and not underwired. Towards the end of treatment some women may find that they stop wearing their bra and choose to wear a crop top or a cotton T-shirt. No adhesive tape should be used in the treatment area and perfumed products such as soap or deodorant should not be used in the treatment area once radiotherapy has started.

Hair follicles and sweat glands are radiosensitive due to their high rate of growth. For this reason patients who receive axillary radiotherapy will lose underarm hair on the treated side and may temporarily stop sweating from that axilla, although the sweat glands usually recover after the treatment. Axillary hair does not normally grow back, which can be seen as an advantage, but if the patient was not expecting it, this can be of concern.

For women who have undergone a mastectomy it is recommended that the permanent breast prosthesis is fitted between four and six weeks after radiotherapy as long as the woman's skin has healed from the radiotherapy. For the 'stick-on' type breast prosthesis a longer period of time is required to ensure that the skin is completely healed. Careful assessment of the woman's skin will need to be made by the prosthetic fitter as some women take longer to heal than others.

When a patient is receiving radiotherapy the treatment area should not be exposed to full sunlight and after treatment the patient should be advised not to expose the treatment area to sunlight until it has completely healed. If after several months the patient wishes to sunbathe she must use a high-factor sun cream on the treated area and should not continue to sunbathe if the area becomes red or sore. The skin will stay sensitive to sun for at least one year post-treatment and caution in future years may need to be taken.

Fatigue is very common among patients who have cancer and this tiredness may be compounded by receiving a course of radiotherapy. There may be many practical reasons why radiotherapy makes the patient tired:

* recovering from surgery;
* receiving concurrent chemotherapy;

- pain;
- frequency of visits to the hospital;
- having to continue parenting or other caring role.

In her research Faithfull (1998) found that patients attending for radiotherapy became very tired. She suggested that this fatigue may be related to the accumulation of metabolites and cell destruction from tissue damage caused by the radiation.

Encouraging the patient to take naps during her treatment can help and pre-treatment explanation will help to prepare the woman for this side effect. Some negotiation of treatment times may be possible although this will depend on the workload of that patient's radiotherapy centre.

Early Effects of Radiotherapy to the Breast

Skin Reactions

The skin is composed of several layers of cells: the normal mature cells which are constantly shed from the skin surface and new cells from the basal layer of the epidermis which move up to replace the mature cells. This continuous cell renewal explains why skin is radiosensitive. Although the skin is not often the primary target, the radiotherapy beams must pass through the skin to treat the underlying breast or chest wall.

Erythema, or a reddening of the skin, may be the only manifestation of mild radiation sensitivity for some women, and may develop two to three weeks after radiotherapy treatment has started. In some women, if their skin is particularly sensitive, the erythema may progress to dry desquamation where there is scaly loss of some of the epidermal layer, or moist desquamation, where there is loss of all of the epidermal layer producing an ulcer. This is more common where skin folds meet, such as the infra-mammary fold beneath the breast.

The College of Radiographers has produced guidelines on the assessment of skin reactions and how to care for them (Glean et al., 2001). These guidelines suggest that the patient is assessed for her potential to develop skin reactions using an approved assessment tool before radiotherapy starts. They make the point that intrinsic factors such as age, infection and coexisting disease may make reactions to radiotherapy worse. Extrinsic factors such as treatment dose, fractionation, adjuvant chemotherapy, site of treatment and energy used also affect how patients react to radiation. Even more complicated is the fact that the same amount of radiation given in the same way can cause completely different skin reactions in different women. Skin sensitivity to radiation differs across the population and cannot be routinely tested for at the moment (Burnet et al., 1998). For all these reasons the patient should be reviewed regularly while on treatment. For the individual, assessment is designed to give appropriate care for her individual reaction. For clinical trials, assessment of normal tissue effects is of great importance, and an agreed skin reaction scoring scale should be used, such as that produced by the Radiation Therapy Oncology Group Criteria (Cox et al., 1995).

Specific Nursing Care for a Patient Undergoing Radiotherapy

Skin Care

Radiation skin reactions can occur in a large number of patients undergoing radiotherapy and there is little evidence to support a particular skin care regime (Porock and Kristjanson, 1999). The following general recommendations are based on guidelines from the College of Radiographers (Glean et al., 2001).

Dry desquamation can be divided into two categories: faint or dull erythema, which can be itchy and uncomfortable but responds well to aqueous cream, and tender or bright erythema, which responds well to aqueous cream and hydrocortisone cream 1%. Hydrocortisone cream must be used sparingly and should be discontinued if there is a likelihood of a fungal infection or if the skin breaks down.

If moist cell desquamation develops, radiotherapy may be interrupted to allow healing, though this is not usually necessary. The moist areas can be dressed using a hydrogel, a hydrocolloid or an alginate dressing. If the area becomes infected a swab should be taken and appropriate antibiotics prescribed. After the radiotherapy has been given, healing may be slow but is usually complete and leaves minimal evidence of the acute damage except for pigmentation or telangiectasia. Telangiectasia is caused by the formation of tiny capillaries in the skin and has no physical consequence apart from the change in appearance of the treated area.

Other immediate problems from radiation may be itchiness of the breast that continues after the radiotherapy has finished, and breast lymphoedema, which is being seen much more frequently in lymphoedema clinics. Keeping the skin of the breast well moisturized with aqueous cream can help the itchiness and irritation. For breast lymphoedema referral to a lymphoedema clinic can provide the patient with advice on lymphatic massage or manual lymph drainage (MLD) and the importance of a well-fitted bra is obvious.

Late Changes of Radiotherapy to the Breast

The use of modern radiotherapy equipment and the delivery of smaller fractions of radiotherapy has reduced the incidence of late skin changes to the breast (Sainsbury et al., 2000). These changes can include some thickening or scarring of the breast tissue and some breast shrinkage.

Despite trying to avoid the lung tissue some may be treated by radiation. Damage to the lung tissue by radiation or radiation pneumonitis may have two components. Acute inflammation, with cough, can occur during or just after a course of radiotherapy but is uncommon with radiotherapy for breast cancer. It is the result of inflammation of the alveolar wall plus an accumulation of exudate in the alveolar air space, similar to pneumonia. Later changes can lead to fibrosis of the lung tissue and thickening of the pleura. Such changes reduce respiratory function in the area treated but the degree of disability is related to the amount and condition of the remaining lung tissue. It is rarely noticeable by the patient after breast radiotherapy.

Damage to the myocardium and the coronary arteries has been recognized as a serious late change caused by radiotherapy to the left side of the chest wall or the left breast (Mangar et al., 2002). With the increased use of anthracycline chemotherapy, which also damages the myocardium, cardiac tolerance can be further compromised. Clinicians are aware of this problem and now make every effort to individualize treatment planning to reduce the amount of heart tissue that is irradiated in order to minimize cardiac toxicity.

The ribs are often treated by adjuvant radiotherapy as they fall within the treatment field. There can be immediate rib tenderness and, over time, the ribs can become more brittle and susceptible to pathological fracture. This is a rare complication.

Swelling of the arm and breast can be caused by radiotherapy, due to fibrosis of the lymphatic channels. This risk of lymphoedema is much increased if the patient has undergone surgery to the lymph nodes and then receives radiotherapy to the same area. For more detail on care of lymphoedema see Chapter 11.

Brachytherapy

Brachytherapy is the use of radioactive material placed within, or near to, the area of the tumour. The radioactive source used to treat breast cancer is usually iridium wire. Empty catheters are placed into the breast by a radiotherapist while the patient is anaesthetized. Two systems are used to deliver the radiation. One option is for the radiotherapist to insert the iridium wires into the catheters manually (manual afterloading). The amount of radioactivity is usually low, and the implants take several days to deliver the required dose of radiation. For the safety of staff and other patients the woman is nursed in a lead-lined room and behind lead shields to minimize exposure to others. The radioactive implants will remain in until the calculated dose of

radiation has been given (usually a few days) and will be removed by a radiotherapist along with the inert tubes.

The second option is to use iridium wire, which has a higher level of
activity, afterloaded into the inert catheters by a remote-controlled machine.
These treatments take a matter of minutes but have to be repeated in a daily,
fractionated way. Using this remote afterloading machine, the radioactive
sources are withdrawn mechanically if the nurse or doctor wishes to enter
the room, so there is no exposure to staff.

Safety Concerns Regarding Brachytherapy

For any staff caring for an inpatient with radioactive implants there are three
watch words to bear in mind: time, distance and shielding (Langmack, 1998).
The nursing care of the patient who is receiving brachytherapy should be
carefully planned before going into the patient's room. The nurse should
spend as little time as possible near the patient while providing for her needs.
The intensity of the radiation reduces as the distance from the radiation
source increases, according to the inverse square law. This means that if a
nurse doubles her distance from the patient she will reduce her radiation
exposure to a quarter. The room in which the patient is cared for is usually
lead-lined and moveable lead shields are placed in front of the patient for
added staff protection. The area where someone is being treated with radiotherapy should be marked very carefully with internationally recognized
radiation symbols and any visitors should also be made aware. The area
should be avoided by pregnant woman, women who think they may be
pregnant and young children. Other adults will usually be allowed to visit for
a short time.

Levels of radiation for individuals can be measured if they wear badges
containing radiation-sensitive film. Each badge is assigned to a specific
individual and assessed for a set time period that is strictly monitored by an
assigned radiation protection adviser, usually a physicist. When this film is
developed the photographic film provides a record of how much and to what
type of radiation that individual has been exposed.

Nursing Care of Patients Treated with Brachytherapy

The patient is isolated when the radioactive implants are in situ and will only
be able to have limited visitors; this should be explained to her before she
embarks on her treatment. The patient should be prepared for the isolation
by being advised to bring in books and other distractions to help pass the
time. A television is usually available in the treatment room. Limited but
sensitive emotional support is essential as the patient is coping with not only
breast cancer but the loneliness of being nursed in virtual isolation. This time

away from normal life may provide her with time to reflect on her situation and to consider her future. When with the patient the nurse should make a little time to listen to her concerns while being mindful of her own exposure to the radiation.

Any sign of a wound infection should be reported to the clinician in charge of the patient's care so that antibiotics may be prescribed. Any pain or discomfort should be assessed and treated with appropriate analgesia. Inactivity may cause the associated risk of thrombo-embolic events. The patient should be encouraged to drink plenty of fluids and may be given anti-coagulation therapy and TED stockings to wear to prevent the formation of deep vein thrombosis.

Safe Practice with Radiotherapy

There are significant and known hazards associated with the insertion and removal of radioactive sources and working around radioactive substances but radiation protection is not within the remit of this chapter. The Ionising Radiation (Medical Exposure) Regulations (HMSO, 2000) stipulate regulations on which local radiation protection policies should be written. These regulations apply to patients who are exposed to radiation, and any other individual who might come into contact with radiation as part of health screening programmes, occupational health surveillance, research or medico-legal procedures (HMSO 2000). All staff working in areas where there is radiation have a responsibility to themselves, their colleagues and their patients to be aware of these and any other local policies that their hospital trust follows, and should practise in strict accordance with them.

Treatment of Recurrent and Metastatic Breast Cancer

Radiotherapy has a very large part to play in the palliation and control of metastatic breast cancer and is generally well tolerated. When used on its own or in conjunction with other treatment modalities, radiotherapy can do much to enhance the quality of life of the patient (Oliver, 1996). External beam radiotherapy can be very effective when treating local/regional disease providing that a substantial dose has not previously been given to the chest wall, remaining breast tissue or supraclavicular nodes as part of the original local treatment. Radiotherapy given to fungating lesions can help to reduce the tumour bulk, reducing the amount of dying tissue and reducing the possibility for infection and odour (Regnard and Tempest, 1998). Painful bone disease can be treated very effectively using standard regimes of 30 Gy in 10 fractions, 20 Gy in five fractions or simply a single fraction (Price et al., 1986;

British Surgeons Group of the BASO, 1995). Radiotherapy can reduce pain and promote calcification of the affected area of bone, so preventing unnecessary fractures. If a bone has been stabilized by surgery, radiotherapy can reinforce the bone around the fixation. Radiotherapy may also give considerable relief from pain in other organs, e.g. liver, with a minimum of side effects. Because fewer fractions of radiotherapy are given than with a curative dose there is less risk of skin side effects such as erythema, and dry and moist cell desquamation.

Single brain lesions can be treated very effectively with specialized stereotactic radiotherapy given in a single high-dose treatment (known as radiosurgery), which may only necessitate an overnight stay for the patient so that steroid cover can be administered and the patient can be monitored carefully (Auchter et al., 1996). Adequate treatment of solitary cerebral metastasis is particularly important when a patient's systemic disease is otherwise controlled. Whole-brain irradiation is particularly useful when treating the patient with multiple brain metastases.

Generally radiotherapy treatment given in these circumstances is well tolerated and provides an effective treatment without compromising the patient's quality of life too much.

Political Issues in Radiotherapy

It is generally recognized that there has been underfunding of the radiotherapy services in this country leading to an insufficient number of radiotherapy machines per capita. There is also a national lack of therapeutic radiographers who manage the radiotherapy machines and treatments on a day-to-day basis. Some patients are now waiting for more than 16 weeks to start their radiotherapy, which was unthinkable five years ago. The literature shows that a wait of three to six months to start radiotherapy is associated with lower patient survival for patients with breast cancer (Richards et al., 1999). The creation of the cancer Tzar, the coordination of cancer services across Britain with the NHS Cancer Plan and the implementation of the Cancer Networks is contributing to the improvement and standardization of cancer care. However, more funding for replacement radiotherapy machines and more recruitment of therapeutic radiographers will have to be implemented if patients are to receive the optimum treatment for their breast cancer.

The Future

Most breast treatment plans in the UK are made in a single two-dimensional (2-D) plane which, when translated into the three-dimensional radiotherapy treatment can lead to variations in radiation dose across the breast. In future, greater accuracy of planning could be achieved using 3-D planning of the breast, incorporating information on the 3-D shape of the breast and the chest wall, for example, using a CT scan (Yarnold, 2002). Some equipment such as the multi-leaf collimator, a mechanism of metal leaves that are able to shape the beam of radiation automatically will, with the addition of computer planning, help to deliver radiation more homogeneously, thus sparing more normal tissue and treating the breast more evenly. More complex treatment techniques such as the use of intensity-modulated radiotherapy (IMRT) may facilitate even more homogeneous dose delivery of radiotherapy, although the planning for each patient could take much longer. Randomized trials of such planning methods will need to be realized if the true value of these methods for giving radiotherapy is to be elucidated.

Radiotherapy treatment of the whole breast following wide local excision could, in some cases, become unnecessary. Targeted intraoperative radiotherapy (Targit) is currently being evaluated at various radiotherapy units in the UK. Targit uses a portable electron-beam emitting device that has been designed to deliver radiation to the tumour bed as one treatment. The radiotherapy machine has a spherical applicator (a little like a lollipop), which delivers radiotherapy directly into the wide local excision at the time of surgery so negating the need for external beam radiotherapy. There are different sizes of applicator for use according to the size of tumour removed but this therapy would only be used for early breast cancers. This radiation, often called 'soft X-rays', attenuates quickly and therefore does not scatter into the surrounding normal tissues or further into the operating theatre, making it a relatively safe treatment to administer (Vaidya et al., 2001). The post-operative care is the same for patients as if they had undergone the usual wide local excision. This is a very new method of delivering breast radiation and is being carefully researched at present for it would have clear resource and patient care implications if it were adopted for wider use in the UK.

Conclusion

Radiotherapy is a crucial component of many patients' treatment for breast cancer. It is an ever-developing treatment modality and its effectiveness continues to be proved. This chapter has aimed to make clear why and when radiotherapy is used and to clarify the importance of caring for patients undergoing this treatment.

Refrences

Auchter RM, Lamond JP, Alexander E, Buatti JM, Chappell R, Friedman WA, Kinsella TJ, Levin AB, Noyes WR, Schullze J, Loeffler JS, Mehta MP (1996) A multi-institutional outcome and prognostic factor analysis of radiosurgery for resectable single brain metastasis. International Journal of Radiation Oncology, Biology and Physics 35(1): 27–35.

Bartelink H, Horiot J-C, Poortmans P, Struikmans Van den Bogaert W, Barillot I, Fourquet A, Borger J, Jager J, Hoogenraad W, Collette L, Pierart M (2001) Recurrence rates after treatment of breast cancer with standard radiotherapy with or without additional radiation. New England Journal of Medicine 345: 1378-87.

Bates T, Evans RG (1995) Report of the Independent Review Commissioned by the Royal College of Radiologists into Brachial Plexus Neuropathy following Radiotherapy for Breast Cancer. London: Royal College of Radiologists.

British Surgeons Group of the British Association of Surgical Oncology (1995) Guidelines for surgeons in the management of symptomatic breast disease in the United Kingdom. European Journal of Surgical Oncology 21 (Suppl. A): 1-13.

Burnet NG, Johansen J, Turesson I, Nyman J, Peacock JH (1998) Describing patients' normal tissue reactions: concerning the possibility of individualising radiotherapy dose prescriptions based on potential predictive assays of normal tissue radiosensitivity. Steering Committee of the BioMed2 European Union Concerted Action Programme on the Development of Predictive Tests of Normal Tissue Response to Radiation Therapy. International Journal of Cancer 79: 606-13.

Cox J, Stetz J, Pajak T (1995) Toxicity criteria of the Radiation Therapy Oncology Group (RTOG) and the European Organisation for Research and Treatment of Cancer (EORTC). International Journal of Radiation Oncology, Biology, Physics 31(5): 1341-6.

Dobbs HJ (2002) What's the rationale for breast cancer irradiation in 2002. Abstract for Breast Cancer: Advances in Radiotherapy Planning and Treatment. IPEM/RCR Meeting. Clinical Oncology 14: 174-7.

Faithfull S (1998) Fatigue in patients receiving radiotherapy. Professional Nurse 13(7): 459-61.

Fisher B, Anderson S, Redmond CK, Wolmark N, Wickerham DL, Cronin WM (1995) Reanalysis and results after 12 years of follow-up in a randomized clinical trial comparing total mastectomy with lumpectomy with or without irradiation in the treatment of breast cancer. New England Journal of Medicine 333(22): 1456-61.

Glean E, Edwards S, Faithful S, Meredith C, Richards C, Smith M, Colyer H (2001) Intervention for acute radiotherapy induced skin reactions in cancer patients: the development of a clinical guideline recommended for use by the College of Radiographers. Journal of Radiotherapy in Practice 2: 75-84.

Hall EJ, Cox JD (1994) Physical and biologic basis of radiation therapy. In Cox JD (Ed) Moss's Radiation Oncology: Rationale, Technique, Results, 7th edn. St Louis, MO: Mosby, pp. 3-66.

HMSO (2000) The Ionising Radiation (Medical Exposure) Regulations, No. 1059. London: Stationery Office.

Langmack KA (1998) Factors influencing occupational radiation doses to brachytherapy nurses. Radiography 4: 141-6.

Late Effects of Normal Tissues Consensus Conference (1995) International Journal of Radiation Oncology, Biology and Physics, 31: 1041-1364.

Mangar S, Kumar S, Shentall G, Kirby M, Massey J (2002) Assessment of cardiac volume in tangential irradiation to the chest wall following mastectomy. Abstract for Breast Cancer: Advances in Radiotherapy Planning and Treatment. IPEM/RCR Meeting, London. Clinical Oncology 14: 174-7.

Oliver G (1996) Radiotherapy for breast cancer. In Denton S (Ed) Breast Cancer Nursing. London: Chapman & Hall. Chapter 6.

Overgaard M, Hansen PS, Overgaard J, Rose C, Andersson M, Bach F, Kjaer M, Gadeberg CC, Mouridsen HT, Jensen MB, Zedeler K (1997) Postoperative radiotherapy in high-risk premenopausal women with breast cancer who receive adjuvant chemotherapy. Danish Breast Cancer Cooperative Group 82b Trial. New England Journal of Medicine 337(14): 949–55.

Porock D, Kristjanson L (1999) Skin reactions during radiotherapy for breast cancer: the use and impact of topical agents and dressing. European Journal of Cancer Care 8(3): 143–53.

Price P, Hoskin PJ, Easton D, Austin D, Palmer SG, Yarnold JR (1986) Prospective randomised trial of single and multifraction radiotherapy schedules in the treatment of painful bony metastases. Radiotherapy Oncology 6(4): 247–55.

Ream E, Richardson A (1996) The role of information in patients' adaptation to chemotherapy and radiotherapy: a review of the literature. European Journal of Cancer Care 5: 131–3.

Regnard CFB, Tempest S (1998)A Guide to Symptom Relief in Advanced Disease. Cheshire, UK: Hochland and Hochland.

Richards MA, Westcombe AM, Love SB, Littlejohns P, Ramirez AJ (1999) Influence of delay on survival in patients with breast cancer: a systematic review. Lancet 353(9159): 1119–26.

Royal College of Radiologists (1995) Management of Adverse Effects following Breast Radiotherapy. London: Royal College of Radiologists.

Sainsbury JR, Anderson TJ, Morgan DA (2000) Breast Cancer. In Dixon JM (Ed) ABC of Breast Diseases. London: BMJ Publishing Group, Ch. 7.

Souhami R, Tobias J (1995) Cancer and its Management, 2nd edn. Oxford: Blackwell Scientific Publications.

START (1998) Standardisation of Breast Radiotherapy Protocol: A Randomised Comparison of Fractionation Regimes after Local Excision or Mastectomy in Women with Early Stage Breast Cancer. London: START Trials Office, Institute of Cancer Research.

Vaidya JS, Baum M, Tobias JS, D'Souza DP, Naidu SV, Morgan S, Metaxas M, Harte KJ, Sliski AP, Thompson E (2001) Targeted Intraoperative Radiotherapy (Targit): an innovative method of treatment for early breast cancer. Annals of Oncology 12: 1075–80.

Yarnold JR (2002) Breast cancer: improvements in treatment planning and dosimetry. Abstract for Breast Cancer: Advances in Radiotherapy Planning and Treatment. IPEM/RCR Meeting, London. Clinical Oncology 14: 174–7.

Yarnold JR, Price P, Steel GG (1995) Treatment of early breast cancer in the United Kingdom: radiotherapy fractionation practices. Clinical Oncology 5: 330–2.

Recommended Reading

Chapman D, Goodman M (1997) Breast cancer. In Groenwald SL Goodman M, Frogge MH, Yarbro CH (Eds) Cancer Nursing: Principles and Practice, 4th edn. Boston, MA: Jones & Bartlett, Ch. 34, pp. 916–79.

CHAPTER 10

Hormones as a Treatment for Breast Cancer

DEBORAH FENLON

Women spend much of their lives aware of the rhythm and influences of their hormonal fluctuations. Within current society it is the custom to blame hormones for women's actions and behaviours, as if there were no other influences in their lives. If they are tired or irritable then it must be their hormones, rather than stress, overwork, lack of sleep or any other possibilities. If men put on weight they say that they do not exercise as much or they are eating or drinking more. If women put on weight, then it is their hormones. Actual information about the way in which hormones work and their effects in the body is sadly lacking. Inevitably when breast cancer occurs, the same beliefs and attitudes will apply. Hormone replacement therapy is often blamed for the occurrence of breast cancer, even if the woman has only been taking it for a few months. Many women automatically attribute weight gain to tamoxifen, irrespective of any other lifestyle changes that take place after breast cancer.

Conversely, healthcare professionals frequently underestimate the impact that hormone therapies might have on an individual with breast cancer. For example, Fellowes et al. (Fellowes et al., 2001) showed that 99 per cent of women had side effects from treatment with tamoxifen or goserelin, but that only 89 per cent were recorded in the medical notes.

It is important, therefore, that nurses and healthcare professionals are properly informed about hormonal treatments and their effects so that they can help women to understand the changes that they observe in their bodies after breast cancer treatment. Proper understanding can help women to make appropriate choices about the treatments they accept and how they cope with any side effects from these treatments.

It will be clear to anyone working in this field that breast cancer is a complex disease. Nowhere is this more apparent than when considering hormonal manipulation as a treatment for breast cancer. This means that logical answers are not always the correct ones and that assumptions cannot be made about the way in which breast cancers will respond to the use of hormones. When answering patients' questions in relation to hormones we must look to the findings of clinical trials. Where trial data are not available then we can only say that we do not know the answer, rather than attempting to extrapolate from what is known.

The development of cancers such as breast cancer can be said to be an evolutionary one (Greaves, 2000). There are a number of barriers that cells need to overcome before they are able to grow and spread around the body. It is unlikely that a single genetic mutation will allow a cell to overcome all these barriers and so there must be a succession of mutations enabling cell populations to evolve until they are ultimately able to establish as a cancer. This process is likely to take many years. Once a cancer has been detected and treated there is no reason to assume that evolution does not continue. On the contrary, in the face of treatments that provide further barriers it is likely that further evolution will be stimulated. As a consequence cancers that initially respond to hormone treatments may change and become resistant to that treatment. Moreover, it is possible that the cancer may evolve to the point where it can use the hormone as a stimulus for growth. Evidence for this comes from clinical practice where it is occasionally seen that a breast tumour will shrink after a hormone treatment is withdrawn.

These principles should be borne in mind when considering the use of hormone treatments. In practice they mean that no assumptions can be made about the safety or efficacy of any hormone in the context of breast cancer. However, the reverse is also true: assumptions cannot be made that hormones are not safe or that they will not be effective.

Breast cancer is nearly always an adult tumour and it becomes more common in older women. Most of the risk factors for breast cancer are related to the amount of oestrogen that the body is exposed to during a lifetime. Breast cancer can occur in men but this is rare. If breast cancer occurs at a young age this points to early genetic damage, either due to an inherited mutation (Easton et al., 1993) or to exposure to other agents that cause genetic damage, such as radiation (John and Kelsey, 1993). The majority of breast cancers occur after the age of 50. The risk factors include early menarche (Brinton et al., 1988), late age at first pregnancy or no pregnancies (Kelsey et al., 1993), late menopause and the use of oral oestrogens, such as the contraceptive pill or hormone replacement therapy (Schairer et al., 2000). Dietary factors and obesity also increase the risk of breast cancer (Mezzetti et al., 1998) but these can be argued to have a hormonal link. Cholesterol is a precursor of the sex hormones and dietary fibre increases elimination of hormones from the body. Sex hormones are made in subcutaneous fat as well as in the gonads and people with a high body mass index have higher levels of circulating oestrogens (Prentice et al., 1990). Thus a link can be demonstrated between high intake of saturated fats and increased hormones, especially oestrogen. All of these indicators point towards the role of oestrogens in the development of breast cancer.

This makes sense when considering the role of oestrogen within the body. The normal function of oestrogen is to cause breast and endometrial tissue to grow. During the first half of the menstrual cycle follicle stimulating hormone (FSH) is released from the pituitary and stimulates the ovary to produce and develop a Graafian follicle. The ovary releases oestrogen at this time, which in turn stimulates the lining of the endometrium and ductal tissue within the breast to grow. Once the Graafian follicle has matured it releases an egg into the Fallopian tube ready for fertilization and the remaining follicle becomes the corpus luteum. This continues to be stimulated by the pituitary under the control of luteinizing hormone (LH) and produces progesterone as the dominant hormone. Progesterone causes maturation of breast and endometrial tissue ready for the development and nurturing of a baby.

If cancers that arise within the breast are similar to the original tissue from which they have arisen, and normal breast tissue is stimulated to grow by oestrogen, then it can be postulated that oestrogen will also stimulate breast cancer to grow. Conversely it might be suggested that depriving breast cancers of oestrogen will cause them to regress. These theories have been upheld in laboratory experiments using rat models.

The rationale for depriving breast tumours of oestrogen has been supported by clinical observation as long ago as 1899, when Beatson demonstrated that women with metastatic breast cancers could achieve remission of disease when their ovaries were removed (Forrest, 1982). In the 1970s the mechanism for this was discovered when it was found that proteins on the surface of tumour cells could selectively bind with oestrogen and facilitate uptake of oestrogen into the nucleus of the cell. These were called oestrogen receptors (Barnes and Hanby, 2001). Receptors have since been found for many other hormones. Oestrogen receptors are a normal part of the cell and are found in cells throughout the body in nearly all the major organs, including the brain, skin, bones and periurethral tract. Not all breast cancers contain oestrogen receptors. Those that are oestrogen receptor negative (ER-ve) are much less likely to respond to hormonal manipulation.

Oestrogen has remained the most important hormone when considering treatment for breast cancer. All the hormonal treatments available are based on reducing the amount of oestrogen or opposing its action in some way.

Reducing Oestrogen

In a pre-menopausal woman, preventing the ovaries from working can eliminate 90 per cent of circulating oestrogen. This can be done by surgically removing them or by destroying them by radiation. In the treatment of breast cancer it is more normal to use drugs that 'switch off' the ovaries. As mentioned above, oestrogen is produced by the ovaries under the stimulation of the gonadotrophic hormones LH and FSH that come from the pituitary gland. In its turn the pituitary is stimulated by luteinizing hormone releasing hormone (LHRH) that comes from the hypothalamus. Synthetic analogues of LHRH have been developed that occupy and block all the receptors in the pituitary, thus rendering it insensitive to further stimulation from the hypothalamus. It then no longer releases any gonadotrophins (Cockshott, 2000). Once the ovary is not being stimulated it ceases to produce any oestrogen. There are a variety of these LHRH analogues, such as goserelin (Zoladex®), buserilin and leuprorelin. They will all induce a temporary menopause and its consequences, such as hot flushes (Matsumoto et al., 2000).

Chemotherapy suppresses ovarian function and may also induce a temporary cessation of menstruation and hot flushes. Those women who are approaching menopause may find that their periods do not return and that menopause is permanent. Younger women usually find that menstruation does return and so they cannot assume that they are not fertile during this time. The probability of menopause after hormone or chemotherapy is illustrated according to age in Figure 10.1.

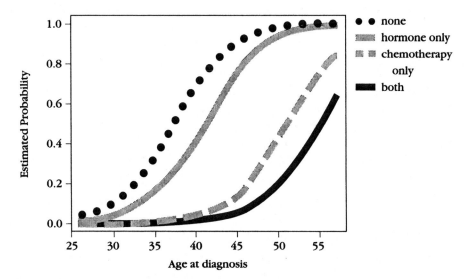

Figure 10.1: Probability of menopause during the first year after diagnosis. Based on: Goodwin et al. (1999b).

Aromatase Inhibitors

Once the menopause is passed, the majority of naturally occurring oestrogens have gone. However, there are still small amounts of circulating oestrogens, which are produced mainly in subcutaneous tissue under the control of the adrenal gland. These are made by the conversion of the androgen androstenedione to oestrogen, by enzymes known as aromatase enzymes (Brodie and Njar, 2000). A variety of aromatase inhibitors have been developed that prevent this conversion from taking place and so further reduce the amount of oestrogen in the body. The first of these was aminoglutethimide, but this was accompanied by high levels of toxicity and so is now rarely used. Anastrozole (Arimidex®), letrozole (Femara®), formestane (Lentaron®) and exemestane (Aromasin®) are now all available. Low levels of toxicity accompany these and most women find them very acceptable. Reduction of oestrogen may result in oestrogen withdrawal symptoms such as hot flushes and dry vagina. Long-term use may be associated with musculoskeletal changes causing aching joints and possibly a loss of bone density. It is not yet known whether this will result in an increase in osteoporosis and higher fracture rate and so long term use is currently not recommended (Baum, 2001).

Opposing Oestrogen

Owing to the complex ways in which oestrogen and progesterone interact with each other, in some situations progesterone may act to inhibit the effect of oestrogen. Synthetic progestogens can be useful in the treatment of breast cancer. The main ones used are medroxyprogesterone acetate (Farlutal® or Provera®) (Pannuti et al., 1993) and megestrol acetate (Megace®) (Powles, 1993). Incidence of side effects is low and some people experience a feeling of well-being when taking progestogens. This makes them particularly useful in palliative care. The main side effect noted is increased appetite and consequent weight gain. Long-term use may also result in Cushingoid changes, such as a redistribution of body fat, which results in a classic moon face and thoracic hump. Earlier changes noted may be increase in sebum production and thinning of hair. Glucose intolerance can be induced so diabetes should be monitored for.

Competing with Oestrogen

The most widely used hormone in the treatment of breast cancer is tamoxifen (Tamofen®, Soltamox®, Nolvadex®) (DeGregorio and Viebe, 1994). This is similar in many ways to oestrogen. It competes with oestrogens to bind to oestrogen receptors. It is then taken into the nucleus of the cell where it stimulates some of the changes in the same way as oestrogen. However, tamoxifen does not have all of the effects of oestrogen and, notably, does not encourage cancer cells to grow. It therefore works as an antioestrogen in relation to breast cancer. However, it continues to stimulate endometrial tissue in the same way as oestrogen and so menstrual irregularities may be seen. Uterine polyps and even uterine cancer may occur (van Leeuwen et al., 1994). A slight increase in deep vein thrombosis and pulmonary embolus has been noted with tamoxifen use (Fisher et al., 2001b). Retinopathy may occur with high doses of tamoxifen use but at the normal dose of 20 mg daily there appears to be no increase in this kind of damage above that which would be expected due to ageing (Lazzaroni et al., 1998). On the whole the risks from tamoxifen are small when weighed against the benefits in terms of cancer treatment and there are other benefits from tamoxifen that should be taken into consideration. It may improve lipid profile and reduce deaths from coronary heart disease (Costantino et al., 1997), although this has not yet been corroborated in long-term studies. It is possible that tamoxifen acts to protect bones from post-menopausal osteoporosis (Love et al., 1994), although bone loss has been observed in pre-menopausal women (Powles et al., 1996). The related drug raloxifene (Evista®) has been licensed for the treatment and prevention of osteoporosis but it does not prevent hot flushes and is not recommended for use either as hormone replacement therapy or for treating breast cancer. It is currently being investigated for its potential to prevent breast cancer (Cummings et al., 1999).

These drugs are known as selective oestrogen receptor modulators (SERMs) because of the way in which they selectively trigger some oestrogen responses and not others (Jordan et al., 2001). Building on the knowledge that this can be done has led to the search for the 'perfect SERM'. This would be a compound that is able to produce all the desired effects of oestrogen and none of the undesirable effects. Desirable effects include protection of bones, cardiovascular system, periurethral tissue, vagina and brain and the prevention of hot flushes. Undesirable effects are the stimulation of endometrial and breast tissue.

Some plants contain compounds that are similar in structure to animal oestrogens and may mimic some of the effects of oestrogen. These are known as phytoestrogens and are available in health food shops with many claims made for their use as 'natural' remedies to 'balance' the body's hormones. If they do have any hormonal effects in the body then it is just as likely that they will have the negative effects as the positive ones. As yet there are few data to support either their safety or their efficacy. As they are classified as foods they are not prepared to the rigorous standards required of

drugs and preparations may contain widely varying amounts of active ingredient. They may also be combined with other ingredients such as steroid
hormones. It is certainly possible that they contain valuable compounds but
caution should be employed when considering their use until more research
is available.

Some of these compounds are found in foodstuffs such as soy protein. It
has been suggested that people who have high levels of soy in their diet have
a low incidence of breast cancer and menopausal hot flushes. It is certainly
true that Japanese women, who traditionally have high intakes of soy, do
have a low incidence of breast cancer and this incidence rises on emigration
to the USA where dietary changes are one of the main changes that occur
(Kliewer and Smith, 1995). It is also the case that hot flushes are rarely
recorded in the literature as a problem for Japanese women. There are some
small studies that show a reduction in hot flushes in women who increase
the proportion of their diet that contains soy (Albertazzi et al., 1998).
However, the role of soy is as yet unclear and there may be other factors that
have not yet been identified that are more important to explain these
phenomena.

Clinical Use of Hormone Manipulation

Prevention

The role of tamoxifen in preventing breast cancer has been explored by a
number of studies with conflicting results. Work in the USA showed a 49 per
cent reduction in the incidence of breast cancer, which was such a strong
preventive effect that the study was discontinued (Fisher et al., 1998).
However, studies in the UK and Italy did not support this finding (Powles et
al., 1998; Veronesi et al., 1998). This could be due to the studies being carried
out in different populations of women. The UK study population was at
much higher risk; many of the subjects had probably inherited a gene
mutation. While it seems possible that tamoxifen has a role to play in
prevention, it is clear that it is not without risk and there are still many
questions to be answered.

Adjuvant Therapy

Once breast cancer has occurred and been treated by surgery, radiotherapy
and chemotherapy, hormonal therapy is considered in order to reduce the
possibility of recurrence. This is known as adjuvant therapy. Tamoxifen has
been shown to reduce the chance of recurrence and mortality from breast
cancer by 47 per cent in those women whose tumours are shown to be
oestrogen receptor positive (Harvey et al., 1999). An additional benefit is to

reduce the incidence of new primaries in the other breast (Nayfield et al., 1991). However, women who have ER-ve tumours do not benefit from tamoxifen (Fisher et al., 2001a). Current guidelines recommend that only women with ER+ve tumours be given tamoxifen as an adjuvant treatment.

It has been shown that there is no additional benefit in continuing tamoxifen for more than five years in those women who have had no axillary lymph nodes involved at primary surgery (Fisher et al., 2001b). There is still some debate as to whether continued tamoxifen should be recommended for women who had disease in the axillary nodes. However, the risks from continued treatment might outweigh benefits if given indefinitely and so current recommendations are to discontinue treatment at five years.

If tamoxifen is given in combination with chemotherapy there may be an increased risk of thromboembolic events (Pritchard et al., 1996) and so it is probably better to reserve tamoxifen use until after chemotherapy has been completed.

Ovarian ablation, either by surgery or by use of LHRH analogues, may also be recommended as an adjuvant treatment for pre-menopausal women (Baum, 2001). The benefit of this has been disputed as it could be argued that chemotherapy that suppresses ovarian function has a hormonal effect as well as a direct cytotoxic effect.

Early results have shown that anastrozole may be at least as effective as tamoxifen in preventing breast cancer recurrence without the risks of endometrial cancer (Baum, 2001). However, some women experience joint aches and pains, and there is a concern that anastrozole may increase the risk of osteoporosis.

Metastatic Disease

Once metastatic disease has been diagnosed in women with breast cancer it is not possible to completely eliminate the disease. The balance of treatment therefore shifts from increasing length of life to maintaining the quality of life. Hormonal therapies can be invaluable in this setting as they have relatively low side effects and may achieve useful responses in ER+ve disease. If the disease is not life threatening, for example it is confined to bone or soft tissue, then hormonal therapy should be regarded as the treatment of choice.

Women who are pre-menopausal should undergo oophorectomy, either surgically or with LHRH analogues. For post-menopausal women tamoxifen has been used for many years as the first-line treatment, although some studies have now demonstrated anastrozole to be equally as effective as tamoxifen (Bonneterre et al., 2000). Hormones can be given sequentially and should be continued until progression. Once tamoxifen and the aromatase inhibitors have been used progestogens may also be useful with the use of androgens, high-dose oestrogen and aminoglutethimide now becoming rare.

The response rate for ER+ve tumours is around 70 per cent and the duration of response is about 20 months.

Hormone Replacement Therapy

Hormone replacement therapy (HRT) remains a contentious issue within breast cancer. It is almost certain that long-term use increases the occurrence of primary breast cancer very slightly (see Table 10.1) (Schairer et al., 2000). This is a small number and most of these tumours are low grade and carry a good prognosis (Holli et al., 1998). There has been no increase in mortality from breast cancer associated with HRT use and the question about the safety of HRT after breast cancer has not yet been answered. Early case control studies show no difference between women with breast cancer who use HRT and those who do not, for either recurrence or mortality (O'Meara et al., 2001). A UK trial has recently been launched to find answers to this question (Marsden, 2000). In the meantime women should be given available information about risks and benefits of HRT so that they can assess for themselves whether they wish to take hormones. For some women menopausal difficulties are severe after breast cancer and they may wish to take on an unknown risk for the future in order to alleviate present suffering. Added to this are the possible benefits in relation to protection from bone loss and heart disease.

Table 10.1: Increased risk of breast cancer with HRT use

Use of HRT	Number of women who develop breast cancer (per 1000)
No use	45
5 years	47
10 years	51
12 years	57

Source: Collaborative et al. (1997).

Male Breast Cancer

There are no controlled studies to determine the most appropriate adjuvant treatment for male breast cancer. However, 85 per cent of male breast cancers are ER+ve and 70 per cent are progesterone receptor positive (Jaiyesimi et al., 1992). As response to hormone therapy correlates to the presence of receptors it is presumed that there is a survival benefit to giving adjuvant tamoxifen to men. It is associated with a high rate of symptoms, such as hot flushes and impotence (Anelli et al., 1994).

In metastatic disease orchidectomy or the use of LHRH analogues may be useful. Tamoxifen, progesterones and aromatase inhibitors may also be used in the same way as for female breast cancer.

Consequences of the Use of Hormonal Therapy in Breast Cancer

Hormone therapies are often given alongside other treatments and so separating out the effects of the hormone therapy from the other treatments can be difficult and sometimes impossible. Women who enter an early menopause due to adjuvant therapy will often assume it is the result of the tamoxifen, as that is a hormonal treatment, rather than chemotherapy. The reverse is usually the case. As seen above (Goodwin et al., 1999b) it is rare to enter the menopause as a consequence of being treated with tamoxifen unless the woman is about to enter menopause anyway. Chemotherapy suppresses ovarian function and can reduce oestrogen levels to less than normal post-menopausal levels. Hot flushes, dry vagina and loss of libido are all more common on chemotherapy than on hormone therapy. Having said that, clinical experience has shown that while chemotherapy may induce menopausal hot flushes, when tamoxifen is added the hot flushes may get worse. Older women who are well past the menopause may find that hot flushes return. Women as old as 82 have been observed to have hot flushes on tamoxifen.

Women who are feeling tired and depressed may blame hormonal imbalances, forgetting that they have been through a major life-threatening illness with aggressive concomitant treatments, all of which frequently result in feeling tired, anxious and depressed. Weight gain is automatically blamed on tamoxifen although it is almost certainly not the culprit (Kumar et al., 1997). One should not dismiss hormones as a possible cause of depression and weight gain but they should not be taken in isolation from other events that are occurring.

The most common side effects with hormonal therapies used in breast cancer can be clustered under the heading of menopausal difficulties and these are addressed below.

Weight Gain

An increase in appetite and subsequent gain in weight are clearly associated with the use of progesterone. However, other weight gain is not clearly related to hormone use. It is the norm for women to increase their weight with age and after menopause the distribution of body fat will change so that it is more concentrated around the abdomen (Astrup, 1999). Davies et al. (2001) showed that weight gain is an age-related effect and not influenced either by cessation of ovarian function or by the use of HRT. A number of studies have shown that it is common to gain weight during the year following a diagnosis of breast cancer, whether or not adjuvant treatment is given (Hoskin et al., 1992; Kumar et al., 1997; Goodwin et al. 1999a), although the use of chemotherapy is closely correlated with weight gain (McInnes and Knobf, 2001). Goodwin et al. (1999a) showed that weight gain is greatest for those who have chemotherapy (1.6 kg) and least for those who have no adjuvant therapy (0.6 kg). Women on tamoxifen gained an average of 1.3kg. Pre-menopausal women gain more weight than postmenopausal women. The most important controlling factor in weight gain is physical exercise (Simkin-Silverman and Wing, 2000). DeGeorge et al. (1990) showed that exercise and dietary measures could be effective in controlling weight gain even after breast cancer treatment.

Body Image Changes

Although the relative contributions of hormone therapy, chemotherapy and menopause are unclear, it is the case that weight gain does occur in women undergoing adjuvant therapy for breast cancer. Western societies put undue pressure on women to conform to the ideal of young, beautiful and slim (Greer, 1991) and so to increase weight is to emphasize change and loss in women who are already undergoing significant change and losses due to facing a life-threatening illness. It may be possible for women to reduce weight by a programme of exercise and dieting but this may also be very difficult in the face of a regime of aggressive treatments with debilitating effects.

Some women also suffer other body image changes such as thinning hair with tamoxifen, and an increase in oily skin with progesterones. If androgens are used in women then virilization will occur. This takes the form of increase in body and facial hair, male pattern hair loss, increase in oily skin and a lowering of the voice. It may also be accompanied by an increase in libido.

The process of undergoing menopause may also contribute to significant body image change in some women. Most cancer treatments last for a defined period, are something to be endured and ultimately come to an end, but menopause is an irreversible change to the body. The woman may feel that she is no longer the person that she used to be. She may now think of herself as an old woman instead of a young woman. Menopause is a constant reminder of all the losses due to the cancer experience (Davis et al., 2000).

Men who are being treated with female hormones may experience gynaecomastia, which can be distressing, especially within the context of a 'female' disease. It is possible to prevent this from occurring by using radiation.

Sexuality

Changes in sexuality can occur with hormone treatments but are more likely to be part of the overall changes that occur at this time. Cancer treatment can have an impact on the quality of sexual relationships owing to the discomfort of breast surgery, the fatigue of chemotherapy and the disruption to sleep caused by hot flushes. Alterations in circulating sex hormones are only one of the contributing factors to changing sexual relations (Greendale et al., 2001). The use of androgens can increase libido in women and the use of oestrogens in men will decrease libido.

Treatments that induce early menopause can cause sexual difficulties due to a dry and painful vagina (see below). Goserelin increases sexual dysfunction during treatment among patients without chemotherapy but the disturbances of sexual functioning are reversible. The use of adjuvant chemotherapy is associated with continued sexual problems, even after three years (Berglund et al., 2001).

Flare

Tumour flare is a rare phenomenon that may happen in patients with metastatic disease. The use of oestrogen, LHRH analogues or, rarely, tamoxifen may cause an initial worsening of the disease due to a temporary surge of circulating oestrogen. In women with bone disease this may cause an increase in pain and a release of calcium into the bloodstream. This can result in hypercalcaemia, which is potentially life threatening. Women should be taught to be aware of the effects of hypercalcaemia and report them immediately.

Thromboembolism

Oestrogens increase the risk of embolism and cause a rise in deep vein thrombosis and pulmonary embolism. A small rise in thromboembolic events has also been observed with tamoxifen (Fisher et al., 1998).

Menopausal Difficulties in Breast Cancer

It has been demonstrated that 60 per cent of all women treated for breast cancer will suffer menopausal difficulties (Canney and Hatton, 1994). These difficulties may be due to the suppression of the ovaries by medical intervention such as goserelin or chemotherapy. Some 30 per cent of all pre-menopausal women will be amenorrhoeic one year after chemotherapy and many more will suffer disruptions to the menstrual cycle (Lower et al., 1999). The nearer to natural menopause, around the age of 50, the more likely it is that menopause will occur and be permanent (Goodwin et al.,

1999b). A further group of women will be undergoing their natural menopause and will be denied the use of HRT. Those who have been taking HRT and are advised to stop when breast cancer occurs will frequently experience hot flushes. It is a commonly held misconception that tamoxifen causes menopause. Unless the woman is near to natural menopause anyway, then this is not the case (see Figure 10.1). However, it is the case that tamoxifen can cause hot flushes in some women (Powles et al., 1994).

Carpenter and Andrykowski (1999) have described the physical effects of menopause experienced by women with breast cancer (Table 10.2).

Table 10.2: Symptoms attributed to menopause by women with breast cancer

Joint pain	77 per cent
Numbness and tingling	40 per cent
Feeling tired	75 per cent
Vaginal dryness	36 per cent
Difficulty sleeping	68 per cent
Dizzy spells	25 per cent
Hot flushes	66 per cent
Pounding heart	25 per cent
Headaches	55 per cent
Painful intercourse	21 per cent
Irritable and nervous	54 per cent
Skin crawls (formication)	18 per cent
Depressed	51 per cent

Source: Carpenter and Andrykowski (1999).

This list is similar to the symptoms given for normal menopause, although Ganz et al. (1998) found that breast cancer survivors experienced an increased incidence of joint pains, headaches and hot flushes when compared with a group of postmenopausal women of the same age who did not have breast cancer. A study by Duffy et al. (1999) showed a very high level of depression, insomnia and hot flushes in women who experienced a premature menopause due to breast cancer treatment.

It may be difficult for women with breast cancer to interpret some of the symptoms that they experience. Some menopausal signs could be confused with effects from treatment or symptoms caused by the cancer itself. For example, sensations of prickling experienced in the upper chest (formication) may be interpreted as cancer recurrence, and the increase in joint aches and pains raises anxiety about bone metastases.

The onset of menopause may also be a reminder for women that they are getting older. They may have hoped not to have to face the menopause for a few more years yet and this represents another change in life. Women experiencing premature menopause interviewed by Singer and Hunter (1999) describe having to redefine themselves: suddenly they are a different person, an older, less attractive person and less of a woman. For some it causes a dramatic loss of self-esteem. Additionally, those women who have never had children, whether by choice or not, may also need to grieve the loss of the possibility of children. It is clear that both breast cancer and menopause cause alterations to body image and may require adjustments in role function. Each human being needs to face her/his own ageing and mortality. However, to have this imposed on one, and to need to address both issues at the same time, may cause particular difficulties with adjustment.

Women undergoing menopause need to be assessed in a holistic fashion so that they can be helped to understand the changes that are occurring in their bodies, and specific interventions may be suggested to help women to adjust to these changes.

Hot Flushes

Hot flushes are a commonly reported sign of menopause but vary widely in their manifestation. They can be frequent and severe and have been reported with up to 240 occurring in a 24-hour period (Levine-Silverman, 1989). Descriptions vary from being a mild feeling of warmth in the upper body and face with mild perspiration through to severe flushes that feel like 'a raging furnace' or 'burning up' (Finck et al., 1998). Carpenter et al. (2002) found that hot flushes in breast cancer survivors were worse than those in women who had not had breast cancer.

Women manage hot flushes with a variety of coping mechanisms. These can be largely divided into physical cooling strategies and cognitive strategies. Cooling strategies that are employed include the use of sprays and fans and choice of appropriate clothing. Cotton is more absorbent than synthetic fibres, layers of thin clothing are easier to adjust, and loose-fitting clothing may be more comfortable than tailored clothes. However, some women may feel disadvantaged by the necessity to wear less feminine clothing and may not wish to alter their clothing but rather maintain their normal social image.

Many women describe how they learn not to fight hot flushes, which can then spiral out of control. They learn to relax and just let the flush wash over them. Concentration may be lost for a few seconds but when this is accepted it is found that it soon passes. Some women describe how they reinterpret the heat as a positive experience, for example reminding themselves of enjoyable summer holidays.

Fears of being unable to cope in social situations are common and are often accompanied by embarrassment and inability to concentrate on tasks at hand. Some women are able to challenge these fears by asking for honest feedback from those they trust about socially embarrassing occurrences such as body odour. Coping strategies such as going back over work done during a flush, or taking a few minutes out for deep breathing, can also help minimize distress.

As well as managing the stress of individual hot flushes, it may be appropriate to lower stress levels in daily life in general. It is known that women who are more stressed experience more hot flushes in a 24-hour period. Relaxation therapy has been shown to be effective in reducing flushing in women who have not had breast cancer (Freedman and Woodward, 1992). Daily relaxation therapy has been shown to reduce anxiety in women with breast cancer and may therefore be beneficial in reducing flushing (Fenlon, 1999). The increased sense of control may reduce intolerable menopausal difficulties to a level that is tolerable. Finally, one of the most distressing problems caused by hot flushes is sleep disturbance and resulting chronic tiredness. Daily relaxation may help to improve sleep and increase feelings of being rested and again increase tolerance of difficult symptoms.

Drugs that are available to treat hot flushes are variable and all have side effects. Clonidine 0.1 mg per day is effective in reducing hot flushes induced by tamoxifen by nearly 40 per cent (Goldberg et al., 1994), although some women have headaches or dry mouth and some experience difficulty sleeping.

Some studies have shown that selective serotonin-reuptake inhibitors (SSRIs) may be effective in reducing hot flushes. Pilot studies have been conducted using venlafaxine (Loprinzi et al., 1998) and paroxetine (20 mg daily) (Stearns et al., 2000). These have shown that 55–67 per cent women show at least a 50 per cent reduction in the incidence of hot flushes and 58–73 per cent reduction in the severity of hot flushes. Unwanted effects of these drugs include dry mouth, nausea, somnolence, nightmares, disorientation and a stimulation of anxiety. While these early studies appear promising, personal experience has shown a high level of side effects that women find totally unacceptable.

Progesterone therapy, such as Megace®, has been found to be effective in reducing hot flushes in women with breast cancer (Loprinzi et al., 1994). However, there are few data on the long-term safety of the use of progesterone after breast cancer.

Many women have used complementary therapies, such as homeopathy and acupuncture, to help hot flushes. Research on these approaches is notoriously difficult and there is very little evidence available to support their use. There is a growing body of anecdotal evidence that supports benefits from these approaches and they may increase a sense of control and well-being in women who use them.

Phytoestrogens in the human diet include many substances classifiable as lignans, isoflavones and coumestrans. Intestinal flora convert inactive plant precursors into compounds active in the human. The biological actions of these compounds are extremely complex and very variable. They are found in a variety of plant food sources, such as red clover, dong quai, liquorice and soy protein. Most studies have not shown any reduction in hot flushes with phytoestrogens either using supplements (Eden, 1998; Baber et al., 1999; Knight et al., 1999) or by incorporating soy flour into the diet (Murkies et al., 1995). One study has shown a reduction in frequency of hot flushes by about 45 per cent by the addition of soy powder (60 g daily) to the diet (Albertazzi et al., 1998). There is some indication that phytoestrogens may have an influence on the maturation of the lining of the vagina (Wilcox et al., 1990) but these are inconsistent and do not correlate with serum levels of phytoestrogen in those who are taking soy supplements (Albertazzi et al., 1999). As suggested earlier, the long-term safety of phytoestrogens is unknown. If they have an oestrogenic effect in the body to prevent hot flushes then it is theoretically possible that they also have an oestrogenic effect in stimulating breast cancer. Until more evidence is available it cannot be assumed that the use of herbal preparations for the relief of hot flushes is safe.

Evening primrose oil is often recommended for hot flushes but there is little evidence to support its efficacy. Vitamin E supplements have been shown to decrease the number of flushes experienced, although the effect is small (Barton et al., 1998). Smoking increases the number of hot flushes that women have (Obermeyer et al., 1999) so smoking cessation should be encouraged.

Vaginal Dryness

While it is clear that vaginal dryness may lead to dyspareunia and thus interfere with sexual relationships, this again cannot be taken in isolation from the other changes that are occurring in a woman's life at this time. Work done by Cawood and Bancroft (1996) showed that the most important predictors of sexuality in menopausal women were not physiological but social. These were other aspects of the sexual relationship, sexual attitudes and measures of well-being. The best predictor of both well-being and depression was tiredness (Cawood and Bancroft, 1996). Therefore while advising on vaginal dryness this should not be taken in isolation from general assessment and discussion regarding general health and well being.

About 36 per cent of women experience vaginal dryness. This may be a mild irritation or can be severe causing pain and inhibiting intercourse. The use of simple moisturisers and gels may be of benefit (see Table 10.3). A polycarbophil moisturising gel such as Replens® can improve vaginal moisture and elasticity and is found to be of benefit in up to 80 per cent of

Table 10.3: Preparations available to use for vaginal dryness

Generic (proprietary) name	Formulation	Regimen	Notes
Astroglide®, Gyne-moistrin®, and Moist Again®	Gel moisturiser	As required	
Vaginal moisturising gel (Replens®)	Polycarbophil gel	Use applicator, insert gel 3 nights per week	
Oestradiol tablet (Vagifem®)	25 µg oestradiol	Insert 1 tablet daily for 2 weeks then reduce to 1 tablet twice weekly Discontinue after 3 months to assess need for further treatment	
Oestradiol ring (Estring®)	Silicone elastomer ring with core that contains 2 mg oestradiol (released as 7.5 µg/ per 24 hours	To be inserted into upper third of vagina and worn continuously; replace every 90 days	Max. duration of continuous treatment 2 years Lack of data regarding systemic absorption

women (Gelfand and Wendman, 1994). Several studies found this to be an effective alternative to local oestrogen therapy (Nachtigall, 1994; Bygdeman and Swahn, 1996).

For some women it may be appropriate to consider the use of local oestrogen. This is very poorly absorbed and indeed when the vagina is particularly dry will not be absorbed at all. Oestrogen preparations should be chosen with care as some contain larger doses which may be absorbed and raise serum oestrogen levels, for example oestrogen creams such as Ovestine® (estriol 0.1 per cent).

Osteoporosis

Some women who experience early menopause due to cancer treatment may be concerned about the possibility of developing osteoporosis in later life, especially if there is a family history of this. Tamoxifen helps to prevent bone loss in post-menopausal women, and aromatase inhibitors increase bone loss. If women are considering using HRT after breast cancer then one of the benefits is the reduction in bone loss and therefore a reduction in the risk of fracture. However, this protection lasts only while hormones are still being taken and the incidence of fractures after the age of 75, when most fractures occur, is unchanged (te Velde and van Leusden, 1994). Weight-bearing exercise will prevent bone loss, although it will not increase bone density (Sharkey et al., 2000). Such exercise can also help to improve fitness and muscle strength, which will contribute to the prevention of falls and a lower risk of fracture (Forwood and Larsen, 2000). In conjunction with advice to increase dietary calcium, exercise plays a significant part in a lifestyle prescription for reducing fractures in later life. Willett et al. (2000) suggest that hormones should not be used routinely even in the non-cancer population for fractures and coronary heart disease because avoidance of smoking, performance of regular exercise and a good diet are effective preventive measures. There are also other non-hormonal drugs that are effective against osteoporosis and so, while HRT could be considered for the relief of menopausal distress it should not be used as a prophylactic against osteoporosis in breast cancer patients.

It has been seen that menopause is a complex phenomenon and that within the context of breast cancer this is even more true. There is much that is still not clearly understood about the way in which women view this transition and the meaning for them when experienced with breast cancer. There is very little reported in the literature about the ways in which women would prefer to manage the difficulties that they may experience. Current advice must be to explore the phenomenon with each individual to help her understand what is happening to her and to identify options and the way in which she will want to manage her difficulties.

Conclusion

While menopause may be a difficult time for some women, most hormone therapies are generally low in side effects (see Table 10.4). Hormone therapies are effective in reducing breast cancer recurrence and can help both to lengthen and to improve the quality of life for women with metastatic disease. As they are not curative, due weight should be given to side effects but many women will find these therapies to be a valuable alternative to other breast cancer treatments. The role of nurses in caring for women on hormone therapies for breast cancer has several components. Nurses need to ensure that they are adequately informed so that they can help the women to understand the changes that are taking place in their bodies. They need to be

Table 10.4: The major hormones used in breast cancer treatment and their side effects

Class of action	Generic name	Trade name	Dose	Route	Side effects and notes
LHRH analogues					
	goserelin	Zoladex®	3.6 mg every 28 days	Intra-muscular Subcutaneous	Menopause induced
Aromatase inhibitors					
	aminoglutethimide	Orimeten®	250 mg daily	Oral	Hot flushes, vaginal dryness, joint aches and pains
					Drowsiness, nausea, lethargy, diarrhoea, ataxia, depression
					Onset of fever and skin rash within 7–10 days, may settle if left
					Needs to be taken with hydrocortisone (withdraw gradually)
	anastrozole	Arimidex®	1 mg daily	Oral	
	letrozole	Femara®	2.5 mg daily	Oral	
	formestane	Lentaron®	250 mg every 2 weeks	Intra-muscular	
	exemestane	Aromasin®	25 mg daily	Oral	

Class of action	Generic name	Trade name	Dose	Route	Side effects and notes
Progestogens					Nausea, fluid retention, weight gain. May experience withdrawal bleeding Prolonged use in high doses may lead to Cushingoid effects Can decrease glucose tolerance – monitor for diabetes
	Medroxyprogesterone acetate	Farlutal® Provera®	500 mg–1 g daily 400–800 mg daily	Oral	
	Megestrol acetate	Megace®	160 mg daily	Oral	
Selective oestrogen receptor modulators					Risk of increased endometrial changes, such as hyperplasia, polyps and cancer. Abnormal vaginal bleeding should be investigated
	Tamoxifen	Tamofen®, Soltamox®, Nolvadex®	20 mg daily	Oral	Hot flushes, vaginal discharge, alterations in menstrual flow Rarely visual disturbances, thromboembolic events Ovarian cysts
	Toremifene	Fareston®	60 mg daily	Oral	Hot flushes, vaginal discharge

prepared to listen to the woman's account of her problems and make a full assessment of her difficulties. They then need to be aware of a range of strategies to help each individual woman work out for herself the best path to take to deal with these problems. Because it is rarely curative, endocrine therapy is one treatment modality where it is clear that the woman being treated needs to make her own decision about quality of life, side effects and the benefits to be gained from treatment.

References

Albertazzi P, Pansini F, Bonaccorsi G, Zanotti L, Forini E, De Aloysio D (1998) The effect of dietary soy supplementation on hot flushes. Obstetrics and Gynecology 91(1): 6–11.

Albertazzi P, Pansini F, Bottazzi M, Bonaccorsi G, De Aloysio D, Morton MS (1999) Dietary soy supplementation and phytoestrogen levels. Obstetrics and Gynecology 94(2): 229–31.

Anelli TF, Anelli A, Tran KN, Lebwohl DE, Borgen PI (1994) Tamoxifen administration is associated with a high rate of treatment-limiting symptoms in male breast cancer patients. Cancer 74(1): 74–7.

Astrup A (1999) Physical activity and weight gain and fat distribution changes with menopause: current evidence and research issues. Medical Science and Sports Exercise 31(11 Suppl.): S564–7.

Baber RJ, Templeman C, Morton T, Kelly GE, West L (1999) Randomized placebo-controlled trial of an isoflavone supplement and menopausal symptoms in women. Climacteric 2(2): 85–92.

Barnes DM, Hanby AM (2001) Oestrogen and progesterone receptors in breast cancer: past present and future. Histopathology 38(3): 271–4.

Barton DL, Loprinzi CL, Quella SK, Sloan JA, Veeder MH, Egner JR, Fidler P, Stella PJ, Swan DK, Vaught NL, Novotny P (1998) Prospective evaluation of vitamin E for hot flashes in breast cancer survivors. Journal of Clinical Oncology 16(2): 495–500.

Baum M (2001) A vision for the future? British Journal of Cancer 85(Suppl. 2) 15–18.

Berglund G, Nystedt M, Bolund C, Sjoden PO, Rutquist LE (2001) Effect of endocrine treatment on sexuality in premenopausal breast cancer patients: a prospective randomized study. Journal of Clinical Oncology 19(11): 2788–96.

Bonneterre J, Thurlimann B, Robertson JF, Krzakowski M, Mauriac L, Koralewski P, Vergote I, Webster A, Steinberg M, von Euler M (2000) Anastrozole versus tamoxifen as first-line therapy for advanced breast cancer in 668 postmenopausal women: results of the Tamoxifen or Arimidex Randomized Group Efficacy and Tolerability study. Journal of Clinical Oncology 18(22): 3748–57.

Brinton LA, Schairer C, Hoover RN, Fraumeni JF Jr (1988) Menstrual factors and risk of breast cancer. Cancer Investigation 6(3): 245–54.

Brodie AM, Njar VC (2000) Aromatase inhibitors and their application in breast cancer treatment. Steroids 65(4): 171–9.

Bygdeman M, Swahn ML (1996) Replens versus dienoestrol cream in the symptomatic treatment of vaginal atrophy in postmenopausal women. Maturitas 23(3): 259–63.

Canney PA, Hatton MQ (1994) The prevalence of menopausal symptoms in patients treated for breast cancer. Clinical Oncology 6(5): 297–9.

Carpenter JS, Andrykowski MA (1999) Menopausal symptoms in breast cancer survivors. Oncology Nursing Forum 26(8): 1311–17.

Carpenter JS, Johnson D, Wagner L, Andrykowski M (2002) Hot flashes and related outcomes in breast cancer survivors and matched comparison women. Oncology Nursing Forum 29(3): E16-25.

Cawood EH, Bancroft J (1996) Steroid hormones, the menopause, sexuality and well-being of women. Psychological Medicine 26(5): 925-36.

Cockshott ID (2000) Clinical pharmacokinetics of goserelin. Clinical Pharmacokinetics 39(1): 27-48.

Collaborative Group on Hormonal Factors in Breast and Cancer (1997) Breast cancer and hormone replacement therapy: collaborative reanalysis of data from 51 epidemiological studies of 52705 women with breast cancer and 108411 women without breast cancer. Collaborative Group on Hormonal Factors in Breast Cancer. Lancet 350(9084): 1047-59.

Costantino JP, Kuller LH, Ives DG, Fisher B, Dignam J (1997) Coronary heart disease mortality and adjuvant tamoxifen therapy. Journal of the National Cancer Institute 89(11): 776-82.

Cummings SR, Eckert S, Krueger KA, Grady D, Powles TJ, Cauley JA, Norton L, Nickelsen T, Bjarnason NH, Morrow M, Lippman ME, Black D, Glusman JE, Costa A, Jordan VC (1999) The effect of raloxifene on risk of breast cancer in postmenopausal women: results from the MORE randomized trial, Multiple Outcomes of Raloxifene Evaluation. Journal of the American Medical Association 281(23): 2189-97.

Davies KM, Heaney RP, Recker RR, Barger-Lux MJ, Lappe JM (2001) Hormones, weight change and menopause. International Journal of Obesity Related Metabolic Disorders 25(6): 874-9.

Davis CS, Zinkand ZE, Fitch MI (2000) Cancer treatment-induced menopause: meaning for breast and gynecological cancer survivors. Canadian Oncology Nursing Journal 10(1): 14-21.

DeGeorge D, Gray JJ, Fetting JH, Rolls BJ (1990) Weight gain in patients with breast cancer receiving adjuvant treatment as a function of restraint disinhibition and hunger. Oncology Nursing Forum 17(3 Suppl.): 23-8; discussion 28-30.

DeGregorio M, Viebe V (1994) Tamoxifen and Breast Cancer. New Haven, CT and London: Yale University Press.

Duffy LS, Greenberg DB, Younger J, Ferraro MG (1999) Iatrogenic acute estrogen deficiency and psychiatric syndromes in breast cancer patients. Psychosomatics 40(4): 304-8.

Easton D, Ford D, Peto J (1993) Inherited susceptibility to breast cancer. Cancer Surveys 18: 95-113.

Eden J (1998) Phytoestrogens and the menopause. Baillieres Clinical Endocrinology and Metabolism 12(4): 581-7.

Fellowes D, Fallowfield LJ, Saunders CM, Houghton J (2001) Tolerability of hormone therapies for breast cancer: how informative are documented symptom profiles in medical notes for 'well-tolerated' treatments? Breast Cancer Research and Treatment 66(1): 73-81.

Fenlon D (1999) Relaxation therapy as an intervention for hot flushes in women with breast cancer. European Journal of Oncology Nursing 3(4): 223-31.

Finck G, Barton DL, Loprinzi CL, Quella SK, Sloan JA (1998) Definitions of hot flashes in breast cancer survivors. Journal of Pain Symptom Management 16(5): 327-33.

Fisher B, Anderson S, Tan-Chiu E, Wolmark N, Wickerham DL, Fisher ER, Dimitrov NV, Atkins JN, Abramson N, Merajver S, Romond EH, Kardinal CG, Shibata HR, Margolese

RG, Farrar WB (2001a) Tamoxifen and chemotherapy for axillary node-negative estrogen receptor-negative breast cancer: findings from National Surgical Adjuvant Breast and Bowel Project B-23. Journal of Clinical Oncology 19(4): 931–42.

Fisher B, Costantino J, Wickerham D, Redmond C, Kavanah M, Cronin W, Vogel V, Robidoux A, Dimitrov N, Atkins J, Daly M, Wieand S, Tan-Chiu E, Ford L, Wolmark N (1998) Tamoxifen for prevention of breast cancer: report of the National Surgical Adjuvant Breast and Bowel Project P-1. Study Journal of the National Cancer Institute 90(18): 1371–88.

Fisher B, Dignam J, Bryant J, Wolmark N (2001b) Five versus more than five years of tamoxifen for lymph node-negative breast cancer: updated findings from the National Surgical Adjuvant Breast and Bowel Project B-14 randomized trial. Journal of the National Cancer Inst 93(9): 684–90.

Forrest AP (1982) Beatson: hormones and the management of breast cancer. Journal of the Royal College of Surgeons of Edinburgh 27(5): 253–63.

Forwood MR, Larsen JA (2000) Exercise recommendations for osteoporosis. A position statement of the Australian and New Zealand Bone and Mineral Society. Australian Family Physician 29(8): 761–4.

Freedman RR, Woodward S (1992) Behavioral treatment of menopausal hot flushes: evaluation by ambulatory monitoring. American Journal of Obstetrics and Gynecology 167(2): 436–9.

Ganz PA, Rowland JH, Meyerowitz BE, Desmond KA (1998) Impact of different adjuvant therapy strategies on quality of life in breast cancer survivors. Recent Results in Cancer Research 152: 396–411.

Gelfand MM, Wendman E (1994) Treating vaginal dryness in breast cancer patients: results of applying a polycarbophil moisturizing gel. Journal of Women's Health 3(6): 427–34.

Goldberg R, Loprinzi C, O'Fallon J (1994) Transdermal clonidine for ameliorating tamoxifen-induced hot flashes. Journal of Clinical Oncology 12: 155-8.

Goodwin PJ, Ennis M, Pritchard KI, McCready D, Koo J, Sidlofsky S, Trudeau M, Hood N, Redwood S (1999a) Adjuvant treatment and onset of menopause predict weight gain after breast cancer diagnosis. Journal of Clinical Oncology 17(1): 120-9.

Goodwin PJ, Ennis M, Pritchard KI, Trudeau M, Hood N (1999b) Risk of menopause during the first year after breast cancer diagnosis. Journal of Clinical Oncology 17(8): 2365–70.

Greaves M (2000) Cancer: The Evolutionary Legacy. Oxford: Oxford University Press.

Greendale GA, Petersen L, Zibecchi L, Ganz PA (2001) Factors related to sexual function in postmenopausal women with a history of breast cancer. Menopause 8(2): 111-19.

Greer G (1991) The Change: Women, Ageing and the Menopause. London: Penguin.

Harvey JM, Clark GM, Osborne CK, Allred DC (1999) Estrogen receptor status by immunohistochemistry is superior to the ligand-binding assay for predicting response to adjuvant endocrine therapy in breast cancer. Journal of Clinical Oncology 17(5): 1474–81.

Holli K, Isola J, Cuzick J (1998) Low biologic aggressiveness in breast cancer in women using hormone replacement therapy. Journal of Clinical Oncology 16(9): 3115-20.

Hoskin PJ, Ashley S, Yarnold JR (1992) Weight gain after primary surgery for breast cancer: effect of tamoxifen. Breast Cancer Research and Treatment 22(2): 129-32.

Jaiyesimi IA, Buzdar AU, Sahin AA, Ross MA (1992) Carcinoma of the male breast. Ann Intern Med 117(9): 771-7.

John EM, Kelsey JL (1993) Radiation and other environmental exposures and breast cancer. Epidemiologic Reviews 15(1): 157-62.

Jordan VC, Gapstur S, Morrow M (2001) Selective estrogen receptor modulation and reduction in risk of breast cancer osteoporosis and coronary heart disease. Journal of the National Cancer Institute 93(19): 1449–57.

Kelsey JL, Gammon MD, John EM (1993) Reproductive factors and breast cancer. Epidemiologic Reviews 15(1): 36–47.

Kliewer EV, Smith KR (1995) Breast cancer mortality among immigrants in Australia and Canada. Journal of the National Cancer Institute 87(15): 1154–61.

Knight DC, Howes JB, Eden JA (1999) The effect of Promensil, an isoflavone extract on menopausal symptoms. Climacteric 2(2): 79–84.

Kumar NB, Allen K, Cantor A, Cox CE, Greenberg H, Shah S, Lyman GH (1997) Weight gain associated with adjuvant tamoxifen therapy in stage I and II breast cancer: fact or artifact? Breast Cancer Research and Treatment 44(2): 135–43.

Lazzaroni F, Scorolli L, Pizzoleo CF, Savini G, De Nigris A, Giosa F, Meduri RA (1998) Tamoxifen retinopathy: does it really exist? Graefes Archive for Clinical and Experimental Ophthalmology 236(9): 669–73.

Levine-Silverman S (1989) The menopausal hot flash: a procrustean bed of research. Journal of Advanced Nursing 14(11): 939–49.

Loprinzi CL, Michalak JC, Quella SK, O'Fallon JR, Hatfield AK, Nelimark RA, Dose AM, Fischer T, Johnson C, Klatt NE et al. (1994) Megestrol acetate for the prevention of hot flashes. New Engand Journal of Medicine 331(6): 347–52.

Loprinzi CL, Pisansky TM, Fonseca R, Sloan JA, Zahasky KM, Quella SK, Novotny PJ, Rummans TA, Dumesic DA, Perez EA (1998) Pilot evaluation of venlafaxine hydrochloride for the therapy of hot flashes in cancer survivors. Journal of Clinical Oncology 16(7): 2377–81.

Love RR, Barden HS, Mazess RB, Epstein S, Chappell RJ (1994) Effect of tamoxifen on lumbar spine bone mineral density in postmenopausal women after 5 years. Archives of Internal Medicine 154(22): 2585–8.

Lower EE, Blau R, Gazder P, Tummala R (1999) The risk of premature menopause induced by chemotherapy for early breast cancer. Journal of Women's Health and Gender Based Medicine 8(7): 949–54.

Marsden J (2000) Hormone replacement therapy and breast cancer. Maturitas 34(Suppl. 2): S11–S24.

Matsumoto M, Miyauchi M, Yamamoto N, Shishikura T, Imanaka N (2000) Investigation of menstruation recovery after LH-RH agonist therapy for premenopausal patients with breast cancer. Breast Cancer 7(3): 237–40.

McInnes JA, Knobf MT (2001) Weight gain and quality of life in women treated with adjuvant chemotherapy for early-stage breast cancer. Oncology Nursing Forum 28(4): 675–84.

Mezzetti M, La-Vecchia C, Decarli A, Boyle P, Talamini R, Franceschi S (1998) Population attributable risk for breast cancer: diet nutrition and physical exercise. Journal of the National Cancer Institute 90(5): 389–94.

Murkies AL, Lombard C, Strauss BJ, Wilcox G, Burger HG, Morton MS (1995) Dietary flour supplementation decreases post-menopausal hot flushes: effect of soy and wheat. Maturitas 21(3): 189–95.

Nachtigall LE (1994) Comparative study: Replens versus local estrogen in menopausal women. Fertility and Sterility 61(1): 178–80.

Nayfield SG, Karp JE, Ford LG, Dorr FA, Kramer BS (1991) Potential role of tamoxifen in prevention of breast cancer. Journal of the National Cancer Institute 83(20): 1450–9.

Obermeyer CM, Ghorayeb F, Reynolds R (1999) Symptom reporting around the menopause in Beirut, Lebanon. Maturitas 33(3): 249-58.

O'Meara ES, Rossing MA, Daling JR, Elmore JG, Barlow WE, Weiss NS (2001) Hormone replacement therapy after a diagnosis of breast cancer in relation to recurrence and mortality. Journal of the National Cancer Institute 93(10): 754-62.

Pannuti F, Martoni A, Zamagni C, Zamagni BM (1993) Progestins I: Medroxyprogesterone acetate. In Powles T, Smith I (Eds)Medical Management of Breast Cancer. Cambridge: Dunitz.

Powles T (1993) Progestins II: Megestrol acetate. In Powles T, Smith I (eds) Medical Management of Breast Cancer. Cambridge: Dunitz.

Powles T, Eeles R, Ashley S, Easton D, Chang J, Dowsett M, Tidy A, Viggers J, Davey J (1998) Interim analysis of the incidence of breast cancer in the Royal Marsden Hospital tamoxifen randomised chemoprevention trial. Lancet 352(9122): 98-101.

Powles TJ, Hickish T, Kanis JA, Tidy A, Ashley S (1996) Effect of tamoxifen on bone mineral density measured by dual-energy X-ray absorptiometry in healthy premenopausal and postmenopausal women. Journal of Clinical Oncology 14(1): 78-84.

Powles TJ, Jones AL, Ashley SE, O'Brien ME, Tidy VA, Treleavan J, Cosgrove D, Nash AG, Sacks N, Baum M et al. (1994) The Royal Marsden Hospital pilot tamoxifen chemoprevention trial. Breast Cancer Research and Treatment 31(1): 73-82.

Prentice R, Thompson D, Clifford C, Gorbach S, Goldin B, Byar D (1990) Dietary fat reduction and plasma estradiol concentration in healthy postmenopausal women. The Women's Health Trial Study Group. Journal of the National Cancer Institute 82(2): 129-34.

Pritchard KI, Paterson AH, Paul NA, Zee B, Fine S, Pater J (1996) Increased thromboembolic complications with concurrent tamoxifen and chemotherapy in a randomized trial of adjuvant therapy for women with breast cancer. National Cancer Institute of Canada Clinical Trials Group Breast Cancer Site Group. Journal of Clinical Oncology 14(10): 2731-7.

Schairer C, Lubin J, Troisi R, Sturgeon S, Brinton L, Hoover R (2000) Menopausal estrogen and estrogen-progestin replacement therapy and breast cancer risk. Journal of the American Medical Association 283(4): 485-91.

Sharkey NA, Williams NI,Guerin JB (2000) The role of exercise in the prevention and treatment of osteoporosis and osteoarthritis. Nursing Clinics of North America 35(1): 209-21.

Simkin-Silverman LR,Wing RR (2000) Weight gain during menopause.Is it inevitable or can it be prevented? Postgraduate Medicine 108(3): 47-50, 53-6.

Singer D, Hunter M (1999) The experience of premature menopause: a thematic discourse analysis. Journal of Reproductive and Infant Psychology 17(1): 63-81.

Stearns V, Isaacs C, Rowland J, Crawford J, Ellis MJ, Kramer R, Lawrence W, Hanfelt JJ, Hayes DF (2000) A pilot trial assessing the efficacy of paroxetine hydrochloride (Paxil) in controlling hot flashes in breast cancer survivors. Annals of Oncology 11(1) 17-22.

te Velde E, van Leusden H (1994) Hormonal treatment for the climacteric: alleviation of symptoms and prevention of postmenopausal disease. Lancet 343: 654-658.

van Leeuwen FE, Benraadt J, Coebergh JW, Kiemeney LA, Gimbrere CH, Otter R Schouten LJ, Damhuis RA, Bontenbal M, Diepenhorst FW et al. (1994) Risk of endometrial cancer after tamoxifen treatment of breast cancer. Lancet 343(8895): 448-52.

Veronesi U, Maisonneuve P, Costa A, Sacchini V, Maltoni C, Robertson C, Rotmensz N, Boyle P (1998) Prevention of breast cancer with tamoxifen: preliminary findings from the Italian randomised trial among hysterectomised women. Italian Tamoxifen Prevention Study. Lancet 352(9122): 93-7.

Wilcox G, Wahlqvist ML, Burger HG, Medley G (1990) Oestrogenic effects of plant foods in postmenopausal women. British Medical Journal 301(6757): 905-6.

Willett WC, Colditz G, Stampfer M (2000) Postmenopausal estrogens: opposed unopposed or none of the above [editorial; comment]. Journal of the American Medical Association 283(4): 534-5.

Chapter 11
Lymphoedema and Breast Cancer

MARY WOODS

Introduction

As a consequence of treatment for breast cancer, or due to advanced disease, patients can view the development of lymphoedema as devastating, debilitating and stressful (Robertson-Squire, 2000). Its presence can have an impact on different aspects of the patient's life, impeding physical ability and affecting body image. The degree to which the patient is affected is not necessarily dependent on the size of the swollen arm but on individual perceptions of the swelling and the coping mechanisms employed to assist in the adaptation to a chronic condition.

In this chapter, the reader will be introduced to the physiology underlying the development of lymphoedema in order to understand how it occurs following treatment for breast cancer and to be able to identify patients at risk of its development. The physical, psychological and psychosocial problems that can occur will then be discussed and an overview provided of the current treatment strategies employed to manage lymphoedema.

Many healthcare professionals come into contact with breast cancer patients during their journey with cancer and all have a role to offer in the education and support of the patient who has developed lymphoedema.

Development of Lymphoedema

Oedema can appear for several reasons and it is important the patient is fully assessed in order to establish the cause of the oedema that is present and to identify the most appropriate strategy of management. Lymphoedema is defined as a chronic, high-protein tissue swelling that can affect one or more limbs (Bianchi and Todd, 2000). Following treatment for breast cancer, lymphoedema may also occur in the breast and adjacent tissues of the trunk.

The lymphatic drainage system serves two main functions:

- the regulation of homeostasis:
  - large molecules, such as proteins, are returned to the circulation;
  - unwanted cellular by-products are removed from the tissues;
  - excess fluid is drained from the intestitium;
- an immunological function:
  - functioning lymph nodes are maintained;
  - foreign material is removed and processed;
  - an appropriate auto-immune response is generated where necessary.
  (Mortimer, 1990)

Larger lymphatic vessels contain smooth muscle and are able to contract. These act as collecting vessels, whereas smaller lymphatics are responsive to pressure changes and propel lymph by muscular movement, arterial pulsation and joint movement (Stanton, 2000). The role of the lymphatic system is to move fluid from within the interstitial spaces into the lymphatics in a unidirectional flow until it reaches the efferent lymphatics, before finally draining into the bloodstream via the thoracic duct (Mortimer et al., 1996).

Lymph drainage can fail when damage or obstruction of the lymph system alters the available drainage routes and results in a reduced lymphatic system transport capacity (Woods, 2000). This may occur following treatment for breast cancer when the lymph node area of the axilla undergoes surgery or radiotherapy treatment. As a result, the lymph flow out of the limb becomes restricted and swelling appears in the tissues of the arm.

Incidence and Prevalence of Lymphoedema

All patients with breast cancer who have undergone axillary intervention are at risk of developing lymphoedema, which may appear many years after the initial breast cancer treatment and in the absence of recurrent disease.

Studies reporting the incidence of breast-cancer-related lymphoedema vary considerably and Keeley (2000) suggests that it is difficult to draw firm conclusions from them because of the different variables used in data collection. A frequently quoted study by Kissin et al. (1986) reports the incidence of lymphoedema among patients who had received axillary surgery or radiotherapy as 25 per cent. Although this study was one of the first to look at the incidence of lymphoedema, it should be acknowledged that treatment for breast cancer is now focused much more on preservation of the axilla (Robinson, 1992; Pressman, 1998) and that this study included only women who had received their treatment within the previous year.

Keeley (2000) suggests that the well-recognized pattern of delay in the appearance of swelling is not acknowledged in studies of patients with a short follow-up period. There are relatively few studies, however, which follow patients at risk of developing lymphoedema for a sufficiently long period to detect its development later on. One such study of the prevalence of arm swelling following treatment for breast cancer (Mortimer et al., 1996) suggested that 28 per cent of women developed lymphoedema at some time following their treatment and that there was a significant increase in prevalence with time since treatment. This indicates that lymphoedema is a significant problem that cannot be ignored.

Risk Factors for the Development of Lymphoedema

Factors that are frequently thought to contribute to the development of lymphoedema include:

- the type of breast cancer treatment the patient receives;
- post-operative events;
- the use and care of the 'at-risk' arm.

Evidence-based support for these assertions, however, is weak and confined to suspected associations experienced primarily in clinical practice. In a systematic review of risk factors associated with lymphoedema, Cole (2000) stated that it is essential to separate the cause of lymphoedema from the risk of its development.

Type of Breast Cancer Treatment

Intervention of the axillary lymph nodes during surgery or radiotherapy results in trauma to the lymphatic system and can alone be responsible for the subsequent development of lymphoedema (Stanton et al., 1996). It is not clear, however, whether the degree of axillary surgery or radiotherapy influences the degree of lymphoedema experienced. Similarly, there is no clear indication that the type of surgical incision used can influence the risk of lymphoedema developing.

Post-operative Events

The development of lymphoedema has been related to several post-operative events including wound complications, seroma formation and cording (Keeley, 2000). It is thought that the occurrence of one or more of these events may place the patient at greater risk of the development of lymphoedema later on. Infection is reported as a significant risk factor (Mozes, 1982) but Cole (2000) suggested that a clearer distinction is required between wound infection occurring at the time of surgery and infection reported as a trigger factor in the later development of lymphoedema.

Additional Trigger Factors

Additional trigger factors that are considered to be related to the development of lymphoedema following treatment for breast cancer include increasing age (Clarysse, 1993), obesity (Segerstrom et al., 1992) and venepuncture in the affected arm (Smith, 1998; Harlow, 2001). However, further research is required in these areas.

Physical Effects of Lymphoedema

Lymphoedema is characterized by visible swelling in a limb, which may influence all or part of the limb. Following breast cancer treatment, lymphoedema may also involve the hand and arm on the affected side, the breast and the adjacent quadrant of the trunk. At an early stage, the swelling may be palpable and soft responding well to treatment designed to reduce the volume of the limb. But as time passes, the tissues can become hardened and fibrosed, making the swelling more difficult to reverse.

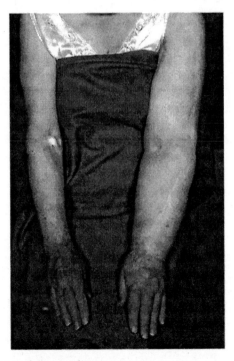

Figure 11.1: Swollen arm following breast cancer treatment.

Effects on the Skin

The connective tissue in the dermis of the skin contains collagen and elastin fibres to give the skin its shape and enable it to move over the subcutaneous tissues (Linnitt, 2000). As stasis of lymph occurs in the limb, fibrin and collagen are deposited in the subcutaneous tissues causing the skin to become hardened and fibrosed. As the swelling progresses further, a loss of limb shape develops, accompanied by skin folds and deep crevices (Hodkinson, 1992). In advanced lymphoedema, a warty, scaly appearance to the skin can develop (hyperkeratosis) and dilated skin lymphatics can give the appearance of blisters on the skin (lymphangiomata) (Veitch, 1993).

Effects on Limb Function

A swollen arm may feel uncomfortable and heavy, presenting difficulties with daily activities. Studies have shown that the weight of a swollen limb can influence shoulder movement (Tobin et al., 1993; Casley-Smith and Casley-Smith, 1994) and larger limbs result in greater physical problems. If the hand and fingers are swollen, fine finger movements may also become impaired.

Psychological Effects of Lymphoedema

Patients with breast cancer who develop arm swelling have been shown to suffer significantly greater depression and poorer adjustment to their illness than patients with breast cancer who have not developed lymphoedema (Tobin et al., 1993). This psychological handicap appears to be related to changes in body image and limb function, coupled with the associated effects that these problems can have on social activities, occupation and personal relationships (Woods et al., 1993). The difficulties experienced by patients, however, are not always related to the size of their swollen limb, with minimal swelling in a limb sometimes causing great psychological distress (Woods et al., 1993).

In a study of women with breast-cancer-related arm swelling, Johanssen (2002) identified two coping strategies that women developed in order to deal with their swelling in everyday life:

- Emotion-focused coping was most commonly used and involved a regulation of the emotions associated with the swelling. Patients described how they tried to adjust their personal values to accept the swelling or 'played down' its influence on their life by trying to carry on as before (Johanssen, 2002).
- Problem-focused coping involved making deliberate changes to the environment where significant problems were being experienced in order to make life easier (Johanssen, 2002).

The visible change in the size and shape of a limb when lymphoedema develops can influence how the patient perceives her/his body image. Although the effects of the original surgery remain hidden by clothing, the swollen arm can attract questions from others and serve as a visible reminder of the cancer and its treatment. Culture, upbringing and the media influence individual perceptions of body image and reactions to an altered body image depend primarily on the person's usual coping mechanisms.

Price (1990) outlines three components to body image:

1. Body reality: how the body is.
2. Body ideal: how we would like our body to look and function.
3. Body presentation: how we present ourselves to the world in order to balance body reality with body ideal.

Lymphoedema can be difficult to disguise and can lead to a negative self-image. Body presentation may require great changes to a preferred style of dress (Woods et al., 1993) and can sometimes lead to a complete loss of interest in dress and appearance (Tobin et al., 1993).

Psychosocial Effects of Lymphoedema

For some patients, the effects of lymphoedema are far reaching, touching many areas of their lives. Studies have shown that relationships and social activities may suffer and that the person's occupation can affect the swelling (Tobin et al., 1993; Woods et al., 1993). In many cases individual adaptation occurs as difficulties arise and the support of family and friends is required to make adaptation possible.

Occupation

Women who have developed lymphoedema following breast cancer treatment and who work outside the home have been shown to have significantly larger swollen arms than women who do not work (Woods et al., 1993). Combining the demands of a chosen occupation with other roles may mean that less time is available to care for the swollen arm. The type of occupation followed may also have an impact on the degree of swelling present, with more sedentary occupations preferable to those requiring exertive, strenuous activities using the swollen arm, which may increase the likelihood of problematic swelling.

Relationships and Social Activities

The uniqueness of each individual may mean that many different problems are encountered by the woman with breast-cancer-related arm swelling. For some, the focus on the swollen arm results in a loss of interest in social activities and as the swelling progresses difficulties in function may influence the work and home environment. The demands of coping with lymphoedema and a loss of self-esteem can place tremendous pressure on relationships of a personal, sexual and social nature. The quality and quantity of understanding and support from others has been shown by Passik et al. (1995) to influence the degree of psychological distress experienced, and Mason (2000) suggests that support received from others can influence how receptive the patient is to a suggested programme of care.

Management of Lymphoedema

Introduction

Foeldi, a German physician, developed an effective strategy of management for lymphoedema in Europe during the 1970s. Based on the experience of Emil and Estrid Vodder, who had developed a technique of lymphatic massage to increase the transport of lymphatic fluid, Foeldi's method comprised four main elements of treatment used in combination, which he termed Complex Decongestive Physiotherapy (Foeldi et al., 1985). Today, this method of treatment can also be termed complex physical therapy (Mason, 1993), complex decongestive therapy (Daane, 1998), and complex lymphoedema therapy (Johansson et al., 1999) but the four elements of skin care, exercise and movement, lymph drainage and external containment continue and are regarded by the British Lymphology Society (BLS) as a desirable approach to the management of lymphoedema in this country (BLS, 2001a).

The treatment of lymphoedema is not curative, due to the disruption that has occurred within the lymph channels. The aim is to maximize lymphatic drainage so that a reduction in the swelling can be achieved based on the potential of the individual patient. Appropriate care of the swollen limb ensures that the likelihood of problematic complications occurring is minimized.

Assessment

Lymphoedema is a long-term chronic condition and the patient should become an active participant in its management. A full and accurate assessment of the patient should therefore include the identification of personal priorities and goals so that the patient and therapist can work together in partnership to achieve maximum improvement and long-term control of the swelling. Mason (2000), in an article which explores rehabilitation in lymphoedema management, suggests that patient-centred decisions regarding treatment should recognize individual experiences, problems and coping mechanisms. Goal setting then becomes relevant and the patient can develop a sense of ownership in the decision-making process, which encourages compliance with treatment (Mason, 2000).

A model for the assessment of the patient with lymphoedema was outlined by Woods (2000) and comprises three areas:

1. General information: This would be acquired from the patient and the case notes to assist in gaining a full understanding of the cause and type of swelling that is present.
2. Physical examination of the limb: This enables the extent of the swelling to be identified and whether any complicating factors are present.
3. Psychological and psychosocial assessment: This enables the influence of the swelling on the individual's circumstances to be assessed.

With the patient's views and wishes fully respected, Woods stresses that the burden of treatment should not exceed the benefit to be gained and that realistic expectations of the outcome of treatment are fully discussed (Woods, 2000).

The Two Phases of Treatment

The four elements of treatment – skin care, exercise and movement, lymph drainage and external containment – are organized into two phases of care described by Jenns (2000) and Todd (1998).

1. The intensive phase

This is a short planned period of therapist-led treatment in which specific goals are mutually agreed between the patient and the therapist. Treatment is usually carried out daily to include multi-layer compression bandaging and additional elements of treatment depending on the patient's needs.

Indications for this phase of treatment include:

- large limbs;
- misshapen limbs;
- severe lymphoedema with skin changes;
- damaged or fragile skin;
- lymphorrhoea;
- support and comfort in the palliative care setting.

Treatment may include some or all of the following elements of treatment:

- skin hygiene and care;
- limb movement and exercise;

- manual lymph drainage;
- external containment using multi-layer compression bandaging.

2. The maintenance phase

The concept of self-care is promoted to enable the patient to become independent in the long-term control and management of the swelling. The therapist provides advice and support for the patient, evaluating progress at regular intervals to ensure that any problems are identified early and that compression garments remain appropriate and are replaced when necessary.

Indications for this phase of treatment include:

- mild/moderately swollen limbs;
- normal limb shape ;
- patient ability to follow a self-care regime.

Treatment may include some or all of the following elements of treatment:

- a skin care regime;
- limb movement and exercise regime;
- simple lymph drainage;
- external containment using compression garments.

Many patients will embark on a maintenance phase of treatment for their swelling without the need for an intensive course of treatment.

Elements of Treatment

1. Skin care

A number of skin conditions are associated with lymphoedema but infection poses a major risk for patients both with, or at risk of, lymphoedema, owing to reduced local immunity when lymph node areas in the axilla have been surgically depleted or irradiated (Maclaren, 2001). Acute inflammatory episodes, also termed cellulitis, can occur following a penetrating skin injury and when skin integrity becomes compromised due to stretching and dryness of the skin.

The aim of skin care is:

- to promote skin integrity;
- to minimize the risks of infection.

Linnitt (2000) suggests that skin care should be carried out daily and include a regime of meticulous hygiene, inspection and observation of the skin, coupled with moisturization with emollients. Patients should also be advised to take precautions to ensure that the integrity of their skin is not compromised during activities likely to place them at risk (Table 11.1).

Table 11.1: Advice to patients with arm lymphoedema

- Wash the skin gently and dry thoroughly
- Moisturize daily with a bland, non-perfumed cream or lotion
- Take care to avoid trauma to the skin when cutting nails and removing unwanted body hair
- Use gloves to protect the hands when gardening, washing up or reaching into a hot oven
- Use an antiseptic cream if trauma to the skin does occur
- Avoid extremes of temperature such a very hot baths and saunas
- Protect the skin from insect bites and sunburn during the summer months and when on holiday
- Avoid any kind of venepuncture in the affected arm through injections or the giving/taking of blood
- Ask for blood pressure recordings to be taken on the other arm

---

Skin problems that can develop are:

- Fungal infections: Common fungal infections include athlete's foot and thrush, which can occur in deep skin folds or between swollen fingers. The skin appears white, scaly and macerated and may be extremely itchy. If left untreated, fungal infections can increase the risk of the development of cellulitis. Treatment is with anti-fungal agents available via the pharmacy.
- Cellulitis: A feature of lymphoedema is attacks of apparent infection in the swollen arm, preceded by symptoms associated with influenza. The patient feels unwell with a fever that progresses to pain and redness in the affected limb coupled with an increase in swelling. Although attacks can occur suddenly and without warning, they are frequently associated with a recent accidental skin injury in the affected arm and can sometimes be severe enough to require hospitalization. Treatment is with antibiotics administered orally or intravenously for a two-week period. The patient should be encouraged to rest during the acute phase of the attack. Recurrent attacks may require control with long-term antibiotics (Mortimer, 2000).
- Dry skin: Stretched skin due to swelling can become inelastic and feel tight and uncomfortable. If left to progress, the skin can become flaky and scaly with an increasing risk of bacterial entry if cracks in the skin

develop. The use of bland, unperfumed emollient lotions or creams soothes and rehydrates dry, irritated skin. A skin care regime of hygiene and moisturizing adopted daily can promote healthy skin.

- Lymphorrhoea: A leakage of lymph through the surface of the skin can develop spontaneously if the skin is tight and fragile. It can also occur following an injury to the skin where skin integrity becomes compromised. Lymphorrhoea poses an infection risk and the persistent leakage of lymph fluid can result in skin excoriation and breakdown. The management of this condition is reported to vary between professionals (Ling et al., 1997) but the use of non-adherent dressings and light compression can achieve some success in terminating the leakage of lymph fluid and allowing the condition of the skin to improve (Gilbert and Mortimer, 2001).

2. Exercise and movement

Joint mobility and lymph drainage can be promoted through movement and appropriate exercise of the swollen arm as the action of the muscle pump stimulates superficial lymphatics to drain. The effect is enhanced when compression garments are worn.

There is little research available to assist the therapist in identifying a safe, effective exercise regime for patients with lymphoedema, but Miller (1996) and Hughes (2000) emphasize the importance of avoiding over-vigorous and static activities such as carrying heavy shopping bags. A gradual, controlled exercise programme, tailored to the patient's lifestyle and interests, appears preferable in order to minimize the risk of sudden, increased blood flow, which can overwhelm the lymphatics and make the swelling worse.

Miller (1996) advocates an exercise programme for patients with breast-cancer-related arm swelling that includes flexibility exercises for the shoulder, a weight-training programme with very light weights and aerobic activity. This combination of exercise aims to restore range of movement, increase functional use of the arm and promote lymph drainage. Normal everyday activities can be incorporated into the programme.

Hughes (2000) identifies swimming as an ideal exercise for the patient with lymphoedema because the water supports the body and provides gentle resistance to the muscles. Isotonic exercises, which stimulate the muscle pump, improve lymph flow (Gilbert and Mortimer, 2001).

The adoption of correct posture during any exercise or movement is also important and Hughes (2000) promotes exercises and activities that encourage the swollen arm to move in the same pattern and range of movements as the unaffected arm. The arm should not be allowed to hang down beside the body as this can encourage fluid accumulation and musculoskeletal problems of the shoulder. When the patient is at rest, the arm should be supported comfortably on pillows or a cushion at heart level to encourage lymph drainage.

3. Lymph drainage

In lymphoedema management, lymph drainage refers to a particular type of skin massage called Manual Lymph Drainage, which has also been adapted into a simplified form called Simple Lymphatic Drainage.

Manual Lymph Drainage (MLD) is a unique method of massage in which specialized movements of the thumbs, fingers and hand are used to exert gentle and smooth pressure on the skin. Originally used by beauticians and masseurs within a framework of classical massage, MLD is now used for a range of medical conditions where lymph drainage routes have not been impaired by medical intervention. In order to treat lymphoedema, MLD therapists must undergo additional specific training in order to understand abnormal or altered lymph flow.

The aim of MLD is:

- to improve the function of the normal lymphatics;
- to encourage superficial lymph channels to find alternative drainage routes;
- to stimulate lymph flow and drainage away from congested areas.

As an aspect of treatment for lymphoedema, there have been reports of significant improvements in swelling following a three-week course of daily treatment (Jackson, 1995; Pearson, 1995). However, MLD is felt to be most effective when used in combination with multi-layer compression bandaging (Jenns, 2000).

There is limited scientific research to support the use of MLD in lymphoedema management but it is frequently used to treat long-standing swelling that has become complex and complicated or where there is congestion evident at the root of the limb, which is impeding the drainage of lymph. It is vital that the therapist performing MLD has undergone appropriate specialist training.

Simple Lymphatic Drainage (SLD) has evolved from MLD to be easily accessible to patients and their relatives. Based on the principles of MLD, with simplified hand movements, it is only used on areas where normal lymph drainage exists (BLS, 2001b).

The aim of SLD is:

- to stimulate normal draining lymphatic;
- to 'milk' fluid away from congested areas;
- to improve superficial lymph drainage.

Most patients with lymphoedema can benefit from using SLD within a self-care programme of management for their swelling. However, the success with which it can be applied is dependent on the ability of the therapist to teach the technique and the motivation and confidence of the patient (Bellhouse, 2000). SLD can be taught to relatives or friends so that they can use it on the patient if there are difficulties with movement which restrict the patient from using the technique independently.

4. External containment (Figure 11.2)

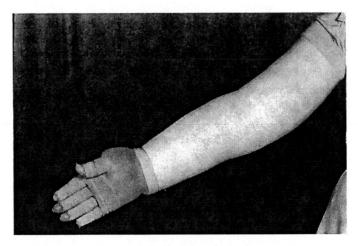

Figure 11.2: Compression sleeve used in lymphoedema management.

In the management of lymphoedema, containment refers to the enclosing of a limb within bandages or compression garments in order to reduce or control swelling. It is a widely used aspect of treatment for lymphoedema, which is acknowledged as particularly beneficial for the majority of patients (Jeffs, 1992; Mortimer, 1995; Todd, 1998; Todd, 2000).

External containment can be applied using support or compression.

- Support, defined as the retention and control of the tissues without the application of compression (Thomas, 1990) is provided by inelastic bandages, which provide a firm outer casing to the swollen tissues. Some rigid inelastic garments also provide support to the tissues. Muscular contraction and relaxation within the inelastic bandages promote lymph flow.
- Compression implies the deliberate application of pressure in order to produce a desired clinical effect (Thomas, 1990). Elastic compression

garments compress the tissues of the swollen arm and increase the flow of lymph out of the arm, while maximizing the effect of the muscle pump.

External support

Low stretch, inelastic bandages provide external support and are used within the intensive phase of lymphoedema treatment to act as a counterforce to voluntary muscular activity. They can provide an effective means of management for lymphoedema where the limb size, shape and condition are compromised or complicated by severe swelling.

The use of bandages within this phase of treatment is a specialist technique requiring skills and knowledge in the application of the bandages and should not be attempted by healthcare professionals without the supervision of an experienced therapist. The therapist has a responsibility to ensure that he/she has a sound knowledge of bandaging theory and a good technique in bandage application as the inappropriate use of bandages or their poor application can result in skin and tissue damage.

The suitability of a patient for a course of bandaging should be carefully considered during a full assessment to ensure that it is appropriate to her/his needs. Education and advice will be required regarding appropriate clothing to accommodate the bulk of the bandages, personal hygiene while the bandages are in place and the impact that the bandages may have on activities of daily living.

For bandaging to be effective in reducing swelling, a number of physical principles must be considered:

- The support provided by the bandages on the swollen arm must be evenly distributed. Where the normal limb shape has become distorted by swelling, it can be corrected by the use of foam and padding underneath the bandages to provide an even profile upon which the bandages can be applied.
- The support must be graduated along the length of the swollen arm to ensure that the most pressure is achieved distally and the least proximally, to aid lymph drainage. This can be achieved by selecting the correct bandage width for the size of the swollen arm and ensuring that the bandage overlap is greatest towards the distal part of the arm and less towards the root of the arm. Graduated pressure can also be achieved by using more that one layer of bandages and controlling the amount of tension applied to the bandages.
- The pressure exerted on the limb must be adequate to counter the limb circumference. When the circumference of the swollen arm is significant, greater pressure will be required in order to influence the swelling. This

can be achieved by the use of more than one layer of bandages and the correct choice of bandage width for the circumference of the arm.

Low-stretch bandages provide a low resting pressure enabling them to be comfortable while the patient is at rest. During muscular activity, however, a high working pressure is provided by the bandages as the muscle works against the support provided by the bandages. For this reason the patient should be aware of the importance of exercise while the arm is bandaged to ensure maximum effectiveness from their use. The bandages should not be painful or uncomfortable but if discomfort occurs at any time they should be removed.

External compression

Graduated compression garments are used in the maintenance phase of lymphoedema management alongside skin care, exercise and simple lymph drainage. By compressing the tissues, they limit the formation of lymph and by maximizing the effect of the muscle pump the flow of lymph towards the root of the limb is increased.

Compression garments are manufactured as either round knit or flat-bed knit. Round-knit garments are produced in one piece and are readily available as 'off-the-shelf' garments at reasonable cost. Synthetic materials are used to produce these garments in order to make them aesthetically pleasing and easy to wear. A wide range of sizes and styles are available to accommodate the needs of most patients.

Flat-bed-knit garments are made as one-piece garments joined with a seam. These are usually specifically 'made-to-measure' for a patient, so accurate measurements of the swollen arm are necessary to ensure that the finished garment fits. These garments can be useful when round-knit garments cannot meet specific patient requirements.

The therapist choosing a compression sleeve for a patient with arm lymphoedema should possess sound knowledge concerning the different types, styles and sizes of the garments available. A full assessment and discussion with the patient should highlight any concerns regarding the safe application and removal of the garments each day and all swollen areas must be included within the garment chosen.

Garments should not be fitted if:

- the limb size is >20 per cent excess volume (Badger et al., 2000);
- the limb shape is irregular, particularly if there are deepened skin folds;
- the skin condition is poor with fragile or damaged areas of skin;
- the patient is suffering an acute infective episode (cellullitis);
- there is arterial or venous insufficiency.

Once it has been chosen, the therapist should evaluate the fitted garment to satisfy him/herself that it will meet the role for which it is intended:

- The garment should fit snugly and be comfortable to wear.
- The garment should not cut into the limb causing a tourniquet effect, or have loose pockets where excess fluid can accumulate.
- The fingers should remain pink and warm with normal sensations.
- The garment should include all parts of the limb where swelling is present.
- The garment should be the correct length and not be allowed to crease or be turned over at the top.

The application of compression garments can be assisted with the use of an ordinary household rubber glove, which facilitates the even distribution of material along the length of the limb. There are also several commercially made aids available if greater assistance is required. The use of creams and oils on the skin should be avoided prior to the application of the garments as these can damage the fabric.

Compression garments are most effective when worn every day, particularly when the arm is most active.

Conclusion

As a chronic condition, which can develop following treatment for breast cancer, the impact of lymphoedema on the patient's life should not be under-estimated. Lymphoedema is not 'a small price to pay' for the cancer treatment received, as some patients are still unfortunately led to believe. The literature discussed in this chapter illustrates how the development of swelling can influence many different areas of the individual's life. Indeed, adaptation to some aspects of daily life is even required by those who are 'at risk' of developing lymphoedema if they are to minimize the risks of problematic swelling occurring in the future.

Individual needs and coping mechanisms are very different and therefore the key to true holistic and patient-centred care for the patient with lymphoedema is not just an assessment of physical symptoms, in order to apply the different physical treatment strategies outlined, but the inclusion of an assessment of psychological and psychosocial needs also. The therapist must seek to understand the patient's individual story in order to adopt an approach to management of the swelling that is acceptable for the patient and promotes independence and confidence in her ability to manage the swelling during everyday life.

References

Badger C, Peacock J, Mortimer P (2000) A randomised controlled parallel-group clinical trial comparing multi-layer bandaging followed by hosiery versus hosiery alone in the treatment of patients with lymphoedema of the limb. Cancer 88(12): 2832–7.

Bellhouse S (2000) Simple lymphatic drainage In Twycross R, Jenns K, Todd J (Eds) Lymphoedema. Oxford: Radcliffe Medical Press.

Bianchi J, Todd M (2000) The management of a patient with lymphoedema of the legs. Nursing Standard 14(40): 51–56.

British Lymphology Society (2001a) Strategy for Lymphoedema Care. Caterham, Surrey: BLS Administration Centre.

British Lymphology Society (2001b) Guidelines for the Use of Manual Lymph Drainage (MLD) and Simple Lymph Drainage (SLD) in Lymphoedema. Caterham, Surrey: BLS Administration Centre.

Casley-Smith JR, Casley-Smith J (1994) Modern Treatment for Lymphoedema. Adelaide: Lymphoedema Association of Australia.

Clarysse A (1993) Lymphoedema following breast cancer treatment. Acta Clinica Belgica Supplementum 15: 47–50.

Cole T (2000) Risk factors associated with lymphoedema. In British Lymphology Society Annual Conference Proceedings 2000 [available at: www.bls.lymphoedema.or/bls (accessed 11 June 2002)].

Daane S (1998) Post mastectomy lymphoedema management: evolution of the complex decongestive therapy technique. Annals of Plastic Surgery 40: 323–7.

Foeldi E, Foeldi M, Weissleder H (1985) Conservative management of lymphoedema of the limbs. Angiology – Journal of Vascular Diseases 36(3): 171–80.

Gilbert J, Mortimer P (2001) Current views on the management of breast cancer related lymphoedema. CME Breast 1(1): 14–17.

Harlow W (2001) Venepuncture – a causative factor in the development of arm oedema following breast cancer treatment. Paper presented at the British Lymphology Society Annual Conference: Innovations in Practice, 1–2 October.

Hodkinson M (1992) Lymphoedema: applying physiology to treatment. European Journal of Cancer Care (2): 19–23.

Hughes K (2000) Exercise and lymphoedema In Twycross R, Jenns K, Todd J (Eds) Lymphoedema. Oxford: Radcliffe Medical Press.

International Journal of Palliative Nursing 4(5): 230–9.

Jackson D (1995) Swollen limbs, helping hands. Independent 28 February.

Jeffs E (1992) Management of lymphoedema: putting treatment into context. Journal of Tissue Viability 2(4): 127–31 .

Jenns K (2000) Management strategies. In Twycross R, Jenns K, Todd J (Eds) Lymphoedema. Oxford: Radcliffe Medical Press, pp. 97–117.

Johansson K (2002) Lymphoedema and breast cancer: a physiotherapeutic approach. Thesis, Lund University, Sweden.

Johansson K, Albertsson M, Ingvar C, Ekdahl C (1999) Effects of compression bandaging with or without manual lymph drainage treatment in patients with post-operative arm lymphoedema. Lymphology 32: 103–10.

Keeley V (2000) Classification of lymphoedema. In Twycross R, Jenns K, Todd J (Eds) Lymphoedema. Oxford: Radcliffe Medical Press.

Kissin M, della Rovere Q, Easton D, Westbury G (1986) Risk of lymphoedema following treatment of breast cancer. British Journal of Surgery 73: 580-4.

Ling J, Duncan A, Laverty D, Hardy J (1997) Lymphorhoea in palliative care. European Journal of Cancer Care 4(2): 50-2.

Linnitt N (2000) Skin management in lymphoedema. In Twycross R, Jenns K, Todd J (Eds) Lymphoedema. Oxford: Radcliffe Medical Press, pp. 118-29.

Maclaren J (2001) Skin changes in lymphoedema: pathophysiology and management options. International Journal of Palliative Nursing 7(8): 381-8.

Mason M (1993) The treatment of lymphoedema by complex physical therapy. Australian Physiotherapy 39: 41-5.

Mason W (2000) Exploring rehabilitation within lymphoedema management. International Journal of Palliative Nursing 6(6): 265-73.

Miller L (1996) The enigma of exercise: participation in an exercise program after breast cancer surgery. National Lymphoedema Network Newsletter OctoberNovember: 15-19.

Mortimer PS (1990) Investigation and management of lymphoedema. Vascular Medicine Review 1: 1-20.

Mortimer PS (1995) Managing lymphoedema. Clinical and Experimental Dermatology 20: 98-106.

Mortimer PS (2000) Acute inflammatory episodes. In Twycross R, Jenns K, Todd J (Eds) Lymphoedema. Oxford: Radcliffe Medical Press, pp. 130-9.

Mortimer PS, Bates D, Brassington H, Stanton A, Strachan D, Levick J (1996) The prevalence of arm oedema following treatment for breast cancer. Quarterly Journal of Medicine 89: 377-80.

Mozes M (1982) The role of infection in postmastectomy lymphoedema. Surgery Annual 14: 73-83.

Passik S, Newman M, Brennan M, Tunkel R (1995) Predictors of psychological distress, sexual dysfunction and physical functioning among women with upper extremity lymphoedema related to breast cancer. PsychoOncology 4: 255-63.

Pearson D (1995) Swell news at last. The Times 22 January.

Pressman P (1998) Surgical treatment and lymphoedema. Cancer 83: 2782-7.

Price B (1990) A model for body-image care. Journal of Advanced Nursing (15): 585-93.

Robertson-Squire M (2000) The patients' perspective In Twycross R, Jenns K, Todd J (Eds) Lymphoedema. Oxford: Radcliffe Medical Press.

Robinson DS (1992) Role and extent of lymphadenectomy for early breast cancer. Seminars in Surgical Oncology 8: 78-82.

Segerstrom K, Bjerle P, Graffman S, Nystrom A (1992) Factors that influence the incidence of brachial oedema following treatment of breast cancer. Scandanavian Journal of Plastic and Reconsructive Surgery and Hand Surgery 26: 223-7.

Smith J (1998) The practice of venepuncture in lymphoedema. European Journal of Cancer Care 7: 97-8.

Stanton A (2000) How does tissue swelling occur? In Twycross R, Jenns K, Todd J (Eds) Lymphoedema. Oxford: Radcliffe Medical Press.

Stanton A, Levick J, Mortimer P (1996) Current puzzles presented by postmastectomy oedema (breast cancer related lymphoedema). Vascular Medicine 1: 213-25.

Thomas S (1990) Bandages and bandaging. Nursing Standard 4(39): 4-6.

Tobin M, Lacey H, Meyer L, Mortimer P (1993) The psychological morbidity of breast cancer-related arm swelling. Cancer 72(11): 3248-52.

Todd J (1998) Lymphoedema: a challenge for all healthcare professionals.

Todd J (2000) Containment in the management of lymphoedema. In Twycross R, Jenns K, Todd J (Eds) Lymphoedema. Oxford: Radcliffe Medical Press.

Veitch J (1993) Skin problems in lymphoedema. Wound Management 4(2): 42–5.

Woods M (2000) Lymphoedema. In Cooper J (Ed) Stepping into Palliative Care: A Handbook for Health Care Professionals. Oxford: Radcliffe Medical Press.

Woods M, Tobin M, Mortimer PS (1993) The psychosocial morbidity of breast cancer patients with lymphoedema. Cancer Nursing 18(6) 467–71.

Chapter 12
Fungating Wounds

RACHAEL KING

Introduction

Fungating wounds are distressing and often complex as there is a need to manage them from both the patient and carer perspective. Fungating wounds present many challenges to nursing staff because they rarely heal and they produce a multitude of problems, which often recur and are difficult to manage (Laverty et al., 2000). They are often an indication that the patient has reached the end stage, or advanced cancer, and that alone is often enough to deal with. There is little research in this area and much of the work is based on anecdotal evidence and case studies. It is imperative to encourage a multidisciplinary approach to care for this group of patients, in order to ensure that the progression in their wound care is optimal.

Radiotherapy, chemotherapy and hormone therapy may have some effect on reducing the size and symptoms of these wounds but the benefits of these treatments need to be balanced against their potential side effects (Naylor, 2001). The main priorities within the assessment and management of this type of wound on this type of patient are to ensure not only that the wound itself is dressed in the most appropriate fashion but that the patient's body image and self-esteem are managed effectively as well.

Definition of a Fungating Wound

A fungating wound develops from the extension of a malignant tumour into the structures of the skin producing a raised or ulcerating necrotic lesion (Moody and Grocott, 1993; Bennett and Moody, 1995; Mortimer, 1998). Fungating wounds are described as 'fungus-like' or 'cauliflower-like' growths because of their appearance (Grocott, 1999). There is some controversy in the available literature in this field as to whether the correct terminology for these types of wounds should be a fungating lesion, malignant lesion or skin ulceration, and all have been identified as being dependent on the stage of the fungating wound (Haargenson, 1971; Petrek et al., 1983; Sims and Fitzgerald, 1985; Bale and Harding, 1987; Carville, 1994). It is important to mention that the appearance and presentation of the wound will significantly differ from patient to patient (Grocott, 1999).

Aetiology of Fungating Wounds

Fungating malignant wounds are a result of the infiltration of the skin and its supporting blood and lymph vessels by a local tumour or of metastatic spread from a primary tumour (Grocott, 2000). They will occur along blood and lymph capillaries and between tissue planes (Moseley, 1998). A reduction in the oxygen diffusion will lead to tissue hypoxia and ultimately lead to tissue breakdown. The consequences of this will be a build-up of anaerobic and aerobic bacteria at the tumour site, which is the cause of the characteristic malodour, and large amounts of exudate production often associated with fungating malignant wounds. There will be an increased level of proteases that will also lead to further breakdown. Regnard and Tempest (1992) claim that the cause of the easy bleeding associated with this type of wound is the fragility of the capillaries contained within the mass. There is high risk to life when the tumour infiltrates into major blood vessels causing a great risk of massive haemorrhage.

Appearance of a Fungating Wound

It is recognized that a fungating wound can appear in the form of a nodule with the appearance of fungus, or it may appear as an ulcerating crater resulting from ignored cancer. Such wounds are generally characterized by the 'lip' that surrounds the margin of the wound and by the nature of their complexity (Naylor, 2001). Fungating wounds are often associated with carcinoma of the breast but can also be the result of sarcoma, squamous cell carcinoma or melanoma (Hallett, 1995).

Incidence of Fungating Wounds

The true incidence of fungating malignant wounds is unknown (Grocott, 1995). A retrospective survey carried out by Thomas (1992) is the most reliable of recent data available. This shows that over a period of a year community nurse practitioners could visit in the region of 2500 patients with fungating wounds, the most prevalent location for this type of wound being on the breast.

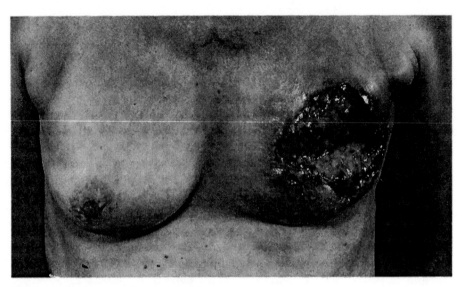

Figure 12.1: Fungating breast wound.

Normal Wound Healing

Wound healing is a complex physiological process that is dependent on a number of interrelated factors. The process of wound healing can be divided into three overlapping phases:

- inflammatory phase;
- proliferative phase;
- maturation phase.

Inflammatory Phase

This is the initial phase that commences the process of wound healing. When the skin becomes subject to trauma, bleeding will occur. The damaged ends of the blood vessels will constrict in order to minimize blood loss, blood clots will occur, allowing a temporary closure of the wound, and a scab will form. The bleeding will also help to cleanse the wound of any debris and bacteria that may have entered the wound as a result of the injury.

Proliferative Phase

During this phase the wound is filled with new connective tissue. There will be a decrease in the wound size as granulation, contraction and epithelialization occur.

Maturation Phase

In healthy individuals this stage begins after about 20 days of injury and may last for months or even years in complex wounds (Clark, 1988). Scar tissue will be formed, reducing in size and colour with time. Scar formation is a normal consequence of the process of wound healing in adults.

Many wounds heal without complications. However, there are many factors that can delay the healing process. Local factors such as wound infection, mechanical stress, use of toxic cleansing agents and the presence of foreign bodies can prolong healing. External factors such as smoking, poor nutrition, age, drug therapy and disease will also slow the wound healing process. Socioeconomic and psychological factors can have a detrimental effect on the rate of repair (Kiecolt-Glaser et al., 1995).

In patients who have a fungating wound, healing will be affected by the concomitant therapies, such as radiotherapy and chemotherapy.

Anaemia may be a common problem in patients who have cancer and this can directly reduce the oxygen supply to the wound bed, ultimately reducing the rate of healing if not corrected.

It has been suggested that stress and anxiety can affect wound healing (Kiecolt-Glaser et al., 1995) and patients who live with fungating wounds often feel the effects of stress and anxiety, along with the psychological impact.

Assessment of Patients with a Fungating Wound

As with all aspects of wound care, it is vital to consider the holistic needs of a patient in order to optimize wound healing. A fungating wound may need additional palliative management, as the wound is often the secondary focus of care.

To ensure that a holistic approach to the care of the wound is taken, it is essential that a thorough assessment be made. Assessment should encompass the following areas (Hallett, 1995):

- history relating to present wound – this will identify factors that may have influenced the disease process;
- cause and stage of disease – may indicate the origin of the cancer and, if appropriate, its expected progression;
- present treatment if any – importantly radiotherapy, chemotherapy, hormone therapy, laser treatment or surgery. It is imperative to have a history of any adverse reactions to any of the treatments;
- physical limitations – the location and range of the wound may affect the dressing choice and the treatment options available;
- nutritional assessment – current nutritional intake is vital information at

this stage as deficiencies in vitamins and minerals will be detrimental to wound care. It will also be important to establish whether there is poor appetite, anorexia, nausea and/or weight loss;

- emotional considerations – depression, social stigma, guilt or shame are often associated with malodorous wounds. Relationships with loved ones and partners can also be affected because of the lack of confidence and sexual expression. Fear of the unknown, pain and death may also be common;
- self-perception of wound and body image – altered body image should be considered, especially when determining dressings that are cosmetically acceptable;
- knowledge of diagnosis – establish amount of knowledge and information patient and family have on the disease process;
- family/carer influences – establish whether family and friends are able to cope with the likely increase in anger vented towards them and that they are aware of the networks available to help them;
- support networks and systems in place – establish whether there is a need for the multidisciplinary team to be involved whenever the patient needs it;
- local wound condition and associated symptoms – a full assessment of the wound should include the size, location, shape, colour of the wound bed, pain, exudate levels, odour, infection and bleeding.

It is vital at this stage that members of the multidisciplinary team are involved and informed of any decisions with regard to treatment. This will ensure that the optimum care can and will be given to the patient.

The use of photography (with patient consent) can be a useful method by which to monitor the condition of the wound. It should be done with caution as it can be an encouragement to the patient if the wound is improving but may be disheartening if the wound deteriorates.

Management of Fungating Wounds

Aims of Managing a Fungating Wound

The aims of wound management for fungating wounds where healing is unlikely should focus on comfort, improving quality of life, controlling the symptoms and promoting confidence and a sense of well-being (Moody and Grocott, 1993). These aims should be met through appropriate use of dressings and interventions.

In many instances it is not possible to provide a cure for the underlying disease. Therefore, the aim of the nursing management of the fungating wound may be palliative and undertaken in an effort to improve the patient's quality of life (Hallett, 1995).

Wound Cleansing

The use of warmed normal saline to cleanse a wound has long been an established and well-recognized method. It can also be useful in the removal of existing dressings that may have stuck and which, if not removed carefully, may cause pain and trauma. Warming the saline before cleansing will be gentler to the patient and it will also ensure that the temperature of the wound does not lower, thus continuing with an environment for optimal wound healing.

In light of the fact that many of this group of patients will be nursed at home, healthcare professionals should encourage patients to shower the wound thoroughly in warmed water. This will enhance the psychological well-being of the patient as well as ensuring the wound is cleaned to the optimum.

Management of Necrotic Tissue

Among the goals for the wound care of patients with fungating wounds is the management of the necrotic tissue caused by the lack of oxygen supply to the tumour area. Surgical debridement may prove beneficial if the patient's condition allows (Fairburn, 1993). If surgical debridement is not suitable, conservative management may be necessary through the use of dressings and other treatments.

Streptokinase and streptodornase have been used in combination to promote debridement of necrotic tissue. There is little evidence to suggest that enzymatic debridement is of greater benefit than other conservative treatments, and it can be quite time consuming to prepare the mixture and to ensure that the treatment is being used appropriately.

Hydrogels and hydrocolloids are useful as they have a high water content and will allow the rehydration of the necrotic tissue.

Hydrogels are available in either sheet or gel format. Hydrogel sheets are used for shallow wounds such as fungating wounds and the gels are more suitable for cavities and dense areas of eschar. A secondary dressing should always be used to keep the dressing in place. There can be problems associated with the use of hydrogels. Peri-wound maceration and excoriation can be experienced as a result of leakage of the gel if an appropriate secondary dressing is not used. The use of a barrier film can combat this. Owing to the high water content of the hydrogel, the wound can be subject to a very wet environment that is conducive to the breeding of infection and in light of this it is imperative that the wound bed is cleansed and inspected frequently.

Hydrocolloids create an environment that encourages the removal of sloughy or necrotic wounds. There is also evidence that hydrocolloids reduce pain in wounds (Rousseau, 1991), which is an important aspect to consider when choosing the correct dressings. The additional advantage of hydrocolloids is their absorptive capabilities, thus ensuring the wound is maintained in a moist environment. These dressings are waterproof, which enables the patient to bath or shower without removing them.

The use of honey, icing sugar and sugar paste has been shown to be effective in encouraging autolytic debridement of necrotic tissue in fungating wounds. These agents also have the benefit of reducing any malodour (Sims and Fitzgerald, 1985; Thomas, 1992).

Larval therapy is a method of treatment that will debride necrotic tissue. The larvae break down and liquefy dead tissue rapidly by depositing powerful proteolytic enxymes. Although larval therapy is back in vogue and is effective at the debridement of necrotic tissue, some patients and nursing staff do not like the thought of it. Its place should be considered carefully for use on necrotic tissue in fungating wounds.

It should be remembered that with the use of any debriding agents on necrotic tissue there is an expected larger area that will remain once the necrotic tissue is removed. This is normal and should not cause concern. It is important that this is considered and that the patient is fully informed to expect it and that it is a sign of improvement to the wound, not deterioration.

Management of a Bleeding or Haemorrhaging Fungating Wound

Haemorrhage may occur as a result of ruptured or eroded major blood vessels local to the tumour, owing to their weakened state. The use of alginates, particularly Kaltostat and sorbsan, is extremely effective in controlling localized bleeding as well as allowing the wound area to continue to be moist (Thomas, 1992).

When carrying out a dressing change it is important to do so gently and with care to reduce trauma and damage. Warmed normal saline will aid the removal of any stuck dressings as well as providing a soothing environment around the wound for the patient.

When the wound is bleeding profusely, more extreme measures may need to be taken but with caution and careful monitoring. Topical adrenaline solution (1 in 1000 for injection) may be used and this may cause localized ischaemic necrosis due to onset of vasoconstriction. Oral or topical tranexamic acid solution (for injection) may be used, as might the cauterization of bleeding vessels. However, owing to the increase and availability of modern dressing products, this method is not used very frequently. Ligation of the bleeding vessels by a surgeon may also be undertaken to stop bleeding (Naylor, 2001).

Radiotherapy, given as a single dose, may also be given. This will reduce the tumour size and bring about a consequent reduction in the symptoms, including bleeding (Young, 1997).

Management of Infection in a Fungating Wound

Infection will often occur as a result of the build-up of aerobic and anaerobic bacteria in the necrotic tissue. Wound infection is a problem as it will prevent a wound from healing. Infection may also lead to further breakdown and extension of the wound. It can also increase patient discomfort, pain, disability, smell and other serious complications that may lead to septicaemia and death.

A swab of the wound should be taken if it shows signs of clinical infection, in order for systemic antibiotics to be administered with the correct sensitivity to that specific organism. The signs of clinical infection could be the presence of pus, increased exudate levels, an increase in pain, a change in appearance, or an increase in any malodour (Cutting and Harding, 1994).

There is some controversy concerning the use of topical antibacterial agents to help treat wound infection. A recent report concluded that: 'Topical antibiotics are inappropriate for wounds and ulcers although they are widely promoted for this purpose' (Drug and Therapeutics Bulletin, 1991). The exception to this is the use of topical metronidazole gel on malodorous wounds, which has been shown to be effective in reducing and preventing odour (Lancet, 1990).

Management of Malodour in a Fungating Wound

Odour at the wound site could possibly be one of the most distressing associated symptoms for a patient with a fungating wound. Patients have described the effect that a malodorous wound has on their lives as being embarrassing, socially isolating and often distressing, as a result of the continuous leaking of exudate that stains clothes and sheets (Neal, 1991; Boardman et al., 1993). There is stigma associated with malodorous wounds that may inhibit sexuality and intimacy (Clark, 1992). There are a number of products available that will reduce such odour. Treatment should depend on the cause of the odour (Haughton and Young, 1995).

Malodour can also be distressing to the nurse, and this distress and fear may be felt by the patient (Hastings, 1993). Odour will often be present in a fungating wound as a result of infection due to the rise in aerobic and anaerobic bacteria. This results in the formation of necrotic tissue on the wound because of the poor tissue oxygenation at the site of the tumour.

The most effective way of managing malodourous wounds is to prevent or eradicate the infection responsible for the odour. The administration of systemic antibiotics and antimicrobial agents may be effective in some cases (Thomas, 1998).

Exudate Management

Wound exudate in a fungating wound is difficult to predict or control. The exudate that is produced by the wound is the result of wound infection/colonization (Gottrup, 1997; Harding, 1997) and the wound type. Lymphatic drainage problems can occur following surgery for cancer, which can increase exudate (Gottrup, 1997). If colonization is reduced, exudate will decrease. It is important to maintain a moist environment while diminishing the need for dressing changes and at the same time ensuring there is no maceration around the wound.

There are a number of dressings available that will cope with moderate to very high levels of exudate. When choosing the dressing, it is imperative that all aspects of the holistic assessment are considered.

Dressings

Where possible, the wound should be kept in a moist environment in order to maximize the healing potential (Winter, 1962). The choice of dressing should limit the frequency of dressing changes while enabling maximum exudate management to prevent peri-wound maceration as well as ensuring that the risk of infection is kept to a minimum.

Odour-absorbing Dressings

The use of the antibiotic metronidazole has been shown to be effective in the treatment of anaerobic infections (Thomas, 1988, 1989). Topical metronidazole gel has been shown to reduce the level of bacteria present in a wound, and is now the preferred treatment for fungating wounds, rather than oral or intravenous metronidazole (Sims and Fitzgerald, 1985; Saunders and Reguard, 1989, Morgan, 1992; Thomas, 1992).

The combined use of metronidazole gel and intrasite gel has been shown to be an effective treatment regime (Thomas, 1992; Boardman et al., 1993). The intrasite gel will encourage autolytic debridement and the metronidazole gel will combat malodour. A non-adherent absorbent dressing should be used as a secondary dressing.

The application of honey is a less conventional method that has been used to manage malodourous wounds. It has been shown in a number of laboratory studies to completely inhibit the wound-infecting bacteria, therefore reducing the malodour associated with the infection produced (Molan, 1999).

The use of sugar paste to control odour has been recommended in the literature (Chirife et al., 1982) because of its antimicrobial properties. Sugar will encourage the removal of exudate and tissue fluid, which will subject the bacteria to an increase in osmotic pressure, resulting in cell injury and death and ultimately inhibition of bacterial growth. The negative aspect of using sugar is that it is most effective after three to four hours of application. This means that the dressing treatment should be applied twice daily, which is something that may be impossible if the patient is being managed in the community. It is not recommended for use on patients who have diabetes. It is however, self-sterilizing, inexpensive and will mould to any wound type.

More recently, larval therapy has been shown to be an effective way of eliminating wound infection and odour from extensive necrotic wounds (Thomas et al., 1996; Evans, 1997; Thomas, 1998).

The use of a charcoal dressing may also be considered to reduce the odour from a fungating wound. This method of combating wound odour was discovered by Butcher et al. in 1976. Since then a number of odour-absorbing dressing have become available, with Actisorb the first manufactured charcoal dressing. A number of dressings containing activated charcoal have been developed and the individual dressing's ability to absorb odour will determine whether it can be used as a primary or secondary dressing. The dressings will dampen the odour and absorb exudate but not treat the cause of the odour. As previously mentioned, some charcoal dressings can only be used as a secondary dressing. This may add bulk to the wound site and give more reason for the patient to be concerned about her/his appearance, which is something practitioners should be avoiding. Many charcoal dressings cannot be cut to size, again restricting the sites at which they can be used and also increasing unnecessary bulk to the dressing.

Since the original charcoal dressing appeared there have been a number of developments that include the use of silver and alginates impregnated within the charcoal dressing. Actisorb Plus and Acticoat are examples of charcoal dressings impregnated with silver, which not only combat malodour but will also fight the levels of bacteria on the wound. This has been seen to be of greater benefit, as the odour will be addressed while combating its cause at the same time.

Carboflex uses a combination of alginate and charcoal. This limits the need for a primary dressing and issues of exudate management and odour absorption have been addressed.

It is imperative to encourage bedding and clothes to be changed once exudate has come into contact with them. The use of aromatherapy should be considered with caution as this will only reduce the smells, not treat the cause, and may leave the patient associating that particular smell with the wound (Haughton and Young, 1995).

Types of Dressings suitable for Fungating Wounds

Hydrofibres

Aquacel(tm) Hydrofibre(tm) stands out as being of exceptional performance in providing an optimum healing environment as well as pain-free removal. It will absorb rapidly and retain exudate, and is highly effective at exudate control without having the risk of maceration. Aquacel has been shown to control the release of bacteria, which may reduce the risk of cross-infection in the clinical setting (Bowler, 2000). This is an important aspect to consider, especially as the patient may be immunocompromised as a result of the adjunctive therapy she/he may be receiving.

Alginates

Alginates were first used in the 1940s (Thomas and Loveless, 1992). They are made from seaweed and can be composed of galuronic acid and mannuronic acid. The amount of each type of acid in the alginate will give rise to the 'gelling' abilities of the dressing; this in turn will reflect the ease of removal of the dressing, an important aspect in reducing pain and trauma to the wound bed. Some alginates have haemostatic properties, which is of additional advantage to the fungating wounds as uncontrolled bleeding is a common problem. Alginates are best used in highly exuding wounds. If the wound is too dry the alginate will adhere to the wound bed and cause trauma to the wound on removal. This could restart bleeding in a fungating wound. A secondary dressing will need to be applied over the alginate to secure it in place. The level of exudate produced from the wound should determine dressing change.

Foams

Foams are formed using a polymer technology. They can absorb large amounts of exudate and are non-adherent to the wound bed. They can be used as a primary or secondary dressing. There are many foam dressings on the market and the amount of exudate that can be absorbed will depend on which one is used and ultimately the length of time needed in between each dressing change.

Allevyn hydrocellular and Allevyn cavity have both been shown to absorb larger amounts of exudate than other low-adherent absorbent padding (Boardman et al., 1993), allowing fewer dressing changes for the patient, which will ultimately increase her/his quality of life.

Two-layer Permeable System

The use of a perforated non-adherent contact layer, Mepitel, protects the wound bed while allowing for inspection of the wound, and enabling exudate to pass through the dressing. It therefore permits the use of cheaper absorbent dressing pads that will absorb the high level of exudate while controlling the expenditure of the total treatment costs. This dressing is gentle on removal and only needs to be changed every seven days, reducing the trauma to the local wound area and ultimately reducing pain at dressing changes for the patient. The negative aspect of Mepitel is that is not recommended for use on bleeding wounds – often a symptom of the fungating wound. However, if used appropriately it has a large number of positive features that other dressings lack.

Drainage Bags

Drainage bags can also be used with a barrier cream to prevent maceration of the surrounding skin (Hallett, 1995). Butterfly drains inserted into the dressings to allow further drainage of exudate have had a limited effect (Grocott, 1991). This would not be considered to be the optimal management as issues associated with body image and self-respect may not have been met.

Cosmetic Appearance

It is imperative that the cosmetic appearance of the dressing used is considered to allow the patient to continue to dress in the same way as she/he did prior to the development of the fungating wound.

Management of Pain

Pain in fungating wounds is frequently the result of the erosion and breakdown of the nerve endings, which often cannot be repaired (Naylor, 2001). Pain may also be due to further invasion or growth of the tumour. The degree of pain will depend on the site of the wound, the degree of the disease and the involvement of nerves, soft tissue damage and past experience of pain. It is imperative that this is established throughout the assessment process.

If pain is continuously felt at dressing change, a review of dressing treatment may be necessary to ensure that the appropriate dressing is being used and that it is not sticking and causing pain on removal. Exudate levels may have reduced over time and therefore pain may be an indication that a change of dressing is required.

Lignocaine gel may be applied directly to the wound surface (Rang, 1995) to help reduce the wound pain. This will act by blocking the message of pain reaching the brain. If this is not adequate, the use of topical opioids, such as diamorphine or morphine, mixed with a soluble medical lubricant or hydrogel and applied topically to the wound may reduce pain at the wound site (Naylor, 2001). This should be used with caution as it may make the wound sensitive to topical opioids (Stein, 1995). It is also unclear as to whether the opioids provide a true analgesia effect or whether they provide a more anti-inflammatory effect that ultimately reduces the pain (Stein, 1995).

It is important to ensure that adequate oral analgesia/opioids have been taken far enough in advance of the dressing change to ensure the analgesia has had time to work.

The use of entinox is short acting and may be effective in reducing pain as a result of dressing change (Naylor, 2001). The use of a barrier film around the wound site will prevent maceration resulting from poor exudate management associated with pain. Non-steroidal anti-inflammatory drugs could be used with caution to reduce the amount of pain that may be a result of localized inflammation.

Management of Itching and Pruritus

Itching may be a further complication as a result of tumour nodules beginning to emerge under the surrounding skin. The stretching of the skin irritates nerve endings and may cause a biochemical reaction leading to local inflammation (Naylor, 2001). The use of oral antihistamines may be of some help. There is documentation which suggests that the use of hydrogel sheets helps in this situation as they have a cooling (especially if they have been refrigerated prior to use) and soothing effect on the irritable skin. They can be covered with a film dressing to prevent them from dehydrating, or they can be used with a secondary absorbent dressing if the wound is exuding (Naylor, 2001). Naylor (2001) also suggests the use of menthol in aqueous cream. The menthol has a cooling effect and can be applied to the itching areas two to three times a day. It should not be applied to any broken areas of skin.

Transcutaneous nerve stimulation (TENS) has been used effectively to relieve pruritis (Grocott, 1999).

Adjunctive Treatment

Radiotherapy

Radiotherapy may reduce the size of the tumour and should therefore reduce the levels of exudate associated with the wound, making the wound more manageable.

Hormone Therapy

Hormonal therapy for breast cancer will be given if the index oestrogen receptor protein is positive, and surgery will not be, or has already been, performed.

Chemotherapy

Chemotherapy may be given immediately after surgery to eliminate micrometastasis. Chemotherapy may also be given pre-operatively to reduce the bulk of a fungating wound in the hope that an inoperable lesion becomes operable.

Nutritional Supplements

Nutritional levels may be depleted/compromised as result of the disease process. Therefore, fluid and nutritional supplements of protein, vitamins and minerals should be encouraged.

Complementary Treatments

Anecdotal evidence exists to support the use of essential oils, and individuals are free to use them for their own benefit (Baker, 1998). It is imperative that a safe and suitable education programme is developed to ensure the safe use of these oils. It is also suggested that a stronger evidence base for the use of essential oils in wound care is established before extending their use in practice (Baker, 1998).

Psychosocial Aspects of Managing Fungating Wounds

Compliance

Involving the patient and family with the decision process for the dressing choice is important to ensure compliance. This should include time needed to carry out dressing changes, frequency of dressing changes and location of dressing changes, whether at home, hospital or doctor's surgery. Importantly, the cosmetic image of the dressing is essential in order to maintain compliance.

Body Image

Illness and radical surgery can directly affect the development and stability of an individual's body image. The breast will carry a special meaning for a woman due to its reproductive and nurturing functions. Wounds resulting from surgery, infection or malignancy to this area have added problems associated with the actual or perceived loss of femininity.

When the wound becomes smelly or unsightly in an area that is not normally exposed, such as the breast, more problems are likely to arise. Touching and exposure of this part of the body would normally only be permitted to those close to the patient. Suddenly this part of the body is expected to be exposed at regular intervals to a large number of medical and nursing staff.

Dressing choice will be fundamental to ensure that the patient is still able to carry on normal activities of daily living and that she is not restricted in what to wear because of the bulkiness of the dressing.

It should never be assumed that it is acceptable to carry out a dressing change. It is essential that the patient be asked if it is a convenient time. If there are any other members of the team who would like to view the wound, it is important that permission is sought from the patient and that her wishes are respected.

When the dressing requires changing it may be an idea to coordinate an appropriate time with other members of the team, as they may wish to monitor the progress of the wound. This will limit the number of dressing changes needed and ensure that the patient's best interests are met. Ultimately, if the whole team is present at this time it is easier to discuss together the next treatment step.

Conclusion

Fungating wound management is a multidisciplinary responsibility. It is imperative that symptom control is managed effectively to ensure all treatment regimes are given the opportunity to be as successful as possible.

There are a number of modern dressings available that have been shown to enhance the healing process of a fungating wound. It is essential that the practitioner is aware of all the advantages and disadvantages of each dressing in order to ensure an optimum wound healing environment.

Effective management of a fungating wound may increase the psychosocial well-being of the patient.

References

Baker J (1998) Essential oils: a complimentary therapy in wound management. Journal of Wound Care 7(7): 355-7.

Bale S and Harding KG (1987) Fungating breast wounds. Journal of District Nursing 9(12): 4-5.

Bennett G, Moody M (1995) Wound Care for Health Professionals. London: Chapman & Hall.

Boardman M, Mellor K, Neville B (1993) Treating a patient with a heavily exuding malodorous fungating wound. Journal of Wound Care 2(2): 74-7.

Bowler P (2000) Infection control properties of wound dressings. In: Aquacel: New Dimensions in the Treatment of Post-surgical Wounds. Proceedings from the 10th Conference of the EWMA Medical Communications, Holsworthy.

Butcher G, Butcher JA, Maggs FAP (1976) The treatment of malodourous wounds. Nursing Mirror 142: 76.

Carville K (1994) Assessment and management of cancerous wounds. Primary Intention 20-26 February.

Chirife J, Scarmato G, Herszage L (1982) Scientific basis for the use of granulated sugar in treatment of infected wounds. Lancet i: 56.

Clark L (1992) Caring for fungating tumours. Nursing Times 88(12): 66-70.

Clark RAF (1988) Overview and general considerations of wound repair. In: Clark RAF, Henson PM (eds) The Molecullar and Cellular Biology of Wound Repair. New York: Plenum.

Cutting KF, Harding K(1994) Criteria for identifying wound infection. Journal of Wound Care 3(4): 194-201.

Drug and Therapeutics Bulletin (1991) Local applications to wounds, 1: Cleansers, antibacterials, debriders. Drug and Therapeutics Bulletin 29(24): 93-4.

Evans H (1997) A treatment of last resort. Nursing Times 9(23): 62-7.

Fairburn K (1993) Towards better care for women: understanding fungating breast lesions. Professional Nurse 9(3): 204-12.

Gottrup F (1997) Is exudate a clinical problem? A surgeon's perspective. In: Cherry C, Harding K (eds) Management of Wound Exudate: Proceedings of Joint Meeting of EWMA and ETRS. London: Churchill Communications.

Grocott P (1991) Application of the principles of modern wound management for complex wounds in palliative care. In: Harding KG, Leaper DL, Turner TD (eds) Proceedings of the First European Conference on Advances in Wound Management: 96-7.

Grocott P (1995) The palliative management of fungating malignant wounds. Journal of Wound Care 4(5): 240-2.

Grocott P (1999) The management of fungating wounds. Journal of Wound Care 8(5): 232-4.

Grocott P (2000) The palliative management of fungating malignant wounds. Journal of Wound Care 9(1): 4-9.

Haargenson CD (1971) Diseases of the Breast, 2nd edn. Eastbourne: WB Saunders.

Hallett A (1995) Fungating wounds. Nursing Times 91(39): 81-3.

Harding K (1997) Is exudate a clinical problem? A specialist physician's perspective. In: Cherry C, Harding K (eds) Management of Wound Exudate: Proceedings of Joint Meetings of EWMA and ETRS. London: Churchill Communications.

Hastings D (1993) Basing care on research. Nursing Times 89(13): 70-4.

Haughton W, Young T (1995) Common problems in wound care: malodorous wounds. British Journal of Nursing 4(16): 959-63.

Kiecolt-Glaser JK, Marucha PT, Malarkey WB, Mercado AM, Glaser R (1995) Slowing of wound healing by psychological stress. Lancet 346: 1194-6.

Lancet (1990) Editorial: Management of smelly tumours. Lancet 335: 141-2.

Laverty D, Cooper J, Soady S (2000) Wound management. In: Mallett J, Dougherty L (eds)

The Royal Marsden Hopsital Manual of Clinical Nursing Procedures, 5th edn. Oxford: Blackwell Science.

Molan PC (1999) The role of honey in the management of wounds. Journal of Wound Care 8(8): 415–18.

Moody M, Grocott P (1993) Let us extend our knowledge base: assessment and management of fungating malignant wounds. Professional Nurse June: 586–90.

Morgan DA (1992) Formulary of Wound Management Products: A Guide for Healthcare Staff, 5th edn. Aldershot: BritCair.

Mortimer P (1998) Skin problems in palliative care: medical aspects. In Doyle D, Hanks G, Macdonald N (eds) Oxford Textbook of Palliative Medicine. Oxford: Oxford Medical Publications.

Moseley JG (1998) Palliation in Malignant Disease. Edinburgh: Churchill Livingstone.

Naylor W (2001) Management of fungating wounds. In: Naylor W, Laverty D, Mallett J (eds) The Royal Marsden Hospital of Wound Management in Cancer Care. Oxford: Blackwell Science.

Neal K (1991) Treating fungating lesions. British Journal of Nursing 4(16): 958–96.

Petrek JA, Glen PD, Cramer AR (1983) Ulcerated breast cancer: patients and outcome. American Surgeon 49(4): 187–91.

Rang H (1995) Pharmacology, 3rd edn. Edinburgh: Churchill Livingstone.

Regnard CF, Tempest S (1992) A Guide to Symptom Relief in Advanced Cancer, 3rd edn. London: Haigh & Hochland.

Rousseau P (1991) Comparison of the various physiochemical properties of various hydrocolloid dressings. Wounds 3(1): 43–8.

Saunders J, Reguard C (1989) Management of malignant ulcers and flow diagram. Palliative Medicine 2: 153–5.

Sims R, Fitzgerald V (1985) Community Nursing Management of Patients with Ulcerating/Fungating Malignant Breast Disease. London: RCN Oncology Nursing Society.

Stein C (1995) The control of pain in peripheral tissue by opioids. New England Journal of Medicine 332(25): 1685–90.

Thomas M (1988) Coping with distressing symptoms In: Wilson J (ed) Nursing Issues and Research in Terminal Care. Chichester: Wiley.

Thomas S (1989) Treating malodorous wounds. Nursing Times (Community Outlook) 85(10): 27–30.

Thomas S (1992) Current practices in the management of fungating lesions and radiation damaged skin. Mid Glamorgan Surgical Materials Testing Laboratories.

Thomas S (1998) Odour-absorbing dressings. Journal of Wound Care 7(5): 246–50.

Thomas S, Jones M, Shutler S, Jones S (1996) Using larvae in modern wound management. Journal of Wound Care 5(2): 60–9.

Thomas S, Loveless P (1992) Observations on the fluid handling properties of alginate dressings. Pharmaceutical Journal 248: 672–5.

Winter G (1962) Formation of the scab and rate of epithelialization of superficial wounds in the skin of a young domestic pig. Nature 193: 293–4.

Young T (1997) Wound care: the challenge of managing fungating wounds. Community Nurse 3(9): 41–4.

Chapter 13
Advanced Disease

ELIZABETH LOMAS

Introduction

Many patients diagnosed with breast cancer, even after treatment, live with the fear that at some point in their lives the cancer will return. For some this fear is unfounded but figures show that for just over half of these patients their fears will come true and despite having surgery and/or radiotherapy they will go on to develop metastatic disease (Smith and de Boer, 2000).

For nurses to provide high-quality, evidence-based care they need to have access to information on advanced breast cancer. This chapter will cover topics that are related to every aspect of the disease. It will discuss local and loco-regional recurrence as well as metastatic disease. It will discuss principles that can be applied when caring for patients with advanced breast cancer. Most importantly it will focus on the symptoms associated with advanced breast disease, looking at what effect these symptoms will have on a patient both physically and emotionally. The help and support that we as nurses can give to the patients and their family/carers will be discussed.

The Pattern of Clinical Spread

It is thought that about 10% of women diagnosed with breast cancer also initially present with metastatic disease (Overmoyer, 1995). Of those remaining, a large proportion will go on to develop metastases, months or even years after being diagnosed.

Advanced disease in breast cancer can take two forms, that of local or loco-regional recurrence and systemic recurrence (i.e. metastases). The two forms are very different and have different implications for the patient, as patients usually die from metastases but not from local recurrence (Souhami and Tobias, 1995).

Local Recurrence

In itself isolated local breast cancer recurrence does not seem to be a threat to survival. However, it is a well-documented fact that local recurrence is a predictor of distant metastases which, although often asymptomatic, should actively be looked for in any presenting patient (Dixon and Sainsbury, 1993). Often, despite optimum treatment, residual tumour cells may remain at the original site or in lymph nodes situated within the local area. These residual cells can lead to a recurrence of the cancer in the remaining breast tissue, in the chest wall, or in the regional lymph nodes. Local recurrence is usually picked up clinically and is confirmed by carrying out a fine-needle aspiration or biopsy.

Once local recurrence has been confirmed there are several different treatment options depending on what treatment has been given in the past, where the secondaries are situated and whether there are singular or multiple nodules. Surgery, chemotherapy, radiotherapy and hormone therapy can all be used individually or in combination to control and treat local recurrence.

Systemic Metastatic Disease

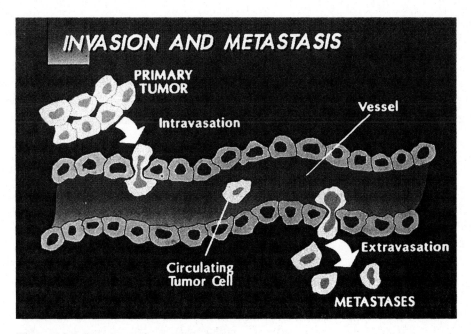

Figure 13.1: Invasion and metastatic disease.

Metastasis means the spread of cancer, and occurs when cancer cells detach from a primary tumour and travel via the lymphatic system or bloodstream to other parts of the body (see Figure 13.1). In breast cancer an obvious route of spread is through the lymph nodes and channels that supply the breast tissue, but it is also possible for the cancer to engulf blood vessels within the breast, thus allowing the cancer cells to enter the bloodstream and spread throughout the body.

Metastatic disease can occur weeks, months or years after an initial diagnosis of breast cancer. Unlike local recurrence, which is commonly asymptomatic, it is often not until the patient presents with a distressing symptom such as bone pain, confusion, and breathlessness that metastatic breast cancer is diagnosed (McGinn and Moore, 2001).

The most common sites of metastatic spread for patients with primary breast cancer are to the lungs, liver, bones and brain, although the heart, adrenal glands, peritoneal cavity and ovaries may also be affected (see Figure 13.2). Various studies put the average survival time with metastases at between eighteen months and three years (Vogel, 1991; McEvilly and Dow, 1998; Leonard et al., 2000). This does of course depend on where the metastases occur. For example, a woman with a single metastasis in her femur may live for many years whereas a woman with multiple metastases affecting her liver may live for a much shorter time.

Common Sites of Metastases in Breast Cancer

Bone Metastases

At any one time in the United Kingdom it is estimated that approximately 25 000 women are living with bone metastases that originate from primary breast cancer (Rees et al., 1994). Metastases can arise in any bone in the body but most commonly occur in the vertebrae, pelvis, ribs and long bones such as the femur or humerus. The incidence of bone metastases among women with advanced disease is thought to be as high as 73%, making the skeletal system the most common site of recurrence.

The prognosis for people with bone metastases is still relatively poor as although bone metastases are not life threatening in themselves, they suggest blood-borne metastatic spread from the original tumour and therefore are often indicative of other soft tissue metastases. The average survival for women with bone metastases is between 20 and 24 months (Rees et al., 1994). Often, even when there is no evidence of other metastatic disease, the complications associated with bone metastases such as spinal cord compression, hypercalcaemia, pathological fractures and musculoskeletal pain all contribute to a reduction in the patient's quality of life and often to that individual's eventual decline (Hoskin and Makin, 1998; Heatley and Coleman, 1999).

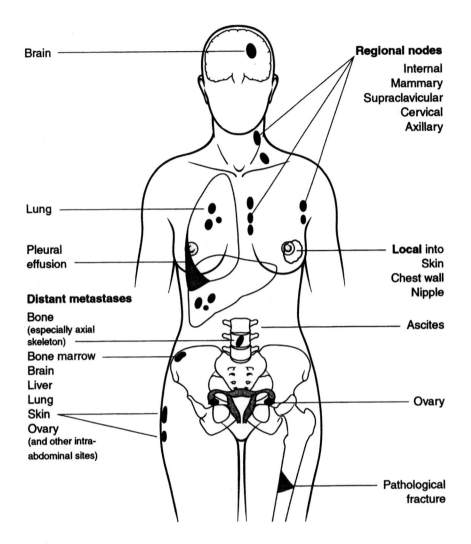

Figure 13.2: Diagram of clinical spread.

Presentation

Some bone metastases are asymptomatic and may only show up on X-rays or scans that are done for other reasons. Often, however, people will present with pain that may be described using the following characteristics:

- dull pain;
- deep aching;

- persistent pain;
- oppressive pain;
- pain worse on movement or when weight bearing;
- pain unrelieved by rest.

If bone metastases are suspected in a woman with breast cancer, initial investigations may include an X-ray of the affected area. The X-ray may show a lytic bony lesion but often a bone scan is required as pain can predate radiological changes and therefore a bone scan is more sensitive and can give more accurate information, often being able to detect bone metastases 2–18 months before changes are evident on plain radiographs (Waller and Caroline, 2000).

When bone metastases are discovered, treatment may be needed over a prolonged period of time. The aim of treatment should be to relieve pain, to strengthen bones and also to try and control further spread. The relatively long prognosis should be taken into account when treatment decisions are being made.

Radiotherapy, hormone therapy, chemotherapy and more recently bisphosphonates (discussed later in this chapter) all have an important role to play in the control and palliation of bone metastases.

Lung Metastases

The lung is the second most common site for metastases in women with advanced breast disease. Metastases can be solitary or multiple and depending on the area of lung affected can be asymptomatic or cause distressing symptoms.

Dyspnoea and cough are usually the most obvious symptoms that patients present with. Breathlessness is indicative of lung tissue infiltration but may also be associated with infection or with infiltration of the lymphatic system, all of which cause reduced lung capacity. The presence of a malignant pleural effusion caused by metastases invading the pleura will also compound symptoms and may cause a degree of pain.

A chest X-ray or CT scan usually confirms lung metastases. Treatment is very much based on controlling the disease and on symptom control. Systemic chemotherapy has been used, and Hoskin and Makin (1998) suggest that in women with metastatic breast cancer its use can increase the median survival rate to 20 months although this is very dependent on tumour response and other sites of disease.

Shortness of breath is probably one of the most anxiety-provoking symptoms a patient can experience, and therefore it is essential that any active treatment given must be used in conjunction with measures to ensure adequate symptom control.

Liver Metastases

Liver metastases are found in approximately 5% of all patients with metastatic breast cancer (Hayes and Kaplan, 1991). The discovery of liver metastases carries with it serious consequences as prognosis is often dramatically cut and if the disease is symptomatic a patient can deteriorate dramatically in a very short period of time.

How people may present with liver metastases can vary; they may have one or more of the following signs:

- enlarged liver on palpation;
- tenderness in hepatic region caused by irritation of stretched liver capsule;
- nausea;
- reduced gastric emptying/feeling of being bloated;
- oesophageal reflux;
- jaundice (this is usually apparent in late stages of liver disease);
- abnormal liver function test (LFTs) – although liver metastases are not the only reason why these may be elevated;
- bruising or bleeding due to impaired production of clotting factors.

Liver metastases are usually confirmed by performing an ultrasound scan and blood tests will normally be taken to assess how much the liver function is impaired.

The best course of treatment for patients with liver metastases must be carefully weighed up both by the doctors involved and by the patient, who should be given specialist support. Treatment more often than not will not extend a person's life but may reduce symptoms.

Systemic chemotherapy is one option that may be discussed with patients but obviously if liver function is impaired the drug type and dosage must be carefully considered. The risk of side effects from the chemotherapy must also be discussed with the patient and often it is this that will put the patient off. For some patients with liver metastases a change in their hormone therapy is an option, especially if chemotherapy is too potent. Very occasionally radiotherapy is given but this is only really done to reduce soft tissue swelling. Whether patients choose to have treatment or not, symptom control and psychological support are essential in maintaining their quality of life.

Brain Metastases

Breast cancer is the second commonest source of brain metastases and cerebral deposits have been found in approx 25% of all patients when a series of post mortems were carried out (Hoskin and Makin, 1998).

Patients may present with a variety of symptoms.

- headache;
- vomiting;
- dizziness;
- visual disturbance;
- impaired intellectual function;
- weakness;
- mood swings;
- fits.

When brain metastases are suspected a CT or MRI scan of the brain will be carried out. Often an MRI scan will prove more sensitive and may detect metastases that do not show up on the CT scan.

Patients with brain metastases will often exhibit very distressing symptoms and first-line treatment is to commence high-dose steroids (12-16 mg dexamethasone daily) even prior to metastases being confirmed by scan. The use of steroids aims to reduce the cerebral swelling, thus reducing symptoms and improving neurological function. Any significant improvement is usually apparent within 24–48 hours.

Steroid treatment is really only a short-term measure and even if improvement is noted initially it is usually only a short-term effect. Depending on the physical condition of the patient and depending on the patient's wishes, other treatment may be considered. For patients with multiple metastases whole-brain radiation is an option. A short course of radiotherapy may be given and would be given with high-dose steroids to reduce excessive oedema. The success of the radiotherapy, however, is limited and it may only be effective for a short period of time. Occasionally an isolated cerebral metastasis may be treated with stereotactic radiotherapy or in some cases surgery but this is only in cases where there is no evidence of any other metastatic disease.

Complications of Metastatic Breast Cancer

The following sections outline some of the more common complications encountered by women with advanced metastatic breast cancer.

Pathological Fracture

A serious pathological fracture is thought to occur in approximately 9% of all patients with bone metastases; of those patients, over half have metastatic breast disease (Waller and Caroline, 2000). Bone affected by metastases is often very unstable and can fracture spontaneously or with relatively little trauma.

Pathological fractures can be prevented and are possible to predict in some cases. High-risk bony lesions can be spotted on bone scan and/or X-ray and may be considered for prophylactic internal fixation to prevent future pain and complications. A sharp increase in pain over days or weeks may be indicative of impending fracture and again surgery may be required. Treatment will obviously depend on the bone involved and the overall condition of the patient.

If internal fixation is performed, the surgery will usually be followed by radiotherapy once the wound has healed. Patients who are too unwell to undergo surgery will be treated with palliative radiotherapy, immobilization and effective pain relief.

For bones such as the ribs and pelvis that cannot be treated with surgery local radiotherapy will be given to relieve pain and promote bone healing.

Spinal Cord Compression

Spinal cord compression is a palliative care emergency and occurs in approximately 5% of all patients with advanced cancer (Waller and Caroline, 2000). It is caused by metastases travelling from the breast to the vertebrae, which develop and thus exert pressure on the spinal canal. Cord compression can occur at any level in the spine but the majority of cases diagnosed (70%) will be found in the thoracic vertebrae (Twycross, 1997).

A patient with spinal cord compression may present with the following symptoms:

- back pain: a constant nagging pain, local to site of lesion or a tight band of pain radiating from front to back;
- limb weakness: a loss of power/strength in limbs, unsteady gait;
- sensory loss: a feeling of numbness/tingling starting in lower limbs;
- sphincter dysfunction: a loss of bowel/bladder control, retention.

It is essential that if patients complain of any of the above symptoms they are investigated immediately. A detailed history will be taken, followed by an MRI scan if at all possible, which will give the most accurate information. X-rays may be taken and in the majority of cases these will show the level of vertebral collapse.

Treatment should start as soon as possible and the commencement of steroids to reduce any swelling (16 mg dexamethasone daily) will often precede an MRI scan. If spinal cord compression is confirmed, urgent radiotherapy will be given to reduce tumour size. Very occasionally there are cases whereby if there is an isolated metastasis causing compression and the patient is deemed fit, surgical decompression may be used (Leonard et al., 2000).

If left untreated, spinal cord compression carries a very real threat of paralysis. Recovery is very much linked to performance status at presentation. Often patients are left with decreased mobility, which can have a significant effect on that person's quality of life. It is important that physiotherapy and specialist palliative care input are offered to all patients with spinal cord compression.

Malignant Hypercalcaemia

Patients with advanced breast cancer are accountable for over 20% of all reported cases of cancer-related hypercalcaemia (Waller and Caroline, 2000).

In the past, a high calcium level in the blood was thought to be linked to patients with bone metastases. However, this is no longer the case and the majority of patients with bone metastases have been found to have a normal calcium reading. What does cause hypercalcaemia is the release of tumour-excreted parathyroid-hormone-related protein into the system. This prompts increased bone resorption, which consequently leads to more calcium entering into circulation.

The symptoms a patient may present with when hypercalcaemic are varied and range from mild to severe. Some symptoms may initially be overlooked as they are common in patients with advanced cancer but they may develop as the calcium level increases.

The symptoms of hypercalcaemia are:

- fatigue;
- weakness;
- anorexia;
- constipation;
- thirst;
- nausea and/or vomiting;
- confusion;
- drowsiness;
- in severe cases coma.

A simple blood test is able to detect the corrected serum calcium level, which normally runs below 2.62 mmol/l. When above 2.62 mmol patients may start exhibiting symptoms.

Hypercalcaemia is treatable but does usually indicate a poor prognosis. Initial treatment involves rehydration, often with intravenous saline, followed by intravenous infusion of a bisphosphonate such as pamidronate. Bisphosphonates work by binding themselves to the exposed surface of the bone and thus interrupting the process of bone resorption. The effect of bisphosponates is usually significant in 2-3 days, with the full effect being seen with in a week (Fleisch, 1995).

Patients will often require repeated treatment with bisphophonates, sometimes as often as every 3-4 weeks.

Pleural Effusion

A pleural effusion is an abnormal volume of fluid in the pleural space. It will occur in approximately 50% of all women with breast cancer (Leonard et al., 2000) and is a sign of advanced, widespread disease.

Symptoms may include a dry, non-productive cough, progressive shortness of breath and pain that may be pleuritic in nature. A simple chest X-ray will initially detect whether there is an accumulation of fluid in the pleural cavity but an ultrasound scan can also be useful in differentiating between fluid and consolidation.

The treatment for a pleural effusion can vary slightly. Pleural aspiration may initially be tried as drainage of as little as 250 ml fluid can prove to relieve symptoms. However, the fluid soon reaccumulates and therefore the insertion of a chest tube and drainage of fluid over 24-48 hrs is far more effective in controlling malignant pleural effusions (Leonard et al., 2000). Pleural effusions are likely to reoccur within a relatively short period of time and therefore, depending on the condition of the patient, a chemical pleuradhesis may be considered. This involves draining the effusion and then introducing a chemical irritant such as bleomycin, tetracycline or talc into the pleural space, which causes the pleural lining to stick together thus preventing a reaccumulation of fluid. In a small majority of cases surgery in the form of a pleurectomy may be considered, but this is a major procedure and the patient would need to be very fit for this to be entertained.

It is important to remember that a patient can be diagnosed with a pleural effusion and yet have no distressing symptoms. If this is the case, no treatment is required. Often patients who are symptomatic with pleural effusions may choose not to have treatment and may prefer instead to have specialist palliative care input.

Palliative Care in Advanced Breast Cancer

Although there have been many advances in the treatment of breast cancer, as of yet there is still no cure for metastatic disease. The main goals of treatment therefore must be to control disease and to palliate symptoms (Powles, 1997).

The World Health Organisation (WHO) (1990) has defined palliative care as 'the active total care of patients whose disease is not responsive to curative treatment'. WHO goes on further to describe the underlying principles which govern what palliative care should be. They are as follows:

Palliative care:

- affirms life and regards dying as a normal process;
- neither hastens nor postpones death;
- provides relief from pain and other distressing symptoms;
- offers a support system to help patients live as actively as possible until death;
- offers a support system to help the family cope during the patient's illness and in their own bereavement.

Palliative care is an area of medicine that has grown and developed considerably over the last decade. The image of palliative care is changing. It is no longer thought of as purely an area specializing in care of the dying. It has now become an area which focuses on how to help people living with cancer live what life they have left to the best of their ability. As Twycross (1997) states: 'the primary aim of treatment is not to prolong life but to make the life which remains as comfortable and as meaningful as possible'.

Quality of life is a term that is often used within palliative care. It will mean many different things to different patients at different times. Ultimately it is about setting realistic goals and standards that are achievable by the patients.

There is still some debate as to when cancer care becomes palliative care but the principles of palliative care are such that they can and often should be applied to a patient's care from the moment of diagnosis.

Symptom Control in Advanced Breast Cancer

Poor symptom control can make patients' lives and that of their families miserable (Waller and Caroline, 2000). In women with breast cancer there is a whole range of symptoms that arise for different reasons and at different stages in their lives. These symptoms may be caused directly by metastases, indirectly from systemic effects of disease, from treatment being given and as a result of medication being taken. It is also important to remember that some patients will show symptoms that may be due to pre-existing conditions, such as arthritis, osteoporosis and heart disease.

WHO (1990) advocates that careful evaluation is the essential basis for symptom management and that this is the responsibility of both doctors and nurses. Nurses at all levels are fundamental in achieving good symptom control for patients. Whether in hospital or in the community, nurses with the ability to assess patients, to identify the possible cause of symptoms and with the knowledge to implement appropriate care will ensure that patients receive a much higher quality of care and thus a greater quality of life.

Pain Control

Pain is often the symptom feared most by patients when they learn they have cancer (Grond et al., 1994). Many see pain as synonymous with cancer, and yet in reality approximately 25% of patients do not experience pain (Twycross, 1997). Of the remainder the pain experienced can in the majority of cases be controlled using effective analgesia and pain-management techniques.

Pain is rarely one-dimensional. There are many different aspects of people's lives that will influence the pain they experience. The concept of 'total pain' recognizes this fact and outlines key components that need to be looked at when assessing the pain.

Components of 'Total Pain' (Saunders, 1996) comprise:

- physical;
- emotional;
- social;
- spiritual.

The intensity of emotions such as anxiety, depression, anger and hostility should always be noted when initially assessing a patient. Such features may often serve to lower a patient's pain threshold and intensify the physical pain (Corcoran, 1991).

Classification of Pain

Pain in cancer patients is usually divided into one of two categories, that of nociceptive pain and that of neuropathic pain. The physiology of pain is somewhat complex and not always fully understood; however, it is important when making treatment choices to be able to classify pain.

Nociceptive pain

Receptors that respond to painful stimuli are called nociceptors. Nociceptive pain usually occurs as a result of tissue damage, as nociceptors respond directly as a result of chemical, physical or thermal stimulation. The pain message travels from the nociceptors that are found in the skin, bone, organs and connective tissue, along intact neurons to the brain.

Neuropathic pain

This is conveyed by similar nociceptive pathways but it occurs as a direct result of injury or abnormal functioning of any nerve in the peripheral or central nervous system.

Classification of Pain

	Category	Characteristics	Examples	Response to Opiates
N	Somatic Pain	Dull, aching, throbbing, or gnawing. Well localized.	Bone Pain Incisional Pain Musculo- skeletal Pain	Excellent
O				
C				
I				
C				
E	Visceral Pain	Results from injury to sympathetically inervated organs	Bowel obstruction Stretching of the liver capsule	Good
P				
T				
I		Caused by infiltration, compression, distention, or stretching of thoracic/ abdominal viscera	Tumour invasion of parietal surfaces Perforation of a hollow organ	
V				
E				
P		Poorly localized, deep dragging, squeezing, or pressure		
A				
I				
N		When acute, colicky associated with autonomic symptoms (nausea, sweating, etc.) Often referred to cutaneous sites remote from lesion		

N			
E	Results from injury to	Brachial/	May be
U	peripheral and/or central	lumbosacral	inadequate
R	nervous system, by tumour	plexopathies	
O	compression or infiltration	Post-herpetic	
P	or damage from surgical	neuralgia	
A	radiation, or chemotherapy	Vincristine or	
T	Superficial burning, stinging	cisplatin	
H	sometimes with lancinating	neuropathy	
I	electric shock-like pain	Diabetic neuropathy	
C	Often associated with		
	sensory changes		
P	There may also be associated		
A	muscle atrophy, autonomic		
I	changes, and trophic		
N	changes in the skin		

Reproduced with permission from Waller and Caroline (2000).

Assessment of Pain

Many patients with advanced cancer will present with more than one pain. Up to 80% of patients will have at least two pains (Grady and Severn, 1999). Often a nurse is one of the first health professionals to assess the patient in pain. Careful assessment of each individual pain, associated signs and symptoms and determination of the underlying cause are essential if appropriate treatment is then to be initiated (Hoskin and Makin, 1998).

Corcoran (1991) outlines four major components which nurses should consider when assessing a patient's pain.

1. A detailed history;
2. Accurate measurement;
3. Consideration of a patient's 'total pain';
4. Repeated review.

A detailed history

The time spent with patients listening to their story is very valuable. It is time in which patients can open up and tell their version of what is happening. It is frequently the first real chance that patients have to express the true extent of the pain and the anxieties that go with it. Patients may try and protect their loved ones by covering up the severity of the pain and therefore the relief at being able to share the burden is often evident. Spending time with the patient, listening to what is being said and being able to interpret what is being communicated are crucial to completion of an accurate assessment. In some cases a patient may not be able to communicate her/his story and therefore the nurse should seek to obtain as much information as possible from someone who knows and is close to the patient.

A detailed history should include the following information:

- Sites of pain: How many? Where are they?
- Referral of pain: Does the pain radiate anywhere?
- Timing: Is the pain continual, intermittent or on movement? What makes it worse?
- Quality: What is the pain like? Burning, stabbing, dull, aching?
- Severity: How bad is the pain? Does it disturb sleep? Does it stop the patient doing normal activities?
- Medical disorders: Are there any conditions other than cancer that could cause pain?

Accurate measurement

It is important when assessing pain that the information received is as accurate as possible. Different methods may be used to measure the severity of a patient's pain. Rating scales such as the ones below are commonly used and can prove very successful in determining whether pain relief is effective.

Visual analogue scale

No pain   *Worst possible pain*

0–10 Numeric pain intensity scale

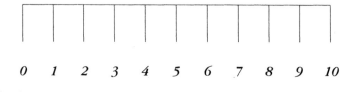

No pain   *Moderate pain*   *Worst possible pain*

Some, although not all, patients may find it helpful to maintain a pain diary. This can be personalized to each individual's needs but can record material such as increased need for breakthrough analgesia, effectiveness of analgesia, development of new pains and sleep disturbance due to pain. Many places will have standardized pain diaries that can be given to the patient.

Whatever method is used to ensure accurate measurement of severity of pain, it must be a method that is patient/carer friendly. There is no point in using a pain intensity scale if the patient is unable to comprehend how to use it.

Consideration of 'total pain'

As has been noted earlier in this chapter, pain is far more that a physical phenomenon. It is important for the nurse to be able to see the patient as a whole and this means identifying signs of psychological, spiritual and social distress. It also means recognizing cultural differences, which can affect the way a patient copes with pain. Anxieties, fears and worries about how family/friends/carers will cope with death, finances and emotional issues are all commonplace and need to be addressed and dealt with if optimum pain relief is to be achieved. If the patient is anxious or depressed, satisfactory pain relief can be delayed by up to 2-4 weeks (Twycross, 1997).

Repeated review

It is more than likely that patients with metastatic cancer will find their situations change regularly. Therefore it is safe to say that new pains will occur and previously controlled pains may worsen. By repeatedly reviewing pain at regular intervals, problems can be identified and dealt with at the earliest possible time.

Complete pain relief may take time to achieve and the patient needs to be reassured about this. Twycross (1997) advocates that it is best to aim for a programme of progressive pain relief. This starts with aiming for pain relief at night, followed by pain relief at rest during the day and finally aiming for pain relief on movement. In a small number of patients the latter aim is not achievable.

Pain Management and Intervention

Analgesia

The World Health Organisation (1996) has outlined six principles which it hopes should be adopted internationally when managing pain and administering analgesia in patients with cancer:

1. By mouth: Whenever possible the oral route of administering analgesia is preferred.
2. By the clock: Analgesics should be given regularly to prevent pain recurring. The patient should not be allowed to feel pain before the next dose of analgesia is given. Analgesia given on an 'as needed' basis is not an effective means of pain relief.
3. By the analgesic ladder: The WHO has developed a three-step analgesic ladder (see Figure 13.3). If analgesia in step one is not effective, move up to the next step.
4. For the individual: Analgesia will affect everyone differently. Therefore there is no correct dose of analgesia. The right dose of morphine is that which controls the pain.
5. Use of adjuvants: Adjuvants are a group of medications that enhance analgesic effects, control adverse side effects of opioids, and manage symptoms that are contributing to a patient's pain.
6. Attention to detail: Do not assume anything. Take an accurate precise history. Explore patient's 'total pain'. Talk about patient's fears and anxieties. Give patient clear verbal and written instructions on how to take prescribed medication.

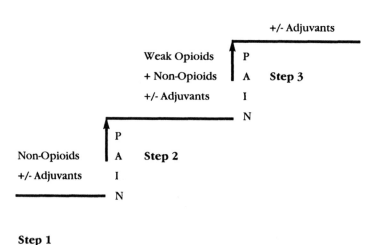

Figure 13.3: World Health Organisation Analgesic Ladder (1996).

Non-opioid Analgesia

This comprises analgesics used in Step 1 of the analgesic ladder and includes aspirin, paracetamol and other non-steroidal anti-inflammatory drugs (NSAIDs).

Aspirin is not the drug of choice in patients with advanced cancer owing to the increased risk of side effects such as gastric irritation and increased bleeding time.

Paracetamol and NSAIDs should be used in particular in patients with metastatic bone disease (common in women with advanced breast disease) and for those with soft tissue pain.

It is important to be aware that many NSAIDs, e.g. diclofenac, indomethacin, ketorolac, should be used with caution. They can cause severe gastric irritation and should never be used in patients with a past history of peptic ulcers. New selective Cox 2 inhibitors such as Refocoxib are now available. They have reduced gastric toxicity and therefore should be considered in patients with bone pain who have previously been unable to tolerate alternative NSAIDs.

Opioids for Mild to Moderate Pain

These are Step 2 Analgesics in the WHO (1996) ladder and may also be known as weak opioids. Often analgesics in this group are combination drugs combining weak opioids with non-opioids. For example, two of the most common drugs prescribed are:

Co-dydramol = dihydrocodeine 10 mg + paracetamol 500 mg
Co-proxamol = dextropropoxyphene hydrochloride 32.5mg + paracetamol
    500 mg

Codeine phosphate, dihydrocodeine and tramadol are also prescribed at this level. Tramadol has a role as an opioid in the upper level of Step 2 and at the lower level of step three and may have some additional activity in neuro-pathic pain. Tramadol works within an hour of taking it and reaches peak plasma concentration within two hours. It is thought to be less constipating than codeine or morphine but has the potential to lower the seizure threshold, especially in patients taking tricyclic antidepressants, and therefore should be used with caution.

If pain is not controlled when opioids at this level are being given regularly and at maximum dosage the next step should be upwards not sideways.

Opioids for Moderate to Severe Pain

This group consists of Step 3 analgesics, which are often called strong opioids. Morphine is the drug recommended for use as a strong opioid in the management of moderate to severe cancer pain (European Association for Palliative Care, 1996).

Oral morphine

Before starting oral morphine it is important that several issues are discussed in depth with the patient. First, there are many misconceptions and fears surrounding the use of morphine, and these need to be explored prior to commencing the drug. For many patients morphine signifies 'the end', i.e. there is no further treatment and death is near. This is not the case. Morphine does not hasten death; it is often used while patients are still undergoing active treatment and generally is given to control pain and thus improve quality of life.

Morphine will not cause patients to become addicts, nor if given correctly will it turn them into 'zombies' or stop them breathing, but these are very real fears for patients and time needs to be spent talking these through.

Second, anticipated side effects should be talked through. Side effects such as nausea and sleepiness can cause a patient to stop taking morphine in the belief that they are allergic to it. Yet if they had persisted for 24–48 hours the side effects may have worn off and effective pain relief been achieved.

Nurses need to educate themselves about the use of strong opioids. Unfortunately, studies have shown that some of the misconceptions and fears held by the patients are also held by some health professionals. Amongst nurses, lack of knowledge, personal beliefs and attitudes towards opiate use, fear of patient addiction and respiratory depression all contribute to ineffective pain management (McCaffrey et al., 1990; Clark et al., 1996; Warden et al., 1998).

Dosage

For patients who have never taken opiates before, or who have been on weak opioids, it is recommended that a starting dose of 5–10 mg immediate-release morphine either in liquid or tablet form be taken four times a day.

If changing to oral morphine from an alternative strong opiate this dose may need to be increased. Additional doses of morphine should be available in between regular doses to allow for breakthrough pain. The dose of morphine should be reassessed every 24 hours and titrated as necessary according to the pain. There is no ceiling dose on morphine and in some cases patients may need 1000 mg or more daily to control pain.

Ultimately, when a morphine dose is reached that provides pain relief, the aim will be to convert patients onto sustained-release preparations that only need to be taken once or twice daily. An immediate-release medication should always be available in case of breakthrough pain.

Diamorphine

Diamorphine is three times more potent than morphine. It is used in palliative care in injection form because large amounts can be given in small quantities. It is most frequently used in advanced cancer when a syringe driver is set up because a patient is unconscious, unable to swallow or when a patient cannot take oral medication due to uncontrolled vomiting.

Alternative Opioids for Moderate to Severe Pain

Transdermal fentanyl has proved increasingly useful in patients who are unable or reluctant to swallow tablets. It is also thought that fentanyl may be less constipating, nauseating and sedating than morphine.

Fentanyl comes in the form of a patch, of which there are four strengths. The patch should be changed every 72 hours and the site of application should be rotated. Appropriate doses of immediate-release morphine should be given for breakthrough pain, especially in the 24 hours following initial application of the patch. If a patient is changing from sustained-release morphine the patch should be applied at the same time as the last tablet is taken, because it will take at least 12 hours to take effect.

Hydromorphone is relatively new in this country but is becoming more widely used in controlling cancer pain. It comes in the form of controlled-release and immediate-release capsules and 1 mg hydromorphone is equivalent to 7.5 mg of morphine. The side effects of hydromorphone are similar to those of morphine but recent studies have shown it to be less sedating in some patients unable to tolerate morphine. It is a useful alternative in patients whose fears about morphine cannot be alleviated.

Other well-known opioids that have a role to play in controlling cancer pain are methadone and oxycodone.

Adjuvant Analgesia

As discussed previously, adjuvants are a diverse groups of drugs whose primary role is not as an analgesic. However, in particular in cases of neuropathic pain, which is rarely sensitive to opioids, they have a successful analgesic effect.

Tricyclic antidepressants are often used to treat the burning, tingling sensations associated with neuropathic pain. Commonly used antidepressants are:

- amitriptyline 10–25 mg nocte;
- lophepramine 70–210 mg nocte.

The role of newer antidepressants (selective serotonin reuptake inhibitors) is still controversial, although work is being carried out to prove their effectiveness (Allen and Taylor, 1999).

Anticonvulsants are again useful in treating neuropathic pain and are particularly useful when pain is shooting or stabbing. Commonly used drugs are:

- carbamazapine – doses vary up to 200 mg four times a day; max 1200 mg/24 hours;
- gabapentin – doses vary up to 900 mg three times a day; max 3600 mg/24 hours;
- sodium valproate 100–200 mg twice a day.

Doses can be titrated up depending on need and whether the patient can tolerate the medication.

Anti-arrhythmics, such as flecainide 50–100 mg or mexiletine 50 mg, may be taken twice a day in neuropathy that does not respond to the above therapies. This group of drugs should only be used under close supervision.

Steroids, especially when given in high doses (dexamethasone 8–16 mg), have an anti-inflammatory analgesic property. They work by reducing swelling and relieving pressure caused by the growth of tumours. They are particularly useful to treat symptomatic cerebral metastases, liver capsule pain and spinal cord/nerve compression. Toxicity from prolonged use should be avoided if possible and alternative analgesics should be considered.

Bisphosphonates were initially used to treat hypercalcaemia in malignant hypercalcaemia. However, they are now being used as the key agents in the analgesic management of pain due to bone secondaries. There is also now evidence that bisphosphonates reduce skeletal complications such as pathological fractures in breast cancer when given to women with known metastatic bone disease (Lipton, 1997).

Bisphosphonates such as pamidronate 90 mg are usually given by intravenous infusion on an intermittent basis. Oral preparations may be given but are poorly absorbed.

Alternative Pain Management in Advanced Breast Disease

Radiotherapy

A short course of palliative radiotherapy is often effective in relieving pain in both primary and metastatic cancer. Often only one fraction of radiotherapy is required to achieve adequate pain relief. Although some patients may experience some pain relief within days, the maximum benefit will usually be seen 2–3 weeks after treatment. Because of this delayed effect adequate alternative analgesia will need to be used initially. Radiotherapy is particularly effective in treating pain caused by bone metastases and gives partial or full pain relief in 80% of patients (Smith, 2001).

Radiotherapy may also be useful in treating pain due to fungating breast tumours, solid growths on the surface of the body and pain due to metastatic liver enlargement that is unresponsive to other medications.

Chemotherapy

Chemotherapy is worth mentioning in regard to pain control as some breast cancers are chemotherapy sensitive. Chemotherapy when given to women with metastatic disease is very often palliative in intent, the hope being that it will reduce tumour size. Therefore pain such as liver capsule pain may reduce as the liver metastases reduce in size. It is always important, however, to weigh up the benefits against the risks and side effects, and to allow patients to make an informed decision about treatment.

Hormone Therapy

Hormone therapy is widely used in the treatment and control of breast cancer and as such has the potential to reduce tumour size in metastatic disease. Reduction in tumour size can lead to effective pain relief and thus hormone manipulation is worth considering as a valid treatment for pain when used in conjunction with analgesic medication.

Anaesthetic Procedures

Nerve blocks

Some difficult cases of cancer pain can be controlled by blocking the nerve pathways along which pain stimuli travel to the central nervous system. Nerve blocks can be short term (using injection of local anaesthetic) or more long term, lasting for several weeks (using chemical injection, e.g. phenol) They should be carried out under specialist supervision and only after a full explanation has been given to the patient.

Spinal analgesia

This is becoming more widely used and can be given either epidurally or intrathecally. These methods are particularly effective in controlling chest wall pain or pain radiating through the lower half of the body. Not all patients will be suitable for this type of analgesia and those that do partake will have to be fully informed and have a close support network.

Physical Therapies in Pain Control

Many women with advanced breast disease will benefit from the use of non-pharmacological approaches to pain control. They are increasingly popular and are used well alongside drug therapy. Nurses need to be aware of these treatments and should be able to offer help and advice to patients.

Superficial heat or cold

The application of heat or cold to an area affected by localized pain can help bring relief.

Heat is particularly effective in pain caused by joint stiffness, muscle spasms or pain relieved by a hot shower or bath. It acts by stimulating nerve fibres, increasing blood supply to the tissues and generally relaxing the patient. Heat pads are available for use in some hospitals and wheat bags can be advocated as a safe alternative for patients to use at home. Care must always be taken to ensure the patient is protected from being burned and heat should not be applied to areas following radiotherapy or to areas where bleeding is likely to occur. Warmth is a great comforter and when used effectively can produce significant pain relief.

The application of cold may often relieve burning pain or muscle spasm. Cold can be applied with ice packs or even with a bag of frozen peas. The cold packs should be wrapped in a soft cloth/towel to protect the patient from skin irritation. Cold packs should not be applied for longer than 15 minutes. Although cold has a more prolonged analgesic effect, many patients find it less comforting than heat and therefore it tends to be used less.

Transcutaneous electrical nerve stimulation (TENS)

TENS works by stimulating large-diameter nerves in the skin and subcutaneous tissues, using small electrodes that are placed on the body surface and connected to a compact battery-operated generator. It is thought to work because these nerve fibres relay the stimuli along the spinal cord, activating an agent called enkephalin, which in turn inhibits painful stimuli being transmitted from the same area at a slower rate along smaller nerve fibres.

TENS can be useful in patients with moderate cancer pain, especially if pain is in the head and neck region, if it is due to nerve compression or if it is bone pain due to metastases.

TENS does not work in every patient. Its success relies on the correct positioning of the electrodes and on accurate adjustment of the electrical output, which will both differ from person to person (Sykes et al., 1997).

TENS has virtually no side effects and if used correctly can give patients a sense of control over their pain. It should not be used in patients with pacemakers or on broken/irritated skin.

Massage

Massage is a treatment that can be used by carers, nurses and trained therapists to provide patients with advanced cancer pleasurable relief from both physical and mental tensions, which can thus decrease pain.

The physical act of massage can relax muscles and increase skin circulation, while the gentle touch can prove to be of great comfort to patients. The intimacy of massage can often lead to a patient opening up and sharing her/his anxieties and fears.

Patients with advanced cancer usually only tolerate gentle massage, and often only to one area of their body. Care should be taken if a patient is known to have clotting disorders or a history of deep vein thrombosis.

The therapies described in this chapter are just a few of those that may prove beneficial in the treatment of pain. More information on additional complementary therapies can be found in Chapter 14.

Nausea and Vomiting

Nausea and vomiting occurs in approximately 60% of patients with advanced cancer at some point in their illness. It is particularly prevalent in women with breast cancer (Waller and Caroline, 2000). Knowledge and understanding about the cause of the symptom can lead to effective management.

The physiological process involved in nausea and vomiting is complex and the causes are multiple. There are two main areas within the brain involved in the process: the chemoreceptor trigger zone (CTZ), which is able to detect blood-borne chemicals, and the integrated vomiting centre (IVC) situated in the lateral medulla, which coordinates incoming impulses and results in the actual vomiting process. Impulses to the IVC can come from higher centres such as memories, sights and smells experienced when in a conscious state and from the balance organs of the inner ear.

The chemoreceptor trigger zone is activated when toxins within the circulatory system or cerebrospinal fluid stimulate receptor cells, which send messages to the IVC. There are also chemoreceptors situated throughout the gut, in the liver and the brain. All are activated by toxins, which cause stimuli to be transmitted via the vagus nerve to the IVC.

Common causes of nausea and vomiting are:

- chemotherapy;
- radiotherapy, especially to brain or GI tract;

- medication – opiates, antibiotics, steroids, NSAIDs, oestrogens, iron;
- electrolyte imbalance;
- uraemia;
- hypercalcaemia;
- gastric hypomotility/stasis;
- constipation;
- brain metastases;
- hepatomegaly;
- pain;
- anxiety/anticipation.

When treating nausea and sickness it is important first of all to identify all possible causes and then correct any that may be reversible. Therefore if sickness is being caused by constipation a laxative should be given; if it is a sign of hypercalcaemia, intravenous bisphosphonates should be used.

Anti-emetics are commonly used to treat nausea and sickness in women with advanced breast cancer. Drugs will usually be given orally and should be taken regularly to achieve the best results. If a patient is vomiting excessively and therefore unable to tolerate oral medications, anti-emetics can be given rectally, intramuscularly or subcutaneously. Often a subcutaneous infusion via a syringe driver is the most effective means of control in prolonged vomiting.

Different anti-emetics work at different points in the vomiting mechanism. It is therefore important that the prescription of anti-emetics is tailored to the potential causes. Often a combination of anti-emetics is required.

Cyclizine 50 mg is a good drug of choice when there are no obvious reasons for vomiting. It works on the histamine transmitters in the IVC and is better at controlling vomiting than it is at nausea.

For vomiting induced by opiates such as morphine, haloperidol 1.5–3 mg, a dopamine anatagonist, can prove very effective and should possibly be prescribed prophylactically when starting patients on morphine.

Metaclopramide 10 mg and domperidone 10–20 mg act on the gut wall. They are useful in the treatment of gastric stasis and in vomiting induced by chemotherapy/radiotherapy.

Explanation and reassurance when a patient is nauseated or vomiting is crucial. Nurses are often the professionals best placed to provide advice and reassurance. Many patients will find mealtimes traumatic if they are feeling nauseated or have recent experience of vomiting. Advice about eating small snacks or portions of food on a more frequent basis should be given to patients and their carers. Often carers may find this difficult to understand as the temptation is to try and 'feed their loved one up'. They may see it as the patient giving up. Carers need time to explore these issues with the nurse's help and may need to be re-educated as to the revised needs of their loved ones. Tastes may change and whereas once patients may have loved hot spicy food, the smell of curry may now make them vomit.

The comfort and dignity of the patient should always be at the forefront of any nursing intervention. Providing quick effective relief of nausea/sickness should be coupled with ensuring patients' privacy, maintaining their hygiene needs and providing a supportive controlled environment.

Weakness and Fatigue

The problem of weakness is probably one of the most commonly reported symptoms in patients with advanced cancer. It is also one of the most difficult to treat. Studies show that up to 82% of patients may experience this symptom (Donnelly and Walsh, 1995).

Weakness is a term difficult to define and many patients will use it synonymously with terms such as fatigue, exhaustion, lethargy and tiredness. Weakness and fatigue are often multifaceted and when complained of should be thoroughly investigated. Anaemia, steroids, biochemical abnormalities, anorexia and cachexia all contribute to the symptom of weakness. Problems such as anaemia and hypercalcaemia can be corrected but for many patients complaining of weakness and fatigue in advanced cancer there is no correctable cause.

The management of weakness and fatigue in most cancer patients is centred on the development of coping mechanisms. Nurses are often looked to for advice on these matters and they should be able to talk on the subject of conserving energy through periods of rest and activity. They should also consider, with the patient's permission, referral to other members of the multidisciplinary team such as the occupational therapist, physiotherapist and care managers, all of whom can offer services that will help maintain a patient's quality of life.

Shortness of Breath (Dyspnoea)

Breathlessness is greatly feared by many patients and is often one of the most distressing and debilitating symptoms experienced. Being unable to breathe will provoke anxiety and fear in both the patient and the family or carers.

The onset of dyspnoea should be carefully investigated. An accurate in-depth history should be taken, if not from the patient then from a carer or family member. The assessment should look at the initial onset, previous attacks, presence of cough, pleuritic pain, sputum colour/amounts, and whether the dyspnoea occurs at rest or on exertion.

Possible causes of dyspnoea in patients with advanced cancer are:

- lung metastases;
- pleural effusion;
- lymphangitis;
- chemotherapy-induced damage;
- radiation pneumonitis;
- obstruction of bronchus by tumour;
- chest infection;
- heart failure;
- pulmonary embolism;
- anaemia.

There are various measures that are simple but will contribute to the effective management of breathlessness. Allowing the patient to assume a comfortable position is extremely important. Most breathless patients do not want to lie in bed but prefer to be sitting semi-recumbent, upright, or sometimes leaning forward supporting themselves on a table. Reassurance should be given at all times and the nurse should act with confidence, giving regular explanation to the patient. Some nurses are trained in basic relaxation techniques and these can be beneficial in preventing a patient from panicking. The patient's room should be well ventilated, either by opening a window or by using an electric fan. In some cases patients may find the use of oxygen helpful but there is little proven benefit to this and in most cases it helps because that is what the patient perceives it will do.

Other interventions for breathlessness include the treatment of reversible causes such as the drainage of pleural effusions or the treatment of a chest infection. Various medications can be used to help control dyspnoea. Steroids can be used for their anti-inflammatory properties to treat lymphangitis or pneumonitis. Nebulizers and inhalers are sometimes worth trying as bronchodilators can be useful in the treatment of airway obstruction. One of the most useful drugs in the management of breathlessness is morphine. Morphine (5 mg starting dose) can reduce the respiratory drive and will ease the sensation of breathlessness in many patients (Boyd and Kelly, 1997). If a patient is very anxious and prone to panic a small dose of a sedative such as lorazepam (0.5–2 mg) given sublingually can help with respiratory symptoms.

Many patients have to adapt to living with dyspnoea for what time they have left. This is often very difficult, affecting both the patient and the family/carers. Psychological, medical and practical support should be offered to ensure that the patient can achieve the optimum quality of life possible.

Constipation

Constipation is a common problem for many patients with advanced cancer. It can be described as 'the evacuation of hard stools less frequently than is normal for the individual' (Twycross, 1997, p. 203) If allowed to go untreated, constipation can cause abdominal pain and swelling, retention of urine, incontinence and faecal overflow/diarrhoea (Fallon and Welsh, 1998).

Constipation can prove extremely uncomfortable for many patients and its effect on quality of life should not be underestimated. The main causes of constipation in patients with advanced cancer are as follows:

- poor fluid and dietary intake;
- low fibre intake;
- medication – especially opioids and also chemotherapy, diuretics, anti-convulsants;
- reduced mobility;
- weakness;
- immobility;
- environmental factors, e.g. poor toilet facilities, lack of privacy. (Maestri-Banks, 1998)

It is important to remember that constipation can also be a symptom of hypercalcaemia, which is a serious condition needing urgent treatment.

The management of constipation can be very much nurse led. On first meeting a patient, the nurse should be able to assess and identify certain factors that may lead to constipation. Simple advice to patients and their family/carers such as increasing fluid and food intake, adding bran to the diet and encouraging consumption of fruit juices may prove an easy solution to constipation. It is recognized, however, that the above measures may be difficult in a patient with far advanced cancer and in fact if the constipation is drug induced they may not actually work. In these cases laxative medication will be needed.

Laxatives are divided into several groups, the most common being:

- Osmotic laxatives: These work by drawing fluid into the bowel lumen, thus softening stool. Lactulose is the most frequently used in this group but can cause abdominal cramps and flatulence. There is a need to ensure an increased fluid intake, which is often difficult if the patient is quite unwell.

- Bulk-forming agents: These work by increasing faecal mass, which increases peristalsis. Fybogel is most commonly used in this group. Again an increased fluid intake is required. The full effect can take days to work. Bran can be used as a natural alternative.
- Stimulant laxatives: These work by increasing intestinal motility. Codanthremer/codanthresate is the most commonly used and is often the drug of choice in opioid-induced constipation. Docusate sodium acts as both a stimulant and a softening agent. Senna is often used in combination with a softener such as lactulose. It can cause abdominal cramps and should not be used in patients with suspected bowel obstruction.
- Rectal measures: These include suppositories and enemas. Approximately a third of patients will need these despite oral laxatives. (Twycross, 1997)

The dose of laxative given should be titrated slowly depending on the patient's response to treatment. Regular assessment (looking at size, frequency and consistency) by a nurse should be carried out and it is often helpful to encourage the patient/carer to keep a stool chart, especially when the patient is at home. The overall aim of laxative therapy is not to achieve a daily bowel action but rather to achieve comfortable defecation (Maestri-Banks, 1998). It is important that the nurse convey this to the patient.

In the majority of patients, constipation can in time be controlled effectively. There are many nursing interventions that can ensure it is dealt with efficiently and sympathetically. Information giving and education of patients and their carers is primary in constipation management. Ensuring privacy and appropriate toilet facilities are available both in hospital and at home is also crucial to the patient's comfort (Maestri-Banks and Burns, 1996). It should never be underestimated how much discomfort and upset constipation can cause to a patient. Its successful management can lead to the patient achieving comfort and therefore a better quality of life.

Psychological and Emotional Impact of Metastatic Breast Cancer

There are many uncertainties faced by women with breast cancer. Living with the knowledge that the cancer may reoccur has a huge emotional impact on the woman and her partner, family and friends. When metastatic disease is confirmed the diagnosis is often more devastating that the original one and invokes all kinds of responses from the patient and those close to her.

Typical responses, as outlined by Haber (1997), are:

1. Personal responsibility: 'I did not do enough to stop the cancer, I have failed, why didn't I do something sooner?'
2. Loss of hope: Many see recurrence as a sign of imminent death, and may become withdrawn and be seen to give up. As previously discussed, prognosis in metastatic breast cancer can be relatively long depending on the extent of the recurrence.
3. Denial: This response is similar to that witnessed at initial diagnosis. Women may put off going to the hospital for routine checks, or may ignore new lumps developing. This type of response is associated with feelings of 'helplessness' (Levy et al., 1985 cited in Haber 1997). Denial is often a valid coping mechanism.
4. Grief: This response may be centred around disappointment that all the efforts made to foster health have not worked. This grief can be worked through and may be short lived if the woman can maintain the perspective that life is not over yet.

Patients with advanced breast cancer will have needs, just as their families and friends will (Rutherford and Foxley, 1991). There is a need to be understood on both a practical and personal level. Patients with breast cancer may want explanations, they may need information, and studies have shown that the better informed the patient the fewer cases of anxiety and depression there are (Fallowfield, 1991). Patients need to be able to make choices. They need, if they so choose, to hold on to some semblance of control in their lives and to feel that they have a role to play. Every patient will cope differently. Some will see the diagnosis as a challenge, using it to enhance their quality of life, and gain a deeper understanding of their life and relationships. Some people will develop a new sense of purpose to their life (Ireland, 1987, p. 28). Some, as we have already said, may see it as the end and despair. Each individual patient will have different emotional needs and therefore her psychological care should be tailored accordingly.

It is very important, especially when following the principles of palliative care, to recognize the emotional needs of the family. When a diagnosis of metastatic breast cancer is given it can have a profound and far-reaching effect on the patient's partner, family and friends. The relationship between the patient and those closest to her can often change. Communication can be hindered between a patient and her loved ones. There is often a sense of wanting to protect one another and this is especially true when looking at communication with children. Family members need to feel listened to. They need to be acknowledged as having emotions, as being involved. At a time when the majority of care centres around the patient, it is easy to forget that the family are equally anxious about what is happening and what the future might hold.

Specialist intervention is often helpful when dealing with problems such as isolation, withdrawal, depression, etc. Often patients and their families will have very specialist needs and this is being recognized by many cancer centres, which employ psychologists, counsellors and social workers as part of the multidisciplinary team. Interventions will be discussed further in Chapter 15.

The Nurse's Role

Nurses have a huge role to play in not only delivering physical care but also in providing emotional support for women with breast cancer. Nurses at all levels will come into contact with patients who have metastatic breast cancer, whether they work in a hospital, in the community or in a hospice. Although many nurses are adept at providing hands-on care, there is still much anxiety associated with providing emotional support for patients and their families. Many junior nurses state how unprepared they feel in their roles as comforters, supporters and bearers of 'bad news' to patients …who are dying of cancer and their families or carers (Costello, 1995).

The dying process, sexual issues, fears and anxieties are all subjects women with breast cancer may want to address and yet it is still often the case that these subjects are made light of, ignored or swiftly brushed aside. Nurses build up very close relationships with some patients and their families. They spend time with them performing often intimate procedures and it is therefore natural that a patient or family member will want to talk to that nurse. Allowing the patient and the family to express themselves is a very important support mechanism. Nurses are often worried about saying or doing the wrong thing but often it is enough for the patient just to be able to talk. A combination of good communication skills and knowledge about cancer is required by the nurse (Tait, 1996). These are skills that will continually develop as the nurse becomes more experienced and more confident.

Nurses need to know where to find support not only for patients and their families but also for themselves. 'If patients and their families are to be helped to cope with the traumas of a life threatening illness in conjunction with unpleasant treatments and uncertain outcomes, support and supervision for nurses must be provided' (Craven, 2000).

Role of the Palliative Care Team

Palliative care has continued to evolve on many levels. It is now feasible that patients, families and staff can access palliative care teams both in hospital and when at home in the community.

The aims of palliative care teams are:

- to concentrate on quality of life;
- to provide effective symptom control;
- to provide psychological and spiritual care;
- to offer a source of support and understanding to the family, friends and carers involved with the patient both before and after death;
- to provide a high-quality, seamless service to patients, family, friends and carers;
- to provide support and education to other health professionals working with patients with palliative care needs;
- to give patients if at all possible a choice in where they want to die.

Palliative care teams vary in size but are usually multidisciplinary. They may consist of consultants, specialist registrars, clinical nurse specialists, occupational therapists, physiotherapists, social workers, counsellors, dietitians and psychologists.

It can be argued that palliative care has a role to play right at the start of a cancer patient's journey. The truth is, however, that patients are often not referred to palliative care teams until the latter stages of their illness.

Hearn and Higginson (1998) carried out some research within the area of specialist palliative care services and concluded that conventional care on its own is not enough for patients with advanced cancer and that a multi-professional approach in hospitals, hospices and the community is most beneficial to patients and their families.

Palliative care teams are happy to discuss referrals at any stage in a patient's illness. Patients do not have to have pain or be in their last few days of life before they can be referred. The team will carry out a thorough holistic assessment of the patient referred and will then offer continued advice and support to enable the patient and family to maintain the optimum quality of life wherever they are. Palliative care teams do not take over from oncologists, GPs, etc., but rather provide a complementary service.

Liaison and communication are key skills within a palliative team whether they are hospital or community based. Palliative care teams should be used as a source of information and support for staff at all levels dealing with patients with cancer.

The role of the palliative care team as discussed is complex and will vary from hospital team to team. However, the overall principles remain the same with each team striving to provide the highest quality care to ensure patients with advanced cancer receive supportive care throughout their cancer journey.

Conclusion

The care and treatment of women with advanced breast cancer has evolved greatly over the past few years. Although there is still no cure for metastatic breast cancer, women are now able to live longer thanks to new treatments.

Caring for patients with advanced breast cancer tests every aspect of holistic nursing care. Nurses are skilled professionals who can provide high-quality care, comfort and support to women with breast cancer and their families as long as they themselves are well supported and given appropriate education.

Patient care should always come first in the treatment of advanced breast cancer.

Multidisciplinary teamwork will enable realistic, patient-centred goals to be achieved.

References

Allen M, Taylor R (1999) Pain control in palliative care. Pharmaceutical Journal 262(7043): 620-4.

Boyd K, Kelly M (1997) Oral morphine in symptomatic treatment of dyspnoea in patients with advanced cancer. Palliative Medicine 11: 277-81.

Clark E B, French B, Bilodeau M L, Capasso V C, Edward A, Empoliti J (1996) Pain management: knowledge, attitudes and clinical practice. Journal of Pain Symptom Management. 11: 18-31 .

Corcoran R (1991) The management of pain. In: Penson J, Fisher R (eds) Palliative Care for People with Cancer. London: Edward Arnold.

Costello J (1995) Helping relatives cope with the grieving process. Professional Nurse 11(2): 89-94. In: Boyle M, Carter E (1998) Death Anxiety amongst Nurses. International Journal of Palliative Nursing 4(1): 37-42.

Craven O (2000) Palliative care provision and its impact on morbidity in cancer patients. International Journal of Palliative Nursing 6(10).

Dixon M, Sainsbury R (1993) Diseases of the Breast. London: Churchill Livingstone.

Donnelly S, Walsh D (1995) The symptoms of advanced cancer. Seminars in Oncology 22: 67-72.

European Association for Palliative Care (Expert Working Group) (1996) Morphine in cancer pain: modes of administration. British Medical Journal 12: 823-6.

Fallon M, Welsh J (1998) The management of gastrointestinal symptoms. In: Faull C, Carter Y, Woof R (eds) Handbook of Palliative Care. Oxford: Blackwell Science.

Fallowfield L (1991) Breast Cancer. London: Routledge.

Fleisch H (1995) Bisphosphanates in Bone Disease, 3rd edn. New York: Parthenon Publishing Group.

Grady KM, Severn AM (1999) Key Topics in Chronic Pain. Oxford: Bios Scientific Publishers.

Grond S, Zech D, Diefenbach C, Bischoff A (1994) Prevalence and pattern of symptoms in patients with cancer pain: a prospective evaluation of 1635 patients referred to a pain clinic. Journal of Pain Symptom Management 9: 372-82.

Haber S (ed) (1997) Breast Cancer. A Psychological Treatment Manual. London: Free Association Books.

Hayes D, Kaplan W (1991) Evaluation of patients following primary therapy. In: Harris JR, Hellman S, Henderson IC, Kinne DW (eds) Breast Diseases, 2nd edn. Philadelphia, PA: Lippincott-Raven.

Hearn J, Higginson I (1998) Do specialist palliative care teams improve outcomes for cancer patients? A systematic literature review. Palliative Medicine 12: 317-32.

Heatley S, Coleman R (1999) The use of bisphosphonates in the palliative care setting. International Journal of Palliative Nursing 5(2): 74-80.

Hoskin P, Makin W (1998) Oncology for Palliative Medicine. Oxford: Oxford University Press.

Ireland J (1987) Life Wish. London: Century. In: Denton S (ed) (1996) Breast Cancer Nursing. London: Chapman & Hall.

Leonard RCF, Rodger A, Dixon JM (2000) Metastatic breast cancer. In: Dixon M (ed) ABC of Breast Diseases, 2nd edn. London: BMJ Books.

Levy S, Herberman R, Maluish A, Schlien B, Lippman M (1985) Prognostic risk assessment in primary breast cancer by behavioural and immunological parameters. Health Psychology 4: 99-113. In: Haber S, ed (1997) Breast Cancer. A Psychological Treatment Manual. London: Free Association Books.

Lipton A (1997) Bisphosphonates and breast cancer. Cancer 80(Suppl. 8): 1668-73.

Maestri-Banks A (1998) An overview of constipation: causes and symptoms. International Journal of Palliative Nursing 4(6): 271-3.

Maestri-Banks A, Burns D (1996) Assessing constipation. Nursing Times 92(21): 28-31.

McCaffrey M, Ferrel B, O'Neil-Page E, Lester M (1990) Nurses' knowledge of opioid analgesic drugs and psychological dependence. Cancer Nursing 13: 21-7.

McEvilly JM, Dow KH (1998) Treating metastatic breast cancer: principles and current practice. American Journal of Nursing 98(Suppl. 4): 26-9.

McGinn K, Moore J (2001) Metastatic breast cancer: understanding current management options. Oncology Nursing Forum 28(3): 507-12.

Overmoyer BA (1995) Chemotheraputic palliative approaches in the treatment of breast cancer. Seminars in Oncology 22(Suppl. 3): 2-9.

Powles TJ (1997) Efficacy of tamoxifen as treatment of breast cancer. Seminars in Oncology 24(Suppl.1): S1-48, S1-52.

In: McGinn K, Moore J (2001) Metastatic breast cancer: understanding current management options. Oncology Nursing Forum 28(3): 507-12.

Rees G, Coleman RE, Brennan JH, Mansel RE, O'Neill WM, Radstone DJ (1994) Supportive care in breast cancer. Journal of Cancer 3: 188-96.

Rutherford M, Foxley D (1991) Awareness of psychological need. In: Penson J, Fisher R (eds) Palliative Care for People with Cancer. London: Edward Arnold.

Saunders C (1996) A personal therapeutic journey. British Medical Journal 313: 274-5.

Smith J (2001) Recurrent breast cancer. In: Burnet K (ed) Holistic Breast Care. London: Baillière Tindall/RCN.

Smith IE, de Boer RH (2000) Role of systemic treatment for primary operable breast cancer. In Dixon M (ed) ABC of Breast Diseases, 2nd edn. London: BMJ Books, Ch. 10.

Souhami R, Tobias J (1995) Cancer and its Management. Oxford: Blackwell Scientific.

Sykes J, Johnson R, Hanks G W (1997) Difficult pain problems. British Medical Journal 315(4 October): 867-9.

Tait A (1996) Psychological aspects of breast care. In: Denton S (ed) Breast Cancer
     Nursing. London: Chapman & Hall.

Twycross R (1997) Symptom Management in Advanced Cancer, 2nd edn. Oxford:
     Radcliffe Medical Press.

Vogel C (1991) Treatment of metastatic breast cancer. Seminars in Oncology Nursing 7:
     194-9.

Waller A, Caroline NL (2000) Handbook of Palliative Care in Cancer, 2nd edn.
     Boston/Oxford: Butterworth-Heinemann.

Warden S, Carpenter JS, Brockopp Y (1998) Nurses' beliefs about suffering and their
     management of pain. International Journal of Palliative Nursing 4(1): 21-5.

World Health Organisation (1990) Cancer Pain Relief and Palliative Care, report of WHO
     Expert Committee, Vol. 804 WHO Technical Report Series. Geneva: WHO: 1-75.

World Health Organisation (1996) Cancer Pain Relief. Geneva: WHO.

Chapter 14
Complementary and alternative therapies

Rosemary Lucey

Introduction

As healthcare professionals we are asked for advice by patients and relatives about a wide variety of complementary and alternative therapies. Some 30% of women with breast cancer visit a complementary therapist after diagnosis (Rees et al., 1999), and 20% of the population of the UK use complementary therapy over the course of a year, spending an average of £14 per month (BBC, 2000). Retail sales of complementary medicine in 1998 totalled £93 million, made up of £50 million from herbal medicine, £23 million from homeopathic medicines and £20 million from aromatherapy essential oils. Sales are rising rapidly and are expected to reach £126 million by the end of 2002.

Nurses have a duty to be aware of the different types of therapies, to be knowledgeable about safety issues and to feel confident about discussing the subject with their patients. Nurses may practise complementary therapies if they have undergone the appropriate training and the therapies are within their competence.

This chapter considers the following issues:

What is complementary and alternative medicine (CAM)?
What is the difference between complementary and alternative therapies?
Regulation and standards for CAM.
The evidence base and research.
How to choose a therapist.
Where to get more information.
Descriptions of therapies commonly used by women with breast cancer.
Brief descriptions of other complementary therapies.
Supplements/herbs, etc., sometimes used by women with breast cancer.

Complementary therapies and menopausal symptoms.
Diet and dietary advice.
Further reading.

Nurses cannot be expected to know everything about complementary
therapies but it is hoped that after reading this chapter they will be able to
ask appropriate questions and give safe, evidence-based advice.

What is Complementary and Alternative Medicine (CAM)?

The term covers a wide range of health-related therapies that are not part of
orthodox medical care. Therapies may have statutory regulations
(osteopathy and chiropractice), a voluntary code (acupuncture, homeopathy,
aromatherapy, etc.) or nothing in place. Doctors, nurses and dentists, etc.,
who practise CAM are also subject to their own professional code. Some
complementary therapies are available on the NHS. A therapy may be
available at a hospital alongside conventional therapies, at a GP's surgery, at a
private health centre, sports club, at an individual therapist's house or in the
patient's own home.

There is no one definition of CAM. The Cochrane Collaboration defines
CAM as 'a broad domain of healing resources that encompasses all health
systems, modalities, and practices and their accompanying theories and
beliefs, other than those intrinsic to the politically dominant health systems
of a particular society or culture in a given historical period'. Edzard Ernst, a
professor of CAM at Exeter University, defines it as follows: 'Complementary
medicine is diagnosis, treatment and/or prevention which complements
mainstream medicine by contributing to a common whole, by satisfying a
demand not met by orthodoxy or by diversifying the conceptual frameworks
of medicine' (Ernst et al., 1995). The British Medical Association (BMA)
described 'non-conventional therapies' and defined them in 1993 as 'those
forms of treatment that are not widely used by the conventional healthcare
professions, and the skills of which are not taught as part of the under-
graduate curriculum of conventional medical and paramedical healthcare
courses' (British Medical Association, 1993).

It is interesting to note that some countries run a dual system of medicine,
e.g. Ayurvedic in India and traditional Chinese medicine in China, both
alongside western medicine. Definitions and explanations are as in the UK.

What is the Difference Between Complementary and Alternative
Therapies?

There is a very important distinction to be made between 'complementary'
and 'alternative' therapies in the way they are used. Complementary

therapies are used alongside conventional medical treatment to help relieve symptoms, increase general well-being and ease side effects from treatment. Alternative therapies are used in place of conventional treatment, often in the hope of a cure. Some therapies can be either complementary or alternative depending on how they are used.

Regulation and Standards for CAM

The status of most complementary therapies will change in the next few years as a result of work currently being undertaken at government level. The recent report of the Science and Technology Committee of the UK House of Lords deliberated the future for regulation and standards. (Osteopathy and chiropractic are the only two complementary therapies currently regulated by Act of Parliament.) The report divides the therapies into three levels, depending on evidence and organization:

Group one: acupuncture, chiropractic, herbal medicine, homeopathy and osteopathy. These are the 'big five' and incorporate diagnosis and treatment within an organized profession. The likelihood is that the other three will join chiropractic and osteopathy in statutory regulation in the next few years.

Group two: these do not have a diagnostic feature, being those practices that complement conventional medicine such as aromatherapy, Alexander technique, counselling, healing, hypnotherapy, massage, meditation and relaxation, reflexology and shiatsu.

Group three:
   (a) therapies that may be long established and traditional with a philosophical approach such as Ayurvedic medicine, Chinese herbal medicine, traditional Chinese medicine and naturopathy;
   (b) therapies that 'lack any credible evidence' (HMSO, 2000) and include crystal therapy, cranio-sacral therapy, dowsing, iridology, kinesiology and radionics.

There is evidence to suggest that therapies in groups one and two are valuable forms of treatment and many have been subjected to scientific study including randomized controlled trials. There is also recognized training and standards, although not necessarily legally enforceable. It is likely that given time this will change. Although the therapies in Group three (a) are traditional and often linked to philosophies or religion, it can be difficult to find an established evidence base by western standards, other than by accumulative observation. This does not mean that they are not effective but rather that they have not been subjected to rigorous scientific research, so cannot be actively recommended.

Nurses should be wary of recommending any of the therapies in Group three (b) for their therapeutic value. It is difficult to find any scientific evidence concerning their efficacy at present.

The Evidence Base and Research

Just because the evidence base for complementary therapies is small does not make them invalid as treatments. Resources are difficult to establish to fund research in an area where there is not a strong track record of research. Methodology is an important subject of debate as conventional research methods may not be suitable to measure the efficacy of CAM owing to the holistic approach. This can make it more difficult to run a randomized controlled trial as standardization of therapy could greatly reduce the effectiveness of that complementary therapy. Different research may require different methodologies with a more flexible design and alternative outcome measures. Research must embrace the holistic and individual approach while remaining scientifically robust.

Although most traditional medical research uses objective measurements, subjective outcome measurements are widely used in many clinical trials, e.g. quality of life, severity of symptoms and structured interviews. The UK Government is to encourage research into complementary therapies in the next few years.

How to Choose a Therapist

Professional organizations exist to protect the public and set standards of education and practice. However, without statutory regulation there is no protection of title (as with the title 'nurse') so in theory anyone can currently call him/herself a therapist as there is no legal registration except for the two mentioned above. Professional organizations will tell you if a therapist is known to them – it is wise to check membership and qualifications. It is also important to consider the following issues before recommending a therapist to anyone:

- What training has she/he undertaken and what qualifications does she/he hold?
- Is she/he a member of an organization that has a code of practice and ethics?
- Does he/she have current insurance?
- What claims does the therapist make for the therapy? (Nurses should not be actively recommending alternative therapies but should be able to support their patients if they decide to go down this route.)
- Could this therapy interact with any conventional treatment the patient is having?

- Does the therapist have experience of treating patients with breast cancer?

Other factors the patient may consider are:

- In what type of premises does the therapist work (e.g. hospital, health centre, private home)?
- Does the therapist make the patient feel comfortable and at ease?
- What is the cost?
- Can this therapy be provided on the NHS?
- Will the therapy involve buying books, videos, supplements, etc.?
- How many sessions are likely to be needed?

If it sounds too good to be true then it probably is!

Where to get More Information

Institute for Complementary Medicine
PO Box 194
London SE16 1QZ, UK
Tel: 020 7237 5165; http://www.icmedicine.co.uk

Professional bodies for each therapy:

The Foundation for Integrated Health
12 Chillingworth Road
London N7 8QJ, UK
Tel: 020 7619 6140; http://www/fimed.org

Research Council for Complementary Medicine
27a Devonshire Street
London W1N 1RJ, UK
http://www.rccm.org.uk (holds the most extensive collection of CAM research references in the UK)

The UK Cochrane Centre has a limited number of reviews.

Magazines such as *Health Which?*

Department of Health information pack on CAM produced for PCGs (2000)

The Internet. The information quality is so variable and vast that it is important only to use good quality sites such as those belonging to cancer information providers; for example:

www.cancerhelp.org.uk
www.macmillan.org.uk
www.cancerbacup.org.uk
www.bristolcancerhelp.org

Both NHS Direct and the National Electronic Health Library plan to have information about CAM available in the near future.

Directories (see under 'Further Reading' at the end of this chapter).
(Owing to the constantly changing organization of CAM in the UK it may be easier to obtain the most up-to-date information from websites.)

Acupuncture

Yes, this is about needles but not as we know them: the 'needles' used are very fine and mostly only inserted subcutaneously. Acupuncture is thought to be at least 2000 years old, originating in China. It was brought to Europe in the nineteenth century. Its modern revival in the West can be traced back to the 1930s when a French diplomat, Soulie de Morant, published a book describing the techniques used in China. There was a further revival of interest when President Nixon visited China in 1972 and saw acupuncture being used as an anaesthetic in surgery and the subsequent public interest in Chinese culture.

There are many types of acupuncture, of which two are most widely available in the UK: one is part of traditional Chinese medicine wherein a practitioner would often also use herbs, acupressure, diet, moxibustion, etc.; the other is medical acupuncture (or western acupuncture) and is practised by medical doctors who have undergone supplementary training in acupuncture. Medical acupuncturists use fewer points (20-30, compared with a traditional acupuncturist who has access to over 300) and tend to use it more for a symptom control, e.g. pain and nausea management, or as an aid to smoking cessation, etc.

A Which? survey conducted in 1995 found that 80% of respondents who had undergone acupuncture in the last 12 months were satisfied with the treatment that they had received. It is the fourth most popular therapy after osteopathy, chiropractic and homeopathy.

Acupuncturists believe that the body has Qi (or Chi), which flows along meridians. Chi is made up of Yin and Yang, which should balance for good health. At times of illness, Yin and Yang are not in balance. Acupuncture needles are inserted at specific points along the meridians in order to restore the balance between Yin and Yang.

For what Conditions is it Useful for Patients with Breast Cancer?

It can be used for just about everything from a symptom point of view and to promote energy levels and general well-being. Acupuncture is used for such things as to alleviate pain (e.g. bone or breast pain); to lessen side effects such as nausea and vomiting with chemotherapy treatment; to reduce or alleviate menopausal symptoms, e.g. for patients on tamoxifen or experiencing depression, headaches and much more.

What is the Experience Like for the Patient/What are the Practicalities?

At the first appointment a full history is taken. Careful note is made of the appearance of the tongue for diagnostic purposes and pulses are taken. Some therapists will perform an abdominal examination. Other questions may involve asking about reaction to temperature, bowel function, emotion, etc. Depending on which points are to be used, the patient may undress. Points can be anywhere on the body according to the condition being treated.

The sensation from the needles is often described as tingling or a dull ache. Needles can be stimulated by heat or electricity. Needle depth is usually less than a centimetre. (In the nail area it would only be a millimetre and in the buttocks it could be deeper.) Needles may be left for an average of up to 20 minutes. (Note: A traditional Chinese acupuncturist may use other therapies in conjunction with acupuncture.)

Sensations vary from no sensation at all, to discomfort and occasionally pain. Sometimes a condition may become worse before it improves. Usually several sessions are needed, the acupuncturist being guided by how the patient feels. Patients describe a mixture of sensations following treatment such as drowsy, relaxed or being full of energy.

Contra-indications/Points to Note

Acupuncture is generally very safe with a qualified practitioner. Research published in 2001 showed that of 34 407 acupuncture treatments there were no serious adverse events (MacPherson et al., 2001). A meta-analysis in 1995 showed that there were only 216 cases of serious complications worldwide (including such things as pneumothorax and tissue damage), over 20 years (Rampes and James, 1995).

A qualified therapist will always use sterile, disposable needles. Care should be taken if patients have a low platelet count or other bleeding disorder. Electro-acupuncture is not recommended for patients with a pacemaker.

Qualifications and Regulations

British Acupuncture Council (BAcC)

The Council holds a register of members who follow a code of practice and ethics and have indemnity insurance. BAcC are aiming for state registration and have set up the British Acupuncture Accreditation Board to determine standards of training. Members must have three years' full-time training or equivalent, which includes western medical sciences, and will have MBAcC after their name.

British Medical Acupuncture Society (BMAS)

This is for members who are also doctors of medicine and is in addition to medical training. There are two levels of membership starting at basic competence gained over several weekends and presentation of case histories. Further training and case studies will gain a certificate of accreditation. Therapists will have BMAS after their name. Some 70% of doctors trained and registered with the British Medical Acupuncture Society are General Practitioners.

Evidence and Research

There is evidence that acupuncture is effective for treating chemotherapy-induced and post-operative nausea and vomiting (Vickers, 1996), as well as pain and menopausal symptoms. There is much anecdotal and observational evidence for many other conditions.

Further Reading

Birch SJ, Felt RL. Understanding Acupuncture. Edinburgh: Churchill Livingstone.
Hicks A. Thorsons Principles of Acupuncture. London: Thorsons.

Aromatherapy Massage

Aromatherapy is the use of essential plant oils for therapeutic purposes. Aromatherapy massage is body massage using essential oils. Different oils have different properties, e.g. relaxing, stimulating, etc. Usually oils are diluted with a base vegetable oil such as sunflower or sweet almond (undiluted they can damage the skin). A massage without essential oils can be enjoyable and beneficial but not as effective. Oils can be massaged and absorbed via the skin, inhaled, or used in a bath or a cold compress.

Aromatherapy was used by the Ancient Egyptians, Greeks and Romans. In the sixteenth, seventeenth and eighteenth centuries, essential oils and perfumes were in great demand in Europe by doctors and herbalists. The term 'aromatherapy' was first used in the 1930s by the French biochemist Gattefosse, who discovered the healing effects of lavender after burning his hand. A French army surgeon, Dr Valnet, used aromatherapy to treat wounds in the Second World War. In France aromatherapy is practised by medical doctors, who prescribe oils to be taken orally. Tisserand, a reputable manufacturer of oils, established training in Britain in the late 1960s.

The smelling of essential oils stimulates the limbic system, which is associated with emotion and affect. Essential oils are absorbed through the skin and are thought to lead to the release of neurochemicals, which affect various parts of the body.

Aromatherapy can also be used by associating a sense of smell with a physiological or psychological function, e.g. relaxing, and is sometimes used with cognitive behaviour therapy or hypnotic suggestion (as in the Queen Elizabeth Psychiatric Hospital, Birmingham, where it has been used to treat epilepsy).

For What Conditions Might it Be Useful for Patients With Breast Cancer?

Aromatherapy is used to promote relaxation and increase general well-being. Other conditions it may help include anxiety, sleeplessness, menopausal symptoms (e.g. those on tamoxifen), pain relief, respiratory congestion and nausea (e.g. anticipatory nausea and vomiting with chemotherapy). Some people describe a release of emotions. MIND (the mental health charity) includes massage and aromatherapy as being possible aids to relieve depression

What is the Experience Like for the Patient/What are the Practicalities?

An aromatherapy massage can be performed on any part of the body, e.g. hand, arm only (useful for patients with mobility problems or skin reactions), but is more commonly done on a wider area (e.g. back, neck). This will involve undressing to uncover the area to be treated.

The first session is usually longer, while the therapist takes a full history, but subsequent sessions would normally be an hour for a full massage. This would be adapted in different circumstances, e.g. in a ward setting, where there may be other constraints, or according to the condition or wishes of the patient.

The approach of aromatherapy is to ensure that the patient feels safe, comfortable and relaxed. After the massage patients may feel any of a range of reactions such as tired, energized, emotionally released or revitalized. The therapist usually discusses with the patient any negative or positive associations with a particular smell and the effect required. For example, lavender or bergamot can be used for relaxation, while geranium or rosemary are used as stimulants.

The patient usually lies on a couch covered by towels or blankets to keep warm and will usually feel relaxed. Following treatment, patients are usually advised to drink extra fluid and to give themselves time before undertaking activity that requires concentration (e.g. driving). Although most of the oil is absorbed by the skin it is best not to wear clothes that may be spoilt by oil getting on to them. Many therapists believe that full benefits are only felt after at least two or more sessions.

Contra-indications/Points to Note

Oils should not be used on broken or sensitive skin or in an undiluted form or taken internally. Cancer patients should go to a recognized practitioner with experience of treating patients with cancer. Oils may interact with sunlight (e.g. citrus oils) and can cause photosensitivity. Certain oils must be avoided if the patient is hypertensive or epileptic. During radiotherapy and until any skin reaction has gone, the area being treated should not be massaged or oils applied. As almond oil is often used, in theory care should be taken if the patient has a nut allergy (although there is no evidence to support this). Aromatherapy massage is contra-indicated for someone with a DVT, and great care should be taken with osteoporosis so as not to damage the bones and cause fractures. Otherwise massage should be only carried out using gentle effleurage, especially if bone metastases are suspected.

Aromatherapy oils are widely available but vary enormously from pure essential oils to synthetic ones or those already mixed with a carrier oil. Toiletries labelled as 'aromatherapy' products may have negligible amounts of essential oil. Price can be a good guide, so it is advisable to compare the same product from different manufacturers. Some oils are very expensive due to their rarity and difficulty of extraction.

Because of the power of some of the oils, it is wise to advise patients to visit a reputable aromatherapist who has experience of dealing with cancer.

Regulatory or Professional Body/Qualifications

Fourteen aromatherapy organizations are represented by the Aromatherapy Organisations Council (AOC). It sets standards of training for schools of aromatherapy. If a therapist has trained at one of the approved schools it indicates an acceptable level of qualification.

The Aromatherapy Trade Council was set up by the AOC and ensures the quality of the oils.

Evidence and Research

Randomized controlled trials have shown a reduction in anxiety (Cooke and Ernst, 2000). Anecdotal evidence is strong.

Further Reading

Tisserand R (1998) Aromatherapy for Everyone. Harmondsworth: Penguin.
Jackson J (1987) Aromatherapy. London: Dorling Kindersley.

Homeopathy

Homeopathy can be traced back as far as Hippocrates. The treatment is based on the premise of treating like with like, i.e. treating with a substance that causes the same symptoms that the disease it is trying to cure. However, the substances are administered in such a diluted form that the original substance is virtually undetectable. Between each dilution stage the remedy is shaken vigorously, a process known as 'succussion'. The dose of the substance is described as 'potency'. Most day-to-day remedies bought over the counter would be a 'sixth potency'.

The modern history of homeopathy started with Samuel Hahnemann, a German doctor who believed that he could help the body overcome health problems by itself, instead of treating symptoms. He published 'The Law of Similars' in 1796 explaining his theories, maintaining that the greater the dilution, the greater the effectiveness of the substance. This meant that one could use potentially fatal substances such as arsenic in such a dilute form as to be undetectable but to produce the effect that he wanted. The first homeopathic practitioner in the UK was Dr Quinn in 1827, who went on to establish the first homeopathic hospital in London in 1850. It gained added credence when the London Homeopathic Hospital had a much lower death rate than other London hospitals during the cholera epidemic of 1854 (16% compared with 60%).

Dr Fisher of St Bartholomew's and the London Homeopathic Hospitals uses the analogy of a computer disk to explain how the dilutions work. A computer disk may contain a large amount of data but in fact it is nothing more than metal. Homeopathic remedies contain only water, the dilution medium and lactose for the tablets. This idea is also known as 'information medicine'.

Nobody really knows how homeopathy works. As previously explained, the remedies are so dilute by the time they are administered that it is not possible to identify the original substance. Homeopathic remedies come in the form of tablets, powder, liquid and also creams. They can be made from plant, mineral or animal sources. The fact that the original substance cannot be detected in what has been given has led some scientists to be sceptical about the effects of this treatment. Research is ongoing although effects have been reproduced in the laboratory at a cellular level. The effects seem to lessen or disappear if the medicine is subjected to a strong magnetic force.

For What Conditions Might it be Useful for Patients with Breast Cancer?

Many women with menopausal symptoms (especially while taking hormone treatments such as tamoxifen) turn to over-the-counter homeopathic remedies or consult practising homeopaths. Remedies such as sepia and pulsatilla are taken to reduce the number and severity of hot flushes and to help general well-being. Anxiety, depression, sleeplessness, itchiness, allergies and promotion of healing may also be helped by homeopathy.

What is the Experience Like for the Patient/What are the Practicalities?

Patients can ask for referral to one of the five National Health Homeopathic Hospitals in this country. There is one in London, Glasgow, Liverpool, Bristol and Tunbridge Wells in Kent. These hospitals are seeing increasing numbers of people as outpatients while retaining very few in-patient beds. Patients can also visit a practising homeopath, who may be medically qualified, or buy remedies over the counter. (Over-the-counter sales were worth £19 million in 1995 in the UK.)

Initial consultation with a homeopath will take up to two hours. Patients would normally be asked questions about their medical history, what sort of person they are, their moods, their sleep pattern, do they feel worse in hot or cold weather, etc., to build a picture before the treatment is chosen. The practitioner would also look at the patient's body type and structure. There are nearly 3000 different homeopathic remedies but usually less than 50 are used. A single homeopathic remedy may be prescribed or several combined into one remedy. Tablets are often placed under the tongue to be dissolved and are generally taken on an empty stomach.

Dosage in the acute stage can mean taking the remedy every two hours. Remedies could be extracted from animal, plant or mineral substances. Initially symptoms may get worse before they get better. Homeopaths believe that one month's treatment is needed for every year that the person has had the imbalance. Patients are asked to return for monitoring before a new prescription is issued.

Many people buy their homeopathic medicines over the counter. This tends to be rather imprecise compared with a full consultation as the homeopathic diagnosis is not made before treatment. However, this probably will cause no harm (but see below), except in the case where conditions are treated that require medical attention. Advice in pharmacies can vary enormously. Many remedies will need to be taken for at least a month to see if they are effective. It is important that any remedies taken are reported to the medical team and recorded in the case notes.

Contra-indications/Points to Note

In about 20% of cases there is a worsening of symptoms before any improvement is seen, so careful monitoring may be needed, e.g. in asthma or epilepsy. Patients need to be aware whether or not the homeopath is medically qualified. It is thought that some conventional drugs may block the therapeutic action of homeopathic treatments but in most cases homeopathic remedies appear safe to take with conventional therapies.

Regulatory or Professional Body/Qualifications

There is at present no statutory regulation so in theory anyone can call him/herself a homeopath. This situation is likely to change in the next few years. Apart from homeopaths with no qualifications, the decision is between medically or non-medically qualified homeopaths. The professional body is the Society of Homeopaths.

Medically qualified homeopaths have completed a six-month postgraduate course and will have MFHom (Member of the Faculty of Homeopathy) after their names.

Non-medically qualified practitioners should belong to the Society of Homeopaths and will have RSHom (Registered with the Society of Homeopaths) or FSHom (Fellow of the Society of Homeopaths) after their name. This indicates an approved three-year training.

A patient must feel confident that the homeopath she chooses understands breast cancer and will not miss signs of serious disease that may need urgent medical treatment.

Research/Further Reading

Ernst E, Hahn EG (eds) (1998) Homeopathy: A Critical Appraisal. Oxford: Butterworth-Heinemann.

Kleijnen J, Knipschild P, Ter Riet G (1991) Clinical trial of homeopathy. British Medical Journal 302: 316–23.

Swayne J (2000) International Dictionary of Homeopathy. Edinburgh: Churchill Livingstone.

Which (1992) Homeopathy off the shelf. Which? Way to Health, October: 158–60.

Reflexology

Reflexology, or reflex zone therapy, was used in India and China over 5000 years ago but its modern history started in the early part of the twentieth century when an American surgeon used it as an anaesthetic for minor ENT surgery. He proposed that the body was divided into vertical zones that could be accessed in the feet. It was further developed by a physiotherapist, Eunice Ingham. It was a pupil of hers, Doreen Bayley, who introduced reflexology to the UK, setting up the Bayley School of Reflexology in 1968, which is still a major influence on the practise of reflexology today.

Reflexology can be used to restore and maintain the body's natural equilibrium and encourage healing. Therapists believe that the body's anatomy and physiology have a corresponding and connecting area on the foot called a reflex, which when stimulated or 'worked' enables the body to promote healing. A reflex showing an area of imbalance is described as feeling like grains of salt under the skin, thought by therapists to be crystal deposits. (The breast reflex is on the top of the foot.) Working the reflexes will rebalance the corresponding area on the body. Similar reflexes are found on the hand. A reflexologist applies gentle pressure to the feet using hands only, encouraging the body to heal itself at its own pace.

Some therapists believe this is connected with meridians and acupressor points.

For What Conditions Might it Be Used by Patients with Breast Cancer?

Reflexogy may be used to reduce anxiety and aid relaxation, to ease sleeplessness, menopausal symptoms, pain relief, depression, nausea and vomiting, headaches, or to aid general well-being.

What is the Experience Like for the Patient/What are the Practicalities?

At the initial consultation the history would be taken with treatment sessions lasting for up to an hour. The patient sits on a comfortable reclining chair exposing only the area below the ankles. The therapist would normally sit in front of the patient on a low stool with easy access to the feet. While working the feet a therapist will often use aqueous cream or cornstarch, using essential oils only if she/he is also an aromatherapist. (If a therapist uses oils see also the section on aromatherapy.) The pressure used on the feet will vary from therapist to therapist and depending on the treatment required. For patients with active disease, a gentle touch is usually recommended. Reactions can vary widely. Some people feel relaxed after treatment or sleepy and some may feel energized, while others report an increase in bowel and bladder function for up to a few days afterwards. Initially treatment is once a week, the frequency reducing as the condition improves. Many people seek 'top up' sessions once a month or once every few months.

Contra-indications/Points to Note

Anyone who does not like their feet being touched is not to be recommended for this treatment! Also contra-indicated is the presence of leg and foot ulcers, and other vascular disease such as deep vein thrombosis, and any infection such as athlete's foot. Therapists will usually avoid any area of active disease or treatment within a few days of patients receiving chemotherapy, although there is little evidence to specifically exclude this.

Qualifications and Regulations

There are two main organizations that both set standards of training and practice and check that their members are insured. Members of the Association of Reflexologists will have MAR after their name while members of the British Reflexology Association will have MBRA.

Evidence and Research

Very little evidence exists to prove the efficacy of reflexology. Research has been inconclusive or weak although there is some evidence to show benefit in premenstrual symptoms (Oleson and Flocco, 1993). Anecdotal evidence is convincing but more research is needed. There is as yet no evidence to prove the theory of reflex zones. For a systematic review of clinical trials see below.

Further Reading

Ernst E, Koeder K. An overview of reflexology. European Journal of General Practice 1997; 3: 52-7.
Hall NM (1991) Thorsons Introductory Guide to Reflexology. London: Thorsons.

Other Complementary Therapies: Brief Overview

Table 14.1 is not intended to be an exhaustive list of therapies but to give guidance on the type of therapies about which the nurse may be asked for advice. I have only given information where it relates to patients with breast cancer - therapies are used for a wide variety of other conditions.

Supplements/Herbs Sometimes Used by Women with Breast Cancer

Many women consider using supplements that can be bought over the counter (Table 14.2). Enquiries about these should be referred to a specialist as there can be interactions with active treatment. It is important that patients understand what they are taking by consulting a reputable therapist or their breast cancer treating team.

With some products it can be difficult to ascertain the strength of the active ingredient, i.e. '100% pure juice' could mean the entire contents or a description before it was added to the finished product. One can usually be guided by the cost.

Table 14.1: Other complementary therapies

Name	What is it	For what conditions do women with breast cancer seek it out	Evidence of effect	Contra-indications/ comment	Professional body
Alexander Technique	Teaching of improved posture to reduce stress on body	General well-being, stress, pain	Yes		Yes
Art	Use of art for communication and emotional therapeutic use	Verbal communication problems		May be used with other psychological methods	
Bach Flower Remedies	Use of plant infusions for correction of emotional imbalances	Anxiety, general well-being	Inconclusive		Yes
Healing (faith healing, spiritual healers, therapeutic touch, psychic healing)	Therapists channel energy to heal people	Well-being; chronic conditions	Yes, some anecdotal	Beware if patient has mental instability	Yes, various
Herbal Medicine	Use of plant remedies taken as tablets, teas, ointments, etc.	Numerous	Yes, but varies with plant, quantity, and condition	Quality control over products; interactions with drugs	Yes
Hypnotherapy	Altered level of consciousness induced by deep relaxation; suggestions are made to enable change	Stress; pain; cessation of smoking; panic attacks	Yes	Exacerbation of psychiatric disorders; abreaction	Yes

Table 14.1: contd.

Name	What is it	For what conditions do women with breast cancer seek it out	Evidence of effect	Contra-indications/ comment	Professional body
Kinesiology	Rebalancing of body's systems to better fight disease using touch	Well-being	No		Yes
Meditation (different types)	Various techniques for inducing relaxation and awareness of body	Well-being; to reduce anxiety and stress; headaches; insomnia; menopausal symptoms; increase self-awareness and confidence	Yes – many studies done by meditation organizations show benefit	No – but be aware of support needed if patient does not have mental stability	Various
Music	Listening to music in a therapeutic way with a therapist	Relaxation; verbal communi-cation problems	Inconclusive		Yes
Naturopathy	Rebalancing the body to better fight illness using methods such as diet, exercise and other CAMs	General well-being; to prevent cancer recurrence	Depends on which therapy used	Depends on which therapy used	Yes
Osteopathy	System of manipulation of musculo-skeletal system	Pain, back problems	Yes for back pain	Osteoporosis; recent fractures; spinal disease (back pain could be undiagnosed metastases)	Yes. Statutory regulation

Table 14.1: contd.

Name	What is it	For what conditions do women with breast cancer seek it out	Evidence of effect	Contra-indications/ comment	Professional body
Reiki	Type of healing	Pain; relaxation; to boost energy	No	None found	Yes
Shiatsu	Massage of points along meridians, positioning and stretching Done through clothes, often on floor	Musculo-skeletal problems etc. stiffness (e.g. arm mobility following axillary surgery	Anecdotal, and some small studies	Osteoporosis; bone metas-tases	Yes
T'ai Chi & Qi Gong	Ancient Chinese forms of gentle rhythmic movements	General well-being; energizing and relaxation	? reduce blood pressure, etc.	None; exercises can be adapted to abilities and function	Yes, various
Yoga	Exercise for posture, stretching, breathing and stamina, and for keeping fit; may be spiritual and meditation	Relaxation; to reduce anxiety; breathing problems	? reduce blood pressure	None; exercise adapted to suit function	Yes, various

The table lists only a few of the products available that are used by breast cancer patients – many of the products have other uses. It is very important that the oncologist is informed of any supplements the patient is taking, especially during the active treatment phase. Patients may also discuss these with their breast care nurse or information centre or one of the specialist organizations listed at the end of this chapter.

Table 14.2: Supplements/herbs available over the counter

Name	Perceived benefit sought by women with breast cancer	Clinical evidence	Comments/safety
Aloe vera	Wound and skin healing General well-being	Conflicting	Some drug interactions
Black cohosh*	Relief of menopausal symptoms	Yes	May interact with anti-hypertensives
Calendula (Marigold)	Anti-inflammatory, healing (used for post-mastectomy lymphoedema)	None found	
Chamomile	Relaxation	None found	Quality of preparations
Cranberry	Prevention of urinary tract infection	Yes RCTs show reduction in incidence	Sugar-free available for diabetics; does not necessarily treat infections
Echinacea	Prevention and shortening of duration of infection, e.g. common cold. General well being	Yes, although some inconclusive	Treatment not usually recommended for longer than a couple of months
Evening primrose oil	Relief of menopausal symptoms	Conflicting results from RCTs. Anecdotal evidence strong!	Examples of trade names = Efamol, Efamast Drug interactions
Garlic	To promote general well-being	Yes, for reducing cholesterol	Interacts with anti-coagulants Discontinue before surgery
Ginger	Nausea and vomiting, e.g. with chemotherapy	Yes	Possible interaction with anticoagulants, cardiac and anti-diabetic therapy

Table 14.2: Supplements/herbs available over the counter

Name	Perceived benefit sought by women with breast cancer	Clinical evidence	Comments/safety
Ginseng (various types) *(some products)	To promote general well-being	Some but more needed	Quality varies Differences with types, e.g. Asian, American, Siberian May interact with MAO inhibitors, anticoagulants, sedatives, hypoglycaemics, etc.
Green tea	Prevention and treatment of cancer	None found	May cause sleeplessness
Lavender	Relaxation	Inconclusive	
Linseed*	Relief of menopausal symptoms	Some, for use in diet with soy products – more information needed	
Mistletoe (Iscador)	Treatment for cancer and side effects	Some evidence for improved quality of life and survival (small)	Drug interactions Local reactions
Phyto-oestrogens*	Relief of menopausal symptoms and osteo-porosis	Yes, seems beneficial to increase in diet but more research needed	
Red clover*	Relief of menopausal symptoms	Inconclusive	Interactions with anticoagulants or hormone treatment possible
Royal jelly	Relief of menopausal symptoms, cancer prevention	No	
Shark cartilage	Cancer prevention	Inconclusive	Do not use with liver disease
St John's wort	Depression	Yes	Drug interactions

Table 14.2: Contd.

Name	Perceived benefit sought by women with breast cancer	Clinical evidence	Comments/safety
Valerian	Sleeplessness	Yes	Note other sedatives
Vitamin E	Relief of menopausal symptoms	Inconclusive	

Substances with an oestrogenic effect are marked * in Table 14.2. These may be inappropriate for women with oestrogen-dependent breast cancer but there is a lack of evidence of this. Most supplements are contra-indicated for pregnant women.

Complementary Therapies and Menopausal Symptoms

One of the most common complaints about side effects from women who have had breast cancer is that of menopausal-type symptoms. Symptoms may include hot flushes and night sweats, mood swings, vaginal dryness, tiredness, and difficulty with confidence and concentration.

These symptoms can be caused by treatments for breast cancer that suppress or stop oestrogen production such as chemotherapy, ovarian ablation or hormonal treatments such as tamoxifen (e.g. Nolvadex, Tamofen,) or an aromatase inhibitor (e.g. Arimidex, Aromasin). They can be further exacerbated if a woman has had to stop hormone replacement therapy (HRT) before receiving treatment for breast cancer. Unfortunately, it is not possible to predict which patients will get these symptoms, their severity or how long they will last. With many hormone treatments likely to last for at least five years, these side effects can have a major impact on quality of life.

Women turn to complementary therapies to treat their symptoms because of the lack of an acceptable effective conventional treatment. HRT is effective but women with breast cancer are not generally offered it because of the theoretical risk of increasing the risk of recurrence, although this is as yet unproved. Drug treatments such as clonidine (Catapres) may be effective in the short term but longer-term studies suggest its effects may wear off. With many women there is also a reluctance to take yet more drugs and the complementary approach is perceived as a more gentle and natural way to tackle the problem.

There are many different types of complementary therapy approaches that women have found helpful. Unfortunately in most cases there is no conclusive evidence from clinical trials that they are effective. However, anecdotal evidence is plentiful from women relating to remedies that have helped them. A holistic practitioner may argue that it is not possible to assess

the effectiveness of these therapies using the assessment methods of traditional conventional medicine. Nevertheless, many patients continue with
hormone treatment and combine it with their choice of complementary
therapy. It is important that patients follow the advice given earlier in this
chapter by asking the right questions, going to a reputable therapist who has
experience in treating cancer patients and keeping their doctor informed.

Treatments for menopausal symptoms may include the following:

- Homeopathy: remedies may include sepia and pulsatilla, sage, rhubarb
  root extract, sulphs and graphites.
- Oriental medicine: Chinese herbs, acupuncture, shiatsu, etc.
- Herbal treatments: for example dong quai, black cohosh, lavender, fennel,
  false unicorn root and wild yam, evening primrose oil, etc.
- Other treatments such as aromatherapy, reflexology or relaxation
  techniques, etc.

A therapist may also give lifestyle advice.

Diet and Dietary Advice

One of the most common questions asked in the Lynda Jackson Macmillan
Centre concerns diet and nutrition. At a time when patients are undergoing
cancer treatments which they feel they have no control over and cannot
influence, making a dietary change can feel like a positive step towards self-help.

Many of us are familiar with dieting food fads and the media focus on food
in general. Scare stories abound! Some women feel that they want to embark
on a complete change of diet at a time of shock after a diagnosis of cancer. It
is perhaps the one thing that they feel they have some control over, perhaps
feeling, like most of us, that our diet could be healthier. It is when perhaps
the body is under stress, e.g. receiving chemotherapy or other treatment, that
people may make sudden changes that can be a shock to the system. Going
down the DIY route of adding supplements or cutting out nutrients may give
patients additional problems.

There has been so much written about cancer and diet that it can be
confusing and difficult for patients and healthcare professionals to determine
what patients should do, if anything. Great care must be taken not to give
advice that could conflict with treatment, e.g. taking vitamin C supplements
that interact with chemotherapy drugs. If a nurse is not cancer trained or a
specialist in the field, the best advice is NOT to give any dietary recommendations. Patients should instead be referred to their oncologist or specialist
nurse or to a hospital dietitian trained in the care of cancer patients.

The following serves as a reminder of the complexities of dietary information. We obtain vitamin A from fish, eggs, milk, etc., and by converting beta-carotene from fruit and vegetables. Beta-carotene is an antioxidant and has long been thought to have a role in cancer prevention. We know from various studies conducted in the 1970s that cancer patients tend to have a lower blood level of beta-carotene and it was thought that raising this level would reduce the incidence of cancer. Two studies found the opposite result. In Finland, 29 000 male smokers took beta-carotene supplements or placebo for an average of six years, which resulted in an increase in cases of lung cancer by 18% in those taking the beta-carotene supplements. A similar trial in the USA showed an increase of 28% in all cancers (ATBC Cancer Prevention Study Group 1998).

It should not be assumed that a naturally occurring substance in food is as good when taken in supplement form. Just because a substance is good for you in your diet does not mean more of it in supplement form is better!

The recent five-year research reported by Oxford University sounds a similar cautionary note. A total of 20 500 individuals were followed to ascertain whether vitamin and mineral supplements could protect patients who are unwell from developing serious illness such as heart disease and cancer. The conclusions were that there was no protection offered at all to people who were already unwell and that people would be better off eating a good diet which includes fresh fruit and vegetables (Heart Protection Study Collaborative Group, 2002).

What is a Healthy Diet?

Remember: the nurse does not have to have all the answers! She/he should not be afraid to involve the dietitian. The following is the standard advice that we should all heed, whether we have cancer or not (individuals may have special needs):

- Aim to eat five portions of fruit and vegetables a day.
- Try not to eat red or processed meats more than once a day.
- Avoid too many high-fat products, e.g. fried foods.
- Try to eat plenty of fibre-rich foods.
- Drink alcohol in moderation.

A healthy diet should include plenty of variety. Table 14.3 is a suitable guide to give to anyone without special dietary needs who asks for advice about healthy eating. Patients with special requirements should be under the guidance of a dietitian or doctor.

Table 14.3: A guide to healthy eating

Food group	Examples	How much to eat	Other comments
Cereal/starchy foods	Bread Rice/pasta Breakfast cereals Potatoes with skins	Plenty from this group Something from this group at each meal	Choose high-fibre cereals
Meat/protein foods	Chicken, beef, lamb etc. Fish, eggs, peas, beans, lentils, nuts	Two choices from this group each day is sufficient.	Not more than one serving a day of red or processed meat (e.g. sausages, meat pies, salami, etc.)
Dairy foods	Milk, cheese, yoghurt, fromage frais	Aim for one pint of milk or equivalent, e.g. 1/3 pint of milk = one carton of yoghurt or fromage frais = 1oz of cheese	Try to opt for low-fat dairy foods such as skimmed or semi-skimmed milk and low-fat cheese
Fruit and vegetables	Fresh, tinned or dried fruit Fruit juice Fresh and frozen vegetables	Choose five a day from this group Examples in next column	Banana with cereal Glass of fruit juice Salad in sandwich Vegetables with meal

It should be remembered that ready-made meals may contain extra salt and sugar.

Alternative Cancer Diets

There are many different types of diets that are recommended as effecting a 'cure' or modifying side effects and it is easy to understand the attraction. We are persuaded that here is a way of regaining control over one's life that promises to make one feel better. The reverse can sometimes be true. Some therapists reject conventional treatment in favour of dietary 'cures'. Although it is of course the right of each patient to accept or reject treatment, it should be done in the full knowledge of all the facts. A diet may involve a new philosophy of life or a complete change of lifestyle. Diets may be time consuming to follow, have little or no scientific evidence or may not include all the nutrients required. There are big profits to be made from selling supplements (one in five of the population takes a multivitamin supplement in the UK) and patients need to be aware of the potential risks.

Questions Patients Should Ask Before Deciding on an Alternative Diet

- What trials have been carried out to prove the success of the diet?
- Is the evidence anecdotal or scientific?
- Who did the research?
- What does the medical team think about this treatment?
- What advantages are there to following this treatment?
- What disadvantages are there to following this treatment?
- What effect will following this diet have on family, friends, social life, etc.?
- What nutrition does the diet provide?
- Is it compatible with conventional treatment?
- How much will it cost in time and money?

Patients should be encouraged to mention any change in diet to their doctor, especially if undergoing current cancer treatment. If patients decide to go against medical advice, it is important that they are able to continue to receive care from nurses as healthcare professionals to support them in the best way possible.

Further Reading

Costain L (n.d.) Super Nutrients Handbook. London: Dorling Kindersley.
Daniel R. (n.d.) Healing Foods. London: Thorsons.
Elliot R. (n.d.) Take Five. London: Cassell.
MAFF (Now DEFRA) (n.d.) Manual of Nutrition. London: Stationery Office.
Stewart M (n.d.) The Phyto Factor. London: Vermillion.
van Straten M, Griggs B (n.d.) Superfoods. London: Dorling Kindersley.

Further Reading About CAM

CancerBACUP (1994) Cancer and Complementary Therapies. London: CancerBACUP.
Cancerlink-Macmillan (2001) Directory of Cancer Self Help and Support 2001/2. London: Cancerlink-Macmillan.
Ernst E (2001) The Desktop Guide to Complementary and Alternative Medicine. St Louis, MO: Mosby.
Glenville M (1997) Natural Alternatives to HRT. London: Kyle Cathie.
House of Lords Select Committee of Science and Technology (2000) Complementary and Alternative Medicine. London: Stationery Office.

Lynda Jackson Macmillan Centre (2002) Breast Cancer, Hormones and HRT. London: LJMC.

Macmillan Cancer Relief (2002) Directory of Complementary Therapy Services in UK Cancer Care 2002. London: Macmillan Cancer Relief.

Mills S, Budd S (2000) Professional Organisation of Complementary and Alternative Medicine in the United Kingdom. Exeter: Centre for Complementary Health Studies, University of Exeter.

Rowlands B (1997) The Which? Guide to Complementary Medicine. London: Which? Books.

Russo H (2001) Integrated Healthcare: A Guide to Good Practice. London: Foundation for Integrated Health [formerly Foundation for Integrated Medicine].

The 2001 Directory of Hospice and Palliative Care Services in the United Kingdom and Republic of Ireland. London: Hospital Information Service at St Christopher's.

Vincent C, Furnham A (1997) Complementary Medicine: A Research Perspective. Chichester: Wiley.

Zollman C, Vickers AJ (2000) ABC of Complementary Medicine. London: BMJ Books.

See also suggestions within each section.

Conclusion

After reading this chapter I hope you are now aware of what a potential minefield CAMs and diet can be for breast cancer patients. The message must be 'beware!'. As nurses we must practise within our competences, and so must be careful about giving advice where we may not have all the facts. It is our duty to facilitate patients making their own choices and to support them, confident in the knowledge that they are making fully informed decisions.

References

ATBC Cancer Prevention Study Group (1998) The effect of vitamin E and beta-carotene on the incidence of lung cancer in male smokers. New England Journal of Medicine 330: 1029-35 .

BBC (2000) BBC Survey of Complementary Medicine Use in the UK. Complementary Therapies in Medicine 8: 32-6.

British Medical Association (1993) Complementary Medicine: New Approaches to Good Practice. Oxford: Oxford University Press.

Cooke B, Ernst E (2000) Aromatherapy: a systematic review. British Journal of General Practice 50: 493-6.

Ernst E, Resch Mills SKL, Hill R, Mitchell A, Willoughby M, White A (1995) Letter: Complementary medicine - a definition. British Journal of General Practice 5: 506.

Heart Protection Study Collaborative Group (2002) MRC/BHF heart protection study of antioxidant vitamin supplementation in 20536 high-risk individuals: a randomised placebo-controlled trial. Lancet 360: 23-33.

HMSO (2000) House of Lords Science and Technology Committee Report. London: HMSO.

MacPherson H, Thomas K, Walters S, Fitter M (2001) The York Acupuncture Safety Study: prospective survey of 34,000 treatments by traditional acupuncturists. British Medical Journal 323: 486-7.

Oleson T, Flocco W (1993) Randomised controlled study of pre-menstrual symptoms treated with ear, hand and foot reflexology. Obstetrics and Gynecology 82: 906-11.

Rampes H, James R (1995) Complications of acupuncture. Acupuncture Medicine 13: 26-33.

Rees R, Feigel I, Vickers A, Zollman C, McGurk R, Smith C, Eade S (1999) Use of Complementary Therapies by Women with Breast Cancer in the South Thames Region: A Short Report. London: Research Council for Complementary Medicine.

Vickers A (1996) Can acupuncture have specific effects on health? A systematic review of acupuncture antiemesis trials. Journal of the Royal Society of Medicine 89: 303-11.

Chapter 15
Psychological issues for the patient with breast cancer

MARY TURNER

Introduction

There is no shortage of literature for nurses interested in psychological aspects of breast cancer. Breast cancer in all its facets is the most researched of all cancers, and the psychological ramifications of the disease that affects almost one in nine women in England and Wales (National Institute for Clinical Excellence, 2002) have been extensively documented. It has long been recognized that a diagnosis of cancer creates a time of crisis for patients and their loved ones, and much has been written about how nurses and doctors can provide psychological support at this critical time (for example, Maguire and Faulkner 1988a; Fallowfield et al., 1990; Faulkner and Maguire, 1994).

However, this vast wealth of relevant and useful work can be somewhat daunting for a nurse new to this field. The purpose of this chapter, therefore, is to provide an accessible introduction to this subject, and highlight some of the key psychological issues that a nurse is likely to encounter when caring for a patient with breast cancer. This chapter aims to:

- discuss some of the common psychological reactions to diagnosis and subsequent treatments;
- explore body image and sexuality;
- consider partner and family reactions to breast cancer; and
- suggest therapeutic nursing interventions to reduce psychological morbidity.

Although psychological reactions can occur at any time, in order to provide some structure to this chapter they will be presented in chronological order, starting with issues around diagnosis and progressing through different treatments to longer-term psychological effects. As the majority of breast cancer patients are women, the female gender will be used throughout this chapter when referring to patients. However, the particular issues facing men with breast cancer will also be considered.

Psychological Reactions to Diagnosis

Haber (1997) contends that breast cancer 'is in many ways the most emotionally loaded of all the cancers', and women who experience it therefore have to deal with huge psychological challenges. When the diagnosis is given, there are as many ways for a woman to react as there are women diagnosed; in other words, everyone will react in an individual and unique way. There are, however, some common reactions, which will be explored, and some of the factors that impact on these will be considered.

Shock

For many women, their immediate reaction to the news that they have breast cancer is one of shock and disbelief. They may also be very fearful and anxious, and it can be some time before these feelings start to diminish. During this initial period of shock, however, the woman is likely to be given a large amount of medical information about treatment options. She is then asked to assimilate this information and make some very difficult decisions while in the midst of a complex psychological reaction to the diagnosis (Haber, 1997). This clearly places a great psychological strain on the woman, who is likely to require a great deal of emotional support.

Anxiety

For a significant number of patients, the shock of a cancer diagnosis will trigger an anxiety state. Faulkner and Maguire (1994) explain that:

> Anxious mood should be diagnosed when patients complain of a persistent inability to relax or stop worrying and are unable to distract themselves from these worries or be distracted by others, and this represents a significant change both quantitively and qualitatively from the patient's normal mood. (p. 3)

Although it can be difficult to diagnose an anxiety state, there are certain symptoms that should alert the nurse. These include: sleep disturbance; irritability and being 'on edge'; sweating; tremor; nausea; palpitations; impaired concentration; indecisiveness; and spontaneous panic attacks (Faulkner and Maguire, 1994; Tait, 1996). Tait (1996) suggests that symptoms need to be present for about four weeks before a diagnosis can be made; however, many women experience acute anxiety on being given a diagnosis of breast cancer, and this may require immediate treatment.

Depression

Like anxiety, depression is another common psychological reaction to a diagnosis of breast cancer. It is known that up to one-third of women develop severe anxiety or a depressive illness within a year of a diagnosis of breast cancer (Maguire, 2000); psychological support must therefore be an integral part of the management of the disease. Common symptoms of depression include: persistent lowering of mood; lack of interest and enjoyment in social activities; poor concentration; low self-esteem and confidence; pessimism and hopelessness; anxiety and irritability; sleep disturbance; loss of appetite; significant change in weight; loss of energy; and constant tiredness (Tait, 1996). Again, symptoms need to persist for a period of about four weeks before a diagnosis of depression can be made.

Loss of Control

In one of many texts written by women who have experienced breast cancer, McCarthy and Loren (1997) describe how important it is for them to be in control of their own lives. They explain that control to them means 'discipline, freedom, self-determination, independence, self-reliance, and choice'. They then add:

> The feeling of being in control deserted us in an instant when we received our diagnoses of breast cancer. (p. 2)

This is a powerful illustration of one of the devastating effects of diagnosis. Patients have to contend with the idea of the disease being in control and then hand their lives over to healthcare professionals, allowing them to take charge of the treatment. It is therefore not surprising that for many women the loss of control associated with a diagnosis of breast cancer is difficult to cope with.

Loss and Grieving

Both the diagnosis of breast cancer and its treatment may represent loss to a woman, from the loss of a breast to the loss of confidence and sense of security. Many women may undergo a grieving process in order to come to terms with their losses (Kubler-Ross, 1978; Parkes and Weiss, 1983). This process can take many months or even years to complete, and can encompass many emotions, including guilt, denial, sadness and anger.

Factors Affecting Psychological Reactions

So far, some of the possible psychological reactions to a diagnosis of breast cancer have been described. However, there are several factors that may influence the extent to which these reactions are experienced. These include a woman's previous experience of breast cancer, the manner in which the diagnosis is given, and the manner and the speed of the diagnosis and first treatment.

Previous Experience

A woman's previous life experience, including her experience of cancer in general and breast cancer in particular may influence her psychological reaction to diagnosis and treatment. If she has for example lost a member of her family to the disease at an early age, she may be more frightened than if she has witnessed a family member make a full recovery. Watson (1991) identifies some important factors that may render a woman more vulnerable to psychological morbidity. These include a history of psychiatric illness; lack of social support; low expectations of the success of the treatment; pre-existing relationship difficulties; and treatment with aggressive chemotherapy. If several of these factors are present, the woman may be even more vulnerable to psychological difficulties.

Breaking Bad News

Dixon and Sainsbury (1998) state that:

> There is no easy way to break bad news. However, it is important to do it in such a way that the patient can bear the news, receive the information that she needs to know and to enable her to express her feelings and concerns. (p. 207)

The way in which the diagnosis is made and the news broken to the patient can have an enormous impact on her psychological reaction (Faulkner and Maguire, 1994). Most experts agree that women who have the news broken to them in a sensitive manner, and are given the opportunity to ask questions, are likely to suffer less long-term psychological morbidity than those who are told abruptly or hurriedly (Maguire and Faulkner, 1988b; Fallowfield et al., 1990).

For this reason, it is clearly stated in breast cancer guidelines (Department of Health, 1996) that protocols and procedures for the breaking of bad news must be in place, and that a specialist breast care nurse should be on hand to support the patient and family. The National Institute for Clinical Excellence has also produced guidance on the management of breast cancer (2002), which includes the recommendation that all members of the breast care team who provide clinical care should have special training in communication and counselling skills.

Screen-detected Cancers

Whether a woman is diagnosed through the NHS Breast Screening Programme or through the symptomatic service may have an impact on her psychological response. The majority (approximately 80%) of women who go to breast clinics for investigation of suspected breast cancer are referred by their GP (National Institute for Clinical Excellence, 2002). These women are symptomatic; in other words, they have discovered a lump or other symptoms and have been concerned enough to seek the opinion and advice of their GP.

On first discovering a change in their breast many of these women immediately fear the worst, and so to some extent start to prepare themselves for a diagnosis of cancer. Women with suspected breast cancer are seen very quickly in a specialist breast clinic as a result of the government's cancer two-week wait guidelines (NHS Executive, 1998). This speed of referral may add to a woman's anxiety pre-diagnosis, as she may feel that she would not be seen so quickly if it were not serious; it may also paradoxically sound a warning note, rendering the actual diagnosis much less of a shock.

However, about 20% of women are referred to breast clinics from the NHS Breast Screening Programme (National Institute for Clinical Excellence, 2002). These women usually have no symptoms, and go for breast screening once every three years expecting to be given a clean bill of health. They may therefore be totally unprepared for a diagnosis of cancer, and it can come as more of a shock to them, precipitating greater psychological morbidity.

One-stop Clinics

The value of one-stop clinics, where a definite diagnosis is made and given to the patient at the first visit, remains controversial. Studies by Harcourt et al. (1999) and Poole et al. (1999) show that women with benign breast disease derive psychological benefit from having a speedy diagnosis, as they are spared the distress associated with waiting.

However, neither of these studies showed reduced psychological distress for women with breast cancer diagnosed in a one-stop clinic. Indeed, Harcourt et al. (1999) showed that eight weeks following diagnosis women with cancer who had been through the one-stop system reported higher levels of depression than women who had experienced the two-stop system. This finding would appear to support Faulkner and Maguire's (1994) contention that bad news needs to be broken slowly in order to avoid the patient having to make too abrupt a transition from 'the perception of being well to that of having a potentially fatal illness'.

Waiting for Treatment

Many women find that the time between being given the diagnosis and having the first treatment seems long, and this waiting can cause anxiety. Many women fear that the cancer might be growing while they are waiting for treatment. For this reason a government target is to cut down the waiting time to four weeks:

> No patient should have to wait more than four weeks for any form of treatment or supportive intervention. (National Institute for Clinical Excellence 2002, p. 8)

For most women the first treatment is surgical. The psychological implications of the different sorts of breast surgery will now be considered.

Surgical Treatments

Mastectomy

It has already been suggested that women react in many different ways to a diagnosis of breast cancer, and similarly there are myriad reactions to mastectomy. Some women regard mastectomy as mutilating surgery, and some find the psychological consequences devastating (see the section on body image and sexuality below). However, many others are not primarily concerned with losing a breast; for example, Fallowfield et al. (1990) found that only 12% of women in their study cited breast loss as their primary concern. Some are far more concerned about the cancer and see mastectomy as a means to improve their prognosis; it can also give them more peace of mind in the long term by helping to assuage the fear of recurrence.

Breast-conserving Surgery

There is an understandable tendency in the literature to focus on mastectomy when considering the psychological effects of surgery. However, breast-conserving surgery also has psychological consequences. The surgery may be disfiguring, altering the shape and size of the breast. In addition, a woman may have fears that the cancer will return in the breast. Fallowfield (1986) found that women who had breast-conserving surgery experienced the same levels of anxiety and depression as those who had mastectomy.

Axillary Node Clearance

It is now common practice to remove the axillary lymph nodes adjacent to the affected breast, both to stage the disease accurately and to treat it adequately. However, removal of these glands carries with it a significant risk of developing lymphoedema of the arm in the future. For some women, this means a reduction in the mobility of their arm, which may in turn lead to a loss of independence. Even those who do not develop lymphoedema can experience high levels of anxiety about their risk of doing so.

Immediate or Delayed Breast Reconstruction

Some women are given the choice of immediate breast reconstruction following mastectomy. A recent study in the UK investigated the psychological advantages of immediate rather than delayed breast reconstruction (Al Ghazal et al., 2000). This study found that most of the women who had delayed reconstruction said they would have preferred immediate reconstruction, whereas the women who underwent immediate reconstruction reported less anxiety and depression, and better body image and self-esteem.

However, immediate reconstruction is not available for every woman. Indeed, some surgeons are reluctant to offer it, because they have concerns that it may delay or compromise adjuvant therapy that they consider to be of paramount importance. A woman who wants this procedure may therefore need to be quite assertive and be prepared to travel to a breast unit where it is available.

Making Decisions about Treatment

When a diagnosis of breast cancer is confirmed, treatment options need to be discussed and decisions have to be made before treatment can commence. In the past, decisions were made by the surgeon alone, and the woman was not consulted. However, there is now research evidence showing that women suffer less psychological morbidity if they are offered a choice of treatments and involved in the decision-making process (Fallowfield et al., 1990; Knobf, 1990). It is therefore now standard practice to involve women in making decisions about their treatment.

However, some women find it very difficult and stressful to make decisions about treatment, and do not want to carry such a heavy responsibility. The National Institute for Clinical Excellence guidelines (2002) point out that:

> There is fairly strong evidence that breast cancer patients benefit from involvement in treatment decisions, but women vary considerably in the amount of responsibility they wish to take and clinicians need to be sensitive to the degree to which individual patients want to become involved in decision making. (p. 29)

Surgeons and other members of the breast care team therefore need to spend enough time with each patient in order to assess her information needs and her willingness to take part in decision making.

Body Image And Sexuality

Defining Body Image

The effect of breast surgery on body image has already been alluded to, but what exactly do we mean by this much-used term? Salter (1997) defines body image simply as 'the way a person sees himself or herself and perceives how he or she is seen by others'. Faulkner and Maguire (1994) identify three components of body image: the loss of physical integrity (feeling no longer whole as a result of the removal of part of the body); a heightened sense of self-consciousness; and feeling less sexually attractive.

Society and the Media

Every day we are bombarded with images in the media that serve to underline the link between breasts and sexual desirability. Tait and Wing (1997) explain that:

> There has never been a time since Adam and Eve when a woman's breasts were not important. Through the ages, the ways in which they were portrayed have changed, but the message remains essentially the same. The female breast is regarded as the symbol of intrinsic femininity, sexual desirability and maternal comfort and succour. Whether breasts are alluded to in a subtle and evocative way or explicitly exhibited, they are central to many people's views about 'being a woman'. It is small wonder, therefore, that any real or potential threat to a woman's breast is stressful. (p. 151)

Given society's preoccupation with breasts, it is hardly surprising that both the surgical treatment and the disease itself can have a devastating impact on a woman's confidence and self-esteem, and make her feel less attractive than before.

Sexuality

Closely allied to body image is the issue of sexuality. Love (2000) contends that sexuality is one of the least discussed subjects in respect of life after breast cancer. This is perhaps not surprising, since the personal and private nature of sex and sexuality can make it a particularly difficult subject to broach. Many healthcare professionals, if they were honest, would probably admit that they find it much easier to focus on issues such as treatment rather than sexuality. Indeed, they may lack both the skills and the confidence to deal with this subject effectively; Salter (1997) points out that communicating about sex is often left out of a health professional's training.

However, many patients want and need to discuss these issues, and they may well choose a nurse rather than a doctor to be their confidante, especially when a good nurse–patient relationship has been established. Nurses should therefore ask patients about their relationships as part of their assessment, and provide opportunities for patients to discuss their concerns about sexuality and body image. Although each patient will, of course, have her own individual concerns, it is worth briefly highlighting some common problems.

Fear of Rejection

Many women fear that their partners will be put off by their appearance following surgery, and that they will no longer find them sexually attractive. Partners too may have fears about how the woman concerned will look, and how this will impact on their sexual relationship. A recent study explored the reactions of husbands to their wives' diagnoses of breast cancer (Woloski-Wruble and Kadmon, 2002). This study revealed that although the husbands described their relationships with their wives as 'excellent', the majority of them experienced a change in their sexual interest, function or satisfaction following their wives' diagnoses of breast cancer. Husbands may also have concerns about hurting their wives, which may deter them from resuming sexual activity. However, it is also worth pointing out that many couples find that the experience of breast cancer brings them closer, particularly if they can share their concerns and reassure one another.

Loss of Libido

Many patients experience a loss of libido in the weeks and months following diagnosis, which may be related both to their psychological reactions and to the effects of treatment. A woman who is experiencing pain following surgery, for example, is perhaps less likely to feel like lovemaking. Many women also find that their sexual relationships are relegated to lower down their list of priorities because they are preoccupied with trying to make a psychological adjustment to their new situation.

Making New Relationships

Of course, many patients are not in sexual relationships at the time of diagnosis and treatment, and this can bring a different raft of problems. A woman on her own may find it harder to embark on a new relationship if she feels that the treatment has impaired her sexual attractiveness.

Nurses can be instrumental in helping patients to cope with all these concerns. As Salter (1997) rightly argues:

> Knowledge about actual and potential problems associated with sexuality and an alteration in body image enables the nurse to assess the meaning of this for the individual patient and family, provide counselling before and after the surgery, and

intervene so that the individual will be able to adapt to an alteration in body image and return to his or her previous activities of daily living and lifestyle. (p. 33)

Adjuvant Therapies

In the past, the only effective treatment for breast cancer was surgery. In recent years, however, there has been a dramatic rise in the number of women given adjuvant therapies for breast cancer, and these carry with them their own potential psychological morbidity. Psychological issues associated with chemotherapy, radiotherapy and hormonal therapies will now be briefly considered.

Chemotherapy

Chemotherapy can bring about many physical changes that can have a negative impact on a woman's body image. One of the most significant and common is hair loss, which for some women is the most distressing part of their cancer treatment. It is relatively easy to disguise the loss of a breast by using a breast prosthesis but, although wigs, scarves and hats can be used, it is sometimes much more difficult to disguise hair loss. Many women are also distressed by the speed with which their hair can fall out. The journalist Ruth Picardie, who was diagnosed with breast cancer when she was 32, describes her experience of hair loss:

> Meanwhile, my hair is falling out with amazing rapidity – I estimate total baldness will be achieved by the weekend, so the whole thing will have happened in a week.... I'm now used to hoovering the bed every morning.... (Picardie, 1998, p. 1)

Even the treatments used to counteract the side effects of chemotherapy can cause side effects of their own, contributing to altered body image. For instance, it is now common practice to give steroids as part of the anti-emetic regime; many women find that steroids increase their appetite, with the consequence that they gain weight and feel less attractive.

Fertility

Although the majority of women are post-menopausal when diagnosed with breast cancer, a significant minority are still of childbearing age, and many of them are given chemotherapy that may affect their fertility. It is therefore very important that an assessment is made of the patient's feelings about future pregnancy, so that her fertility is preserved if at all possible.

Fatigue

Fatigue can occur with all forms of cancer treatment but there is now clear evidence that it is the most common side effect for patients receiving chemotherapy (Richardson, 1995a, 1995b). The exact physiological mechanisms that lead to fatigue are not fully established but research shows that patients relate it to treatment, as well as to other symptoms, levels of activity and psychological concerns. There is little doubt that psychological reactions and physiological fatigue are closely linked, and it can be difficult to untangle them. For example, if a patient is depressed it may be hard to tell whether this is a cause or a consequence of fatigue. Fatigue can have a detrimental effect on all aspects of a woman's quality of life, including her interpersonal relationships, and as such can be very difficult to cope with.

Radiotherapy

Radiotherapy is another widely used treatment that can induce fatigue. It can also have other side effects. One of the most common side effects of radiotherapy to the breast is a sunburn-like skin reaction that, although temporary, can nevertheless result in significant psychological morbidity.

Women who have radiotherapy following breast-conserving surgery face two additional psychological challenges. First, the treatment can alter the shape, texture, sensation and appearance of the breast, and can therefore alter the woman's perception of herself; in other words, her body image. Second, the treatment sometimes brings about changes within the breast tissue that make radiological assessment of the breast difficult in the future. This means that each time the woman has follow-up mammography there may be uncertainty and increased anxiety about whether or not the disease has returned.

Hormone Therapy

Hormonal therapies have been used to treat breast cancer for many years now and are widely considered to be both effective and well tolerated. However, they can have side effects that can be very distressing for some women. For example, menopausal symptoms such as hot flushes, night sweats, mood changes, vaginal dryness, vaginal discharge and weight gain can all have an adverse effect on a woman's psychological well-being, her body image and sexuality. Once again, the nurse needs to be able to assess the psychological effect of these therapies in order to provide supportive care.

Male Breast Cancer

Approximately one in two hundred breast cancers occur in men (Dixon and Sainsbury, 1998). The clinical features, treatments and prognosis are all similar to those of female breast cancers. However, there is a tendency for them to present later, perhaps due to the common misconception that breast cancer can only occur in women.

Because the vast majority of people with breast cancer are women, there is still a tendency in the literature to ignore male breast cancer, or at best to pay it scant regard. Even the recently published National Institute for Clinical Excellence guidelines (2002) make no attempt to deal with male breast cancer, merely making the statement: 'This manual update deals only with services for women with breast cancer'. Although it may of course be legitimate to deal with male breast cancer separately, nevertheless its omission from a major government document may only serve to further isolate and marginalize those affected by it.

As well as having to face many of the same issues as women, a man may experience specific psychological ramifications of having what is widely considered to be a female disease. The effect of mastectomy on body image can be every bit as traumatic for a man as for a woman, and just as a woman might struggle with her femininity a man may feel his masculinity is compromised by both the disease and its treatment. For example, it might be difficult for him to explain to his friends in the pub that he is experiencing menopausal symptoms as a result of hormonal therapy. All of these issues need to be considered by the nurse caring for a male breast cancer patient.

Living With Uncertainty

For many people, a diagnosis of cancer is a life-changing event. Life as it existed before the diagnosis can never be the same again, and a process of psychological adaptation needs to take place. Many people during the recovery phase express the desire for life to 'get back to normal'. This is in fact not possible, because what was 'normal' has now changed. However, with the passage of time, psychological adaptation takes place which allows the new, at first very frightening, situation to feel gradually more familiar and less frightening, and a new sort of 'normal' develops.

Long-term Adaptation

Carter (1993) studied the process of adaptation that long-term survivors of breast cancer undergo, and she offers some useful insights from this research. She identified a six-phase survival process that involves interpreting the diagnosis, confronting mortality, reprioritizing, coming to terms, moving on and flashing back. To begin with, informants first interpreted the meaning of the cancer diagnosis for them. Many then experienced an 'existential realization of being mortal', which caused them to experience high levels of anxiety. In the third phase, many women made changes in their priorities concerned with their lifestyles and life goals. The author then describes what happens in the fourth phase, coming to terms:

> Informants commonly recognized that they were reconstituted or changed in some way by their cancer experience. Some informants accepted the fact of having had cancer, accepted changes that resulted from cancer, and integrated the changes into their lifestyles in healthy and productive ways. (p. 358)

In the next phase, moving on, the informants proceeded with life after cancer, having placed the cancer experience into the background and the past. However, many women also revisited and relived their previous experiences in the final phase, flashing back, as a way of 'tying the past, present and future together in a meaningful context'. This work offers a useful explanation of the process that many women undergo in the months and years following the diagnosis and treatment of breast cancer.

Recurrent Disease

Although many women have to learn to live with the fear of breast cancer recurrence, most will never have to face the disease again. Unfortunately, however, for a proportion of women such fears will become reality, as at least one-third of patients develop recurrent disease, sometimes many years after the initial treatment (National Institute for Clinical Excellence, 2002).

When breast cancer recurs, women may go through similar psychological reactions to those they experienced the first time round. However, there may be additional emotional challenges to be faced. Tait (1996) explains that:

> It can be a shattering blow to a patient to find that all the effort, skill and courage used to cope with the primary disease has not been effective in stopping the disease spreading. (p. 21)

As a consequence, some women experience feelings of failure when the cancer returns. However, perhaps surprisingly, Fallowfield (1991) contends that some women actually feel relieved to discover the cancer is back, because they have remained anxious that it would, and the diagnosis allows their uncertainty to end.

Partner and Family Reactions

A diagnosis of breast cancer affects not just the person diagnosed but also the people surrounding her: her partner, children, grandchildren, parents, siblings, friends and work colleagues. (For reasons of simplicity the term 'relative' will be used to encompass all these relationships.) It is therefore not uncommon for relatives to experience their own psychological reactions.

Tait (1996) points out that breast cancer can jeopardize a patient's close personal relationships, because it can be difficult for patients and relatives to talk about both the disease and their psychological reactions to it. Some of the more common reactions will now be considered.

Fear

Fear is a very common response amongst relatives, and can be related to many different issues. The most obvious is the fear that the patient will die. Children in particular may harbour this fear, and may also be afraid that their mother will be too ill to look after them.

Depending on their age, children may have great difficulty in understanding what is happening to their mother, and therefore need to be given information and support in a manner appropriate to their age. Of course, a child of fifteen can understand a great deal more than a child of five, but even very young children need to have explanations they can understand. They also need to feel they can voice questions and concerns, and that they will be listened to and answered honestly.

Relatives may have fears about the effects of treatment, and be worried that the woman will change in some way and no longer be the person they knew. They may also be very apprehensive about how she will look, for example if she experiences hair loss during chemotherapy.

Guilt

Guilt is another common emotion amongst relatives, often arising from the fact that the disease has struck the woman rather than the relative. Parents of breast cancer patients may feel that in the natural order of things it should be them and not their child facing a potentially life-threatening disease. This guilt may be particularly intensified if the patient is a member of a 'breast cancer family' and has inherited a faulty gene from a parent.

Children sometimes feel guilty as they wrongly believe they caused the disease by misbehaving or upsetting their mother. And partners can feel guilty, possibly because they believe the patient is a better person than they are and therefore less deserving of cancer. It may be particularly difficult for same-sex partners, especially in the case of screen-detected cancers where one partner is given the all-clear and the other is told she has cancer.

Feeling Protective

Some relatives react by being protective, and in some cases over-protective. It is, of course, a natural instinct to want to protect our loved ones from pain and suffering. However, this can seem suffocating for the patient, as many do not want to be handled with kid gloves or treated any differently from usual.

Some relatives even try to prevent health professionals giving the patient full information about her diagnosis and prognosis in an effort to protect her, and this can require skilful handling by the breast care team.

Although the nurse's primary concern is the patient, if she is offering truly holistic care then she will need to take the relatives into account. Brewin (1996) believes that by helping the relatives we help the patient, and that therefore nurses need to pay more attention to how they communicate with and support relatives.

Nursing Implications

So far, this chapter has considered the psychological consequences of breast cancer and its treatment for the patient. It is clear that nurses have a crucial role in helping patients to deal with their psychological reactions, and some aspects of the nurse's role will now be considered.

Communication Skills

In 1996 the United Kingdom Central Council for Nursing, Midwifery and Health Visiting (UKCC) published a document entitled 'Guidelines for Professional Practice' in which it is stated that:

> Communication is an essential part of good practice... Effective communication relies on all our skills. Building a trusting relationship will greatly improve care and help to reduce anxiety and stress for patients and clients, their families and their carers. (UKCC, 1996, p. 15)

It is hard to imagine a more stressful and anxiety-inducing experience than being given a diagnosis of cancer; therefore good communication from the point of diagnosis onwards is of paramount importance.

However, the ability of nurses to communicate effectively with cancer patients should not be taken for granted. Some research evidence suggests that nurses specializing in cancer nursing lack appropriate skills in communication (for example, Wilkinson, 1991; Faulkner and Maguire, 1994). Indeed, many cancer nurses use communication strategies (such as closed questions) that actually block effective communication (Wilkinson, 1991). The reasons for this are complex, and may include lack of training, lack of confidence, inadequate support, lack of time and pressures of workload. Nevertheless, it is clear that if the UKCC guidelines are to be implemented nurses need to be able to communicate well with their patients.

Non-verbal Communication

Northouse and Northouse (1991) describe communication in oncology settings as 'a complex and multifaceted process', and make the important point that a large part of the communication that takes place between nurses and patients is non-verbal. Begley (1996) notes that non-verbal communication is thought to be five times more effective than verbal. It is therefore essential that nurses learn to be aware of their own body language and what messages they are tacitly sending to patients, so they can use non-verbal communication in a therapeutic way to promote the nurse–patient relationship, rather than to block effective communication.

Assessment

Faulkner and Maguire (1994) contend that although the diagnosis and treatment of cancer is associated with a significant psychological morbidity, this often remains unrecognized and unresolved:

> Patients and relatives are reluctant to disclose any problems, while health professionals are loath to enquire actively about them. (p. 1)

Faulkner and Maguire (1994) recommend that, when assessing patients, nurses should try and keep the discussion focused on the patient's feelings, and they suggest some skills which promote disclosure, such as open directive questioning, prompting, responding to cues, using silence, and encouraging the expression of emotions. It must be acknowledged, however, that such assessments require time and privacy, and for this reason may not be practicable in for example a busy surgical ward. The breast care specialist nurse can therefore play a key role in assessing the patient, and this will be discussed further below.

Giving Information

It is also important for health professionals to understand that at the time of diagnosis a patient who is in shock is unlikely to be able to absorb very much information. For this reason, many women need to go over the information several times, and some experts advocate the practice of tape-recording the initial consultation so that the patient can take the tape home and reconsider the information in the days following the diagnosis (Hogbin et al., 1992).

The importance of written information is also widely acknowledged, and it is now viewed as an essential part of good practice to give the patient written information suited to her needs at each part of the treatment process. The National Institute for Clinical Excellence guidelines (2002) state that:

> At every stage, patients should be offered clear, objective, full and prompt information in both verbal and written form. Each patient should receive information relevant to her case about the disease, diagnostic procedures, treatment options and effectiveness. The amount and timing of the information should take each patient's preferences into account. (p. 26)

The nurse therefore needs to be skilful in assessing the patient in order to ascertain her information needs.

Common Assumptions about Psychological Reactions

The literature abounds with assumptions about how women react to a diagnosis of breast cancer. For example, Love (2000) states that:

> The first thing a woman thinks of when diagnosed with breast cancer is: 'Will I die?' This is quickly followed by 'Will I have to lose my breast?' (p. 347)

Although not denying that many women may indeed experience such fears, it is dangerous to assume that all women will react this way. Not all patients will be distressed at losing their breast; some will be hugely relieved, as they will be much more concerned about having cancer (Fallowfield, 1990).

Others may focus on what some might regard as more trivial concerns. For instance, a woman who wears dentures may be very concerned about having to remove them in order to undergo surgery, because of the alteration this makes to her facial appearance; this may be the body image issue she focuses on at that time. It is therefore very important that nurses do not make assumptions about patients' psychological reactions to breast cancer.

It should also be pointed out that despite the literature exhorting nurses to explore the feelings of cancer patients (Faulker and Maguire, 1994), not every patient will want to share her deepest feelings with relative strangers when diagnosed. Even if a patient does experience feelings of fear about dying or losing a breast, this may not be what she chooses to divulge. Not all patients will want to unburden themselves emotionally; some will want to cope privately, or within their own support network. The challenge for nurses is to assess each patient on an individual basis without prejudice, and then endeavour to meet her needs.

Other Resources

It is important for nurses to be aware of other resources that are available both locally and nationally to support patients with breast cancer. Many patients derive benefit from the support of others who have been through the experience of breast cancer, and for this reason many breast cancer support groups exist. Of course, some patients prefer not to participate in such groups; nevertheless, all patients should be informed about what is available to them and how to participate if they so wish.

In recent years there has also been a huge increase in the number and variety of complementary therapies that are available (Barnett, 2002), many of which can play a part in the psychological support of people with breast cancer and their families. However, the array of complementary therapies can be quite bewildering for patients, and nurses can help by knowing what is available in their locality and how to access it.

Caring for the Carers

Since the advent of primary nursing in the 1980s nurses have been encouraged to develop relationships with patients in order to enhance care and reduce the patient's fear and anxiety (Pearson, 1988; Salvage, 1990; Wright, 1994). Indeed, there is a large body of literature on caring, which extols the virtues of interpersonal relationships between nurses and patients. Watson (1985), for example, believes that through interpersonal relationships nurses can help patients achieve a higher degree of harmony within the mind, body and soul.

Some writers, however, sound a note of caution. Van Hooft (1987) believes that it is not possible for nurses to sustain this level of caring:

> If the nurse is to be responsible for the growth in a holistic sense of the client as a total person, or if the nurse has to open with every client a depth of communication that allows for the sharing of the most intimate levels of existence, then the practical professional life of that nurse will become impossible. And this is not just because there will not be enough time; it's just not going to be psychologically possible either. (p. 33)

In other words, forming relationships with patients can have negative consequences for nurses. Caring can be stressful; indeed, Benner and Wrubel (1989), despite being strong advocates of caring, acknowledge that it is inevitably stressful. The National Institute for Clinical Excellence guidelines (2002) also warn that:

> Health care workers may come to treat patients in detached or even dehumanised ways as a way of reducing their own emotional stress. (p. 28)

Each nurse therefore needs to be aware of how she is affected psychologically by caring and forming relationships with patients. Turner (1999) suggests that nurses have to go through a process of learning how to manage their involvement if they are to become proficient at establishing and sustaining relationships with cancer patients. They also require both educational and emotional support if they are to learn how to manage their involvement in a positive and constructive way (Turner, 2001). It is therefore vitally important that adequate support is available to nurses, through education, guided reflection, mentorship and clinical supervision. The breast care nurse also has a part to play in the provision of support for less experienced staff.

Role of the Breast Care Specialist Nurse

The breast care nurse is now viewed as an essential member of the breast team, and therefore every woman with breast cancer should have access to a breast care nurse who has appropriate post-registration qualifications and is trained in counselling and communication (National Institute for Clinical Excellence, 2002).

Traditionally, the primary focus of the role has been to provide support and information to breast cancer patients and their families. Faulkner and Maguire (1994) describe the competences they expect of specialist nurses. These include the ability to identify patients with anxiety states, depressive illness, body image problems, sexual difficulties, or interpersonal problems. They also suggest that breast care nurses:

> ... should be aware of signs of over-involvement or over-identification with patients, and be familiar with the concepts of transference and counter-transference. They should be comfortable with empowering patients rather than trying to act for them. They should be encouraged to continue their education, evolve their own working methods, and accept ongoing supervision, as well as to scrutinize their time-management. (p. 183)

The role is therefore multi-faceted and complex. In addition, in recent years roles have started to expand and develop in diverse ways in different breast units across the UK, and are continuing to do so. For example, some breast care nurses now hold their own clinics for triple assessment, breast cancer follow-ups, or family history risk assessment; such clinics were once the exclusive domain of the medical staff.

At the same time as focusing on patients, breast care nurses also have a key role in educating and supporting other staff. In the past, specialist nurses have sometimes been accused of undermining other nurses, because they assume all the responsibility for psychological care of patients, leaving other nurses in both the hospital and the community feeling they are not allowed to contribute as much as they would like (Faulkner and Maguire, 1994). Alternatively, other nurses may choose to leave psychological care in the province of the specialist nurse, because it prevents them from having to risk involvement. However, it is more beneficial for both patients and staff if part of the specialist nurse's role is to support other staff in developing self-awareness, confidence and communication skills.

Conclusion

With the incidence of breast cancer rising to one in nine (National Institute for Clinical Excellence, 2002) it is safe to assume that most nurses will care for women with this disease at some point in their career. It is therefore incumbent upon all nurses to acquire sufficient knowledge of the psychological issues faced by these patients, together with the necessary skills to build therapeutic relationships, in order to improve the quality of the care they can offer.

References

Al Ghazal S, Sully L, Fallowfield L, Blamey RW (2000) The psychological impact of immediate rather than delayed breast reconstruction. European Journal of Surgical Oncology 26(1): 17-19.

Barnett H (2002) The Which? Guide to Complementary Therapies. London: Which? Books.

Begley CM (1996) Triangulation of communication skills in qualitative research instruments. Journal of Advanced Nursing 24: 688-93.

Benner P, Wrubel J (1989) The Primacy of Caring: Stress and Coping in Health and Illness. Reading, MA: Addison-Wesley.

Brewin T (1996) Relating to the Relatives: Breaking Bad News, Communication and Support. Oxford: Radcliffe Medical Press.

Carter BJ (1993) Long-term survivors of breast cancer. A qualitative descriptive study. Cancer Nursing 16(5): 354-61.

Denton S (ed) (1996) Breast Cancer Nursing. London: Chapman & Hall.

Department of Health (1996) Guidance for Purchasers: Improving Outcomes in Breast Cancer: The Manual. London: NHS Executive.

Dixon M, Sainsbury R (1998) Handbook of Diseases of the Breast, 2nd edn. London: Churchill Livingstone.

Fallowfield L (1991) Breast Cancer. London: Routledge.

Fallowfield LJ (1986) Effects of breast conservation on psychological morbidity associated with diagnosis and treatment of early breast cancer. British Medical Journal 293: 1331-4.

Fallowfield LJ, Hall A, Maguire GP, Baum M (1990) Psychological outcomes of different treatment policies in women with early breast cancer outside a clinical trial. British Medical Journal 301, 575-80.

Faulkner A, Maguire P (1994) Talking to Cancer Patients and their Relatives. Oxford: Oxford University Press.

Haber S (ed) (1997) Breast Cancer. A Psychological Treatment Manual. London: Free Association Books.

Harcourt D, Rumsey N, Ambler N (1999) Same-day diagnosis of symptomatic breast problems: psychological impact and coping strategies. Psychology Health and Medicine 143: 57-71.

Hogbin B, Jenkins VA, Parkin JA (1992) Remembering 'bad news' consultations. Psycho-oncology 1: 147-54.

Knobf T (1990) Early stage breast cancer: the options. American Journal of Nursing November, 28-30.

Kubler-Ross E (1978) On Death and Dying. New York: Macmillan.

Love S (2000) Dr Susan Love's Breast Book. Massachusetts: Perseus Publishing.

Maguire P (2000) Psychological aspects. In: Dixon M (ed) ABC of Breast Diseases. London: BMJ Books.

Maguire P, Faulkner A (1988a) How to do it: improve the counselling skills of doctors and nurses in cancer care. British Medical Journal 297: 847-9.

Maguire P, Faulkner A (1988b) How to do it: communicate with cancer patients, 1: Handling bad news and difficult questions. British Medical Journal 297: 907-9.

McCarthy P, Loren JA (eds) (1997) Breast Cancer? Let Me Check My Schedule! Oxford: Westview Press.

National Institute for Clinical Excellence (2002) Guidance on Cancer Services: Improving Outcomes in Breast Cancer: Manual Update. London: National Institute for Clinical Excellence.

NHS Executive (1998) Breast Cancer Waiting Times - Achieving the Two Week Wait Target, Health Service Circular. London: NHS Executive.

Northouse LL, Northouse PG (1991) Interpersonal communication systems. In: Baird SB, McCorkle R, Grant M (eds) Cancer Nursing: A Comprehensive Textbook. Philadelphia, PA: WB Saunders.

Parkes CM, Weiss RS (1983) Recovery from Bereavement. New York: Basic Books.

Pearson A (ed) (1988) Primary Nursing: Nursing in the Burford and Oxford Nursing Development Units. London: Croom Helm.

Picardie R (1998) Before I Say Goodbye. Harmondsworth: Penguin.

Poole K, Hood K, Davis BD et al. (1999) Psychological distress associated with waiting for results of diagnostic investigations for breast disease. Breast Journal 8: 334-8.

Richardson A (1995a) Fatigue in cancer patients: a review of the literature. European Journal of Cancer Care 4(1): 20-32.

Richardson A (1995b) The pattern of fatigue in patients receiving chemotherapy. In: Richardson A, Wilson-Barnett J (eds) Nursing Research in Cancer Care. London: Scutari Press.

Salter M (1997) Altered Body Image: The Nurse's Role, 2nd edn. London: Bailliere Tindall.

Salvage J (1990) The theory and practice of the 'new nursing'. Nursing Times 86(4): 42-5.

Tait A (1996) Psychological aspects of breast cancer. In: Denton S (ed) Breast Cancer Nursing. London: Chapman & Hall.

Tait A, Wing M (1997) Whole or partial breast loss and body image. In: Slater M (ed) Altered Body Image: The Nurse's Role, 2nd edn. London: Balliere Tindall.

Turner JM (2001) Managing Involvement: A Grounded Theory of Nurses' Personal Involvement in Relationships with Cancer Patients. Unpublished PhD thesis, University of London.

Turner M (1999) Involvement or over-involvement? Using grounded theory to explore the complexities of nurse–patient relationships. European Journal of Oncology Nursing 3(3): 153-60.

United Kingdom Central Council for Nursing, Midwifery and Health Visiting (1996) Guidelines for Professional Practice. London: UKCC.

Van Hooft S (1987) Caring and professional commitment. Australian Journal of Advanced Nursing 4(4): 29-38.

Watson J (1985) Nursing: Human Science and Human Care: A Theory of Nursing. New York: National League of Nursing Press.

Watson M (1991) Breast cancer. In: Watson M (ed) Cancer Patient Care: Psychosocial Treatment Methods. Cambridge: Cambridge University Press.

Wilkinson SM (1991) Factors which influence how nurses communicate with cancer patients. Journal of Advanced Nursing 16: 677-88.

Woloski-Wruble A, Kadmon I (2002) Breast cancer – reactions of Israeli men to their wives' diagnoses. European Journal of Oncology Nursing 6: 93–9.

Wright SG (1994) My Patient – My Nurse: The Practice of Primary Nursing, 2nd edn. London: Scutari Press.

Chapter 16
The Differing Roles of Specialist Nurses

Emma Pennery

Introduction

As the world around us changes, nursing practice is, of course, not immune to evolution, and within the specialty of breast care, nursing change has been inescapable over recent years. Inevitably, losing sight of what we find familiar is both rewarding and challenging. Perhaps the rewards include witnessing the emergence of new facets of breast cancer care, new options for role development and the advancement of specialist breast care nurses as an influential professional group. However, challenges of implementing change are also ongoing and relate predominantly to role definition and significantly increased demands on individual post holders in all spheres of breast care.

Prior to exploring the diversity of advanced nursing roles within breast cancer care and appraising the contribution that they make, it is essential to appreciate the factors that have influenced their evolution and subsequent direction in recent years. Advances in breast disease management and increased medical technology generally have resulted in a corresponding increase in the expectations of users of healthcare. There is a noticeable and often politically driven trend towards acceptable minimum standards of care. Patient involvement and consumer rights are integral to this and the consequence has been enforced changes in the provision and organization of breast care services. Finally, the sociocultural positions of women in society generally are altering and a corresponding change in the professional status and ambitions of nurses as a professional group has ensued. These factors are discussed in turn below.

Breast cancer care is a rapid and evolving specialty and recent years have witnessed numerous changes in the approach to and outcome of many facets of this area of clinical care. For example, a greater understanding of cancer genetics has resulted in more women having prophylactic mastectomy with the intention of maximum risk reduction. Greater emphasis has also been focused on preventing breast cancer with the use of drugs such as tamoxifen and toremifene. The national screening programme is evolving to include more women and more detailed surveillance. Once diagnosed with breast cancer, patients face a greater array of treatment options than ever before. Chemotherapy and endocrine therapy have replaced surgery as the primary treatment in some clinical scenarios, sentinel node biopsies may serve as an alternative to axillary dissections, traditional chemotherapy regimens have been replaced by superior ones and new endocrine therapies appear every year. Novel therapies and discoveries, as discussed in earlier chapters, have represented completely new ways of approaching the detection and management of breast cancer and have extended survival even in people with widespread metastases. Amid all of the above, the incidence of breast cancer is increasing worldwide every year, although mortality rates are beginning to fall (Cancer Research UK, 2002), resulting in greater numbers of patients undergoing routine follow-up after their treatment is over. If one takes time to consider these immense changes in our clinical patterns and effectiveness, it is unsurprising and perhaps inevitable that these have, in turn, resulted in changes to nursing roles. In particular specialist nurses require new levels of knowledge and new skills if they are to organize and deliver optimum care to individuals affected by breast cancer.

Changes in provision of healthcare generally have had an irreversible effect on how the management of breast cancer is organized. People experience shorter stays in hospital after operations, often returning home with wound drains still in situ, and rapid access to services is to be the norm rather than the exception. Increasingly, in an attempt to mandate safe and effective care, the Government has imposed standards that relate to expeditious management of patients with breast cancer; for example a maximum two-week wait for a hospital appointment following urgent referral by the general practitioner and a maximum one-month wait from diagnosis to commencement of treatment (Department of Health, 2000). All such initiatives are monitored and enforced by the newly set up Commission for Health Improvement, which aims to improve the quality of patient care across England and Wales (Department of Health, 2002).

These global changes in the culture of the National Health Service with regard to implementation of minimum standards of care and assuring an acceptable quality of practice have also contributed to the evolution of specialist nursing roles. Clinical Governance is 'an umbrella term for everything that helps to maintain and improve high standards of patient care' (RCN, 2000). It serves as a framework and encompasses various components such as clinical audit, clinical effectiveness and quality assurance. The combined aim of these is to ensure quality of care is both demonstrable and

applicable to all healthcare providers from all disciplines. In accordance with
the principles of Clinical Governance, documents specifically related to
breast cancer care detail mandatory aspects of service delivery and, rather
encouragingly, these commonly make reference to the pivotal role of
specialist nurses, thus recognizing the integral contribution that experienced
nurses make in achieving quality of care for people with breast cancer. For
example, the British Association of Surgical Oncology (BASO) Breast Group
produces regularly updated guidelines for surgeons on the management of
breast disease (1998) that aim to represent targets for clinical excellence and
that are evidence based wherever possible. These guidelines encompass
primary care and diagnostic services, quality assurance and multidisciplinary
working, medical therapies, recurrent and metastatic disease, and workload
and training issues. They reiterate the consensus opinion that all patients
diagnosed with breast cancer should be offered the opportunity to access a
breast care nurse specialist throughout the disease trajectory. Similarly, the
Clinical Outcomes Group guidance on improving outcomes in breast cancer
(NHS Executive COG, 1996) details recommendations for improving the
process and consequence of numerous aspects of breast cancer care,
including diagnostics, treatment modalities and patient-centred care. Again,
the suggestion that nurses invaluably contribute to team working and inter-
professional communication is decisive.

Although all of the above initiatives may be undeniably virtuous, they
inevitably place pressure on resources for the provision of care and, as such,
have also been a motivating factor in changing nursing roles. It can be
supposed that political expediency imposed change on us. As individual
breast teams struggle to enforce Department of Health Standards, there has,
in turn, been greater emphasis on blurring professional boundaries with the
intention of devolving some aspects of medical care to professionals other
than doctors. However, as standards of healthcare improve, people in general
are both more informed and more vociferous about their rights to quality
healthcare. The document Your Guide to the NHS (Department of Health,
2001), which superseded The Patient's Charter (Department of Health, 1992)
declares its intention of providing a comprehensive and high-quality health
service, shaped around the needs and preferences of patients, their families
and carers. An increasing number of patient welfare groups, coupled with
more stringent complaints procedures, ensure there are penalties to getting it
wrong. Interestingly, in the United States breast care as a specialty (and
specifically delays in diagnosis) rates as second highest in the number of
litigation episodes it attracts (Physician Insurers Association of America,
1995). All this means that specialist nurses within breast cancer care, like
all other healthcare professionals, are increasingly held accountable not
just for their own professional practice but also for their contribution as a

professional group to the multidisciplinary approach to management of breast disease.

Another inescapable influence on nursing role development may be broadly attributed to changes in society generally. We now live in an age of greater technology, with higher standards of general education and widespread access to the Internet. The changing sociocultural position of women impacts on nursing as an essentially female-dominated professional group. Women are more educated and there are greater opportunities for combining a career with marriage and raising children. As women increasingly contribute to household income, nursing has had to respond with better opportunities for promotion and recognition of expertise in a bid to stop experienced nurses seeking enhanced job satisfaction and salaries outside the profession. It could be presumed that the development of autonomous nurse practitioner roles (to be discussed later in this chapter) might have arisen partly because nurses were no longer content with their traditional roles as handmaidens for doctors, but instead aspired to greater involvement in the organization and delivery of care. Indeed employers have little choice but to recognize this desire on the part of senior nurses for autonomous, advanced and better paid roles if they are to reverse the pattern of recruitment problems and poor retention of experienced staff that has been so prolific and so alarming in recent years.

Finally, another altogether reasonable facet of breast cancer care is our increased recognition that quality encompasses far more than just survival rates from the disease. Equally as crucial as mortality figures is the acknowledgement of the unique impact of breast cancer and its treatment and hence the importance of individualized care. Recent years have seen an upsurge in research studies which demonstrate the very real psychosocial, emotional and informational needs of people with breast cancer at all stages of their treatment and subsequent recovery (for example Irvine et al., 1991; Luker et al., 1995; Ferrell et al., 1997; Burstein and Winer, 2000; Maguire, 2000). This has had immense and extensive implications for nursing role development, not least because patients are exposed to whole new areas of care that are particularly geared towards their psychosocial needs and are highly relevant to specialist nursing input. Examples include multiple treatment options at diagnosis, selection of and preparation for breast reconstruction (immediate or delayed), management of treatment-induced menopausal symptoms, learning to live with the fear of recurrence, concerns regarding their children's risk of developing breast cancer and treatment-induced fertility issues. In summary, the necessity for psychosocial support for people with breast cancer (men and women) and the importance of having a specialist nurse to provide this is now widely accepted (Expert Advisory Group on Cancer, 1994; Richards et al., 1994; Jary and Franklin, 1996; McArdle et al., 1996).

All of the above have represented key driving forces for the evolution of specialist nursing roles both generally and in breast care. The next sections will examine specifically the development of clinical nurse specialist (CNS) and nurse practitioner (NP) roles and aim to critique both models in terms of their application to enhancing the care of people with breast cancer.

Clinical Nurse Specialists

In the United Kingdom (UK) between the 1940s and 1970s, it became increasingly noticeable that nurses with ambition moved towards education or management because of the lack of career opportunities and remuneration in clinical care. This led Clarke to advise that:

> The present structure in nursing in Britain demands that if a successful nurse wishes to advance beyond the grade of a ward sister ... she must devote all her energies to either administration or teaching and forget about contributing directly to patient care, i.e. clinical work. (Clarke, 1967, p. 331)

Subsequent endorsement of Clinical Nurse Specialist (CNS) roles (a title adopted by the Royal College of Nursing in 1975) served as an attempt to retain and promote the value of clinical experts within practice while also raising the profile of nursing as a whole. At the same time, changes in medical manpower and working hours (NHSME, 1991) resulted in the gradual process of nurses adopting more clinical responsibility. Thus the evolution of CNS roles aimed at keeping successful and ambitious nurses in clinical care while also improving standards of specialist nursing input. Ensuing employment opportunities increased in a widening variety of settings and CNSs have existed in numerous clinical areas (including breast cancer care) since the late 1970s, with their numbers proliferating throughout the 1980s and 1990s.

Initially application in the area of breast care was somewhat narrow in its focus, demonstrated by early references to post holders as merely 'mastectomy nurses'. However, the last 10 years or so have witnessed an explosion, both in the numbers of CNSs in breast care and in their profile as a professional group. In a survey of specialist and advanced practice conducted in England during the mid-1990s, breast care was found to be the sixth most common clinical area for CNSs out of 19 fields of practice cited (McGee et al., 1996). Broadly, traditional CNSs in breast care support people with benign breast disease, and those who are at high risk of or already have breast cancer and their carers. They provide information, monitor physical and psychological progress, provide emotional support and counselling, and give practical advice at all points in the disease trajectory about all aspects of the diagnosis, management and impact of breast cancer (Royal College of

Nursing, 1999), thus facilitating continuity and coordination (Armstrong et al., 2002).

Central to the development of CNS roles was the notion that they would encompass more than just clinical work and their multi-faceted nature has been repeatedly described in the literature, with core components including clinical practice expertise, education/teaching, management/consultation and research (RCN, 1988). However, while clinical nurse specialism in theory offers an ideal opportunity to combine clinical and academic expertise (Hamric, 1989), the emerging reality is that CNSs struggle to fulfil the role in its entirety (specifically the research elements) and the clinical role predominates over all others (McCreaddie, 2001; Armstrong, 2002).

Hence ongoing criticism of CNSs relates to the somewhat haphazard way in which they developed as a professional group, with development of posts perhaps more influenced by the capabilities of existing nursing staff, rather than as a result of following a consistent approach to the core components of the role. The amount of time assigned to each sub-role and the level of practice development achieved by post holders is vastly different (Armstrong, 2002), resulting from an apparent lack of standardization of role inception, responsibility, activity and performance (Bousfield, 1997).

Consequently, in breast cancer care, as in all nursing specialties, there has been increasing concern with regard to inequity and inconsistencies among post holders regarding the use of titles, the function and the preparation of specialist nurses (Ball, 1997; Read et al., 1999). In addition, substantial variations in the grades associated with such posts (from 'E' to 'I') have resulted in unjust remuneration for work undertaken (both over- and under-payment of post holders relative to experience and qualifications).

In recognition of this, the RCN Breast Care Nurses Forum declared that consensus and clarity are vital to ensure optimum standards of specialist nursing care for individuals with breast cancer. Thus they propose definitions of advanced nursing practice roles and minimum educational and practice requirements for those aspiring to them (RCN, 2002). Of course, some diversity in role function will always be apparent because of several influencing factors. The type of setting worked in will determine overall numbers of referrals and treatment modalities offered. For example, not all centres offer specialist services such as cancer genetics or breast reconstruction. Some CNSs will not be involved with chemotherapy or radiotherapy on site and some have no input into palliative care. Also there is diversity in nursing practice according to the availability and extent of the local multidisciplinary team. For example, some CNSs will be actively involved in lymphoedema management and prosthesis fitting, whereas others will benefit from the availability of physiotherapists, lymphoedema nurse specialists and appliance officers who undertake the majority of such tasks. Finally, different practice settings will require the CNS to have different levels of input regarding outpatients versus inpatients, private versus NHS patients and on-site versus home visits. A comprehensive list of clinical fields of practice associated with the traditional CNS role in breast cancer care is presented in Table 16.1.

Table 16.1: Fields of clinical practice associated with the role of traditional CNS in breast care

- Family history and genetics (includes prevention and prophylactic mastectomy)
- Benign breast disease
- National Health Service Breast Screening
- Patients newly diagnosed with breast cancer
- Patients undergoing chemotherapy (and related side effects)
- Patients undergoing radiotherapy (and related side effects)
- Patients on endocrine therapy (and related side effects)
- Breast surgery
- Breast reconstruction
- Prosthesis fitting
- Management of menopausal symptoms
- Management of lymphoedema
- Management of fungating wounds
- Treatment-induced fertility issues
- Metastatic disease
- Social issues and finance
- Recovery, rehabilitation and follow-up (including lifestyle changes)

Predictably, evolution of CNS roles has implications for inter- and intra-professional working. Generally speaking, CNSs have not attracted the same ferocity of inter-professional power struggles because they more closely represent traditional mainstream nursing rather than radical change and as such are potentially less threatening to doctors. However, CNSs have not completely escaped intra-professional resistance, largely because other nurses perceive that they commonly work in isolation (rather than being team players) and de-skill/devalue other nursing staff, leading to suspicion and hostility (Bigbee, 1996).

Nurse Practitioners

The UK in the 1970s and 1980s also witnessed an increasing number of Nurse Practitioner (NP) roles, which focused on expansion of nursing tasks, especially related to domains traditionally regarded as medical, and traditional nursing roles began to extend and expand. Earlier examples of expanded roles included administering intravenous drugs, cannulation and giving chemotherapy. Even today there is still no universally accepted defin-ition of an NP, although the RCN has detailed general principles (see Table 16.2) (RCN, 1997). Essentially, NPs should retain the capacity for advanced level practice, but whereas CNSs are more traditionally placed within a nursing model of care, NPs commonly undertake tasks more akin to those of medicine. Most NP models encompass assessment (seeing the patient and eliciting data); treatment (making decisions without a doctor); carrying one's own caseload and receiving direct referrals. Examples of extended role tasks more specific to breast cancer care are detailed in Table 16.3.

Table 16.2: What do Nurse Practitioners do? (RCN 1997)

- Make professionally autonomous decisions, for which they have sole, responsibility
- Receive patients with undifferentiated and undiagnosed problems. An assessment of healthcare needs is made based on highly developed nursing knowledge and skills, including specials skills not usually exercised by nurses (such as physical examination)
- Screen patients for disease risk factors and early signs of illness
- Develop with the patient a nursing care plan for health with an emphasis on preventive measures
- Provide counselling and health education
- Have the authority to admit or discharge patients from their caseload and refer to other healthcare providers as appropriate

Source: RCN (1997).

Table 16.3: Extended nursing role tasks in breast cancer care

- Family history screening and surveillance
- Accepting direct referrals (for example for breast pain)
- Diagnostics (palpation, fine-needle aspiration cytology, ultrasound)
- Admitting/discharging
- Seroma drainage
- Implant inflation/deflation
- Prescribing
- Nipple tattooing
- Follow-up consultations and examinations

NP roles have also attracted intra- and inter-professional opinion. The publication of the UKCC document *The Scope of Professional Practice* (1992) lent support to autonomous and flexible nursing practice by providing a framework for nurses wishing to undertake additional tasks, specifically those more traditionally performed by doctors, and allowing them responsibility for their own competence. However, it also fuelled tensions between those who recognized and welcomed opportunities for practice and professional development and those who were concerned about the medicalization of nursing and therefore the loss of its intrinsic value (Finlay, 2000). As NP roles become more visible, concerns have continued as to whether these roles maintain the essence of nursing and always incorporate nursing care within them or merely represent nurses as substitutes for doctors and result in fragmentation and devaluing of nursing (Edwards, 1995). The motives for adopting such roles have also been questioned, in terms of them representing legitimate areas for the advancement of nursing versus nurses being seen as the cheaper alternative. Hence the use of NPs might be regarded as a cost-saving exercise aimed at ameliorating service deficiencies (Edwards, 1995; Weston, 1975; Castledine, 1996).

The literature reveals supporters of both camps: those that recognize the potential for NPs to pioneer new aspects of nursing versus those that suspect anyone can be trained to perform mechanical tasks with a view to replacing the necessity for doctors to do them. This latter view is typified in the following quotation:

> The attempt to persuade professionally educated nurses that they should take on medical tasks and function at a lower level in the field of medicine represents an unbelievable human and intellectual waste. (Castledine, 1997, p. 265)

In contrast, supporters of NPs recognize that the potential weaknesses may lie not in the philosophy behind the role but in poor individual interpretation and execution. It would seem prudent for consummate implementation to involve post holders being aware that they need authority and competence in both the medical management of breast cancer and specialist nursing care issues. If one were to perform only the medical and perhaps mechanical tasks without integrating the substance and core of nursing care, there would be no difference between NPs and doctors and no apparent qualitative improvement in the service offered to women with breast cancer. In fact, evidence suggests that such differences do exist and that the skills of NPs enable them to add strength and diversity to nursing care (Lawson and Emmerson, 1995).

Elder and Bullough (1990) undertook a comparison of CNS and NP roles, which included questioning post holders about their role activities, the percentage of time spent on direct and indirect care, supervision and job satisfaction. They found that significant differences between the two groups emerged in only eight out of 25 activities specified. Predictably, NPs were more likely than CNS to conduct physical examinations, order laboratory tests, prescribe medication and treatments and make referrals as part of their everyday work role. CNSs, on the other hand, were more likely to teach staff and conduct support groups. However, both groups were involved in teaching patients and their families, counselling and psychosocial assessments. CNSs spent more time in indirect care than NPs and more commonly had nurses as their supervisors, whereas NPs had doctors. The authors concluded that the professional views of CNSs and NPs are strikingly similar and that there was little difference in many clinical areas commonly described as components of the CNS role, with large areas of overlapping functions.

A recently published meta-analysis reveals patients are more satisfied if NPs rather than doctors provide care. It seems NPs offer longer consultations, compile more complete records and are associated with offering more detailed and helpful advice to patients (Horrocks et al., 2002). Such themes have also been demonstrated in studies on NPs specifically in breast cancer care. NPs working in breast clinics commonly take histories, examine, request imaging, perform fine-needle aspiration cytology and give patients test results. This has been demonstrated to be safe, acceptable to patients and is associated with better satisfaction, less anxiety, more information provision, equal decision-making skills and a lower percentage of inadequate cytology specimens when compared with doctors in a breast clinic (Hammond et al., 1995; Garvican et al., 1998).

Indeed, my own experience of providing nurse-led follow-up after treatment for breast cancer substantiates the above, with greater satisfaction reported in women seen in the nurse-led clinic when compared with traditional medical follow-up. A randomized controlled trial comparing follow-up by the two professional groups revealed that key advantages of the nurse-led clinic include improved continuity and greater attention paid to emotional needs and answering questions, thus attending to the issues that women perceive to hinder rehabilitation and recovery. Although not always easy to articulate why, women noticed a shift of emphasis from the traditional medical model of physical examination of the breast, to a consultation that focused on the individual patient and the unique impact of breast cancer on their lives. According to the study, areas that specifically benefit from attention in the nurse-led clinic include management of menopausal symptoms, information regarding lifestyle changes and the opportunity to revisit prognosis and individual likelihood of disease recurrence (unpublished thesis).

A major difficulty with standardization of NP roles relates to training and qualifications. Unfortunately, education and courses for specific extended roles may not be available and certainly within breast care there is no nationally accredited course that prepares one for extended role activities such as breast examination. General programmes of study for NPs are beginning to emerge from diploma to master's level and largely include a greater focus on anatomy and physiology, comprehensive physical assessment, diagnostics, pharmacology, pathophysiology and disease management. Professional bodies suggest that recognized NP qualifications should be undertaken if extended role tasks are a major focus of the individual job description. However, it is arguable as to what extent possession of core physical assessment skills, such as percussion and auscultation, will be relevant to NPs in very specific clinical areas such as breast care.

Commonly, new nursing roles akin to those of medicine are often undertaken with informal training and without a record of competence or measurement of ongoing development. Learning 'on the job' does not automatically result in explicit documentation. This relates not only to initial training but, equally importantly, to maintenance of the skill through ongoing practice. Therefore, training and proficiency in extended role tasks must be clearly documented and such tasks should be practised continuously to maintain competence. It is essential that, if NPs are to be accountable for clinical decisions and making professionally autonomous decisions for which they have sole responsibility, there is documentation of practical experience and training in order to demonstrate competence to perform extended role tasks.

CNSs versus NPs

The term Advanced Nurse Practitioner (ANP) is now widely accepted as an umbrella title that encompasses within it the roles of both Clinical Nurse Specialists (CNS) and Nurse Practitioners (NP). The UKCC describes advanced nursing practice as follows:

> Advanced nursing practice is concerned with adjusting the boundaries for the development of future practice, pioneering and developing new roles responsive to changing needs and with advanced clinical practice, research and education to enrich professional practice as a whole. (UKCC, 1994, p. 1)

Experienced clinical nurses have probably embraced ANP roles in recent years because they have recognized their potential to increase professional status, pay and job satisfaction. Some people refer to CNS versus NP roles within breast cancer care, implying that the roles are in opposition to each other and that debate should focus on proving one is more legitimate than the other. In fact, the reality is not so straightforward and ANPs in breast care should not be considering one role versus the other, but enforcing minimum standards for both. Ball (1999) suggests that although the distinctions between the two roles may continue to be contested, perhaps a common core of knowledge, skills and sub-roles should be required of both, and as such any differences between the two will be based only on the focus of service they offer. NP posts may exist alongside CNS posts but must be subject to development of the same sub-roles (expert clinical practice, education, management and research) and orderly progression of level (from apprenticeship upwards) (RCN, 2002).

Overlap of both roles is already apparent within breast cancer care and considerable ambiguity regarding them remains, as it is sometimes difficult to clarify precisely the differences between CNSs and NPs within the specialty. This is not least because, as well as discrete NP post holders, many traditional CNS roles have developed to include NP functions (such as nurse-led follow-up) thus further blurring role boundaries and resulting in blended CNS and NP roles. A concern with a model that merges both roles relates to increased pressures that will inevitably accompany this, specifically in terms of time. With traditional posts already evolving to reflect breast cancer treatment advances, an obvious concern is that further expansion of duties to incorporate even some extended role activities may result in compromised standards of care or individual burnout of the post holder! As the traditional role is already largely validated, it seems counterproductive to sacrifice any aspects of this arguably invaluable contribution to service provision.

Instead it may be appropriate for post holders to consider the needs of their local area when planning implementation of advanced nursing practice posts. CNSs with a predominant focus on surgery rather than chemotherapy and radiotherapy, for example, may consider surgically related role extensions, such as seroma drainage, to be facilitative of legitimate improvements in patient care. Selection of CNS, NP and blended skill mix according to post holders, local service needs and delivery gives further support to the concept of both posts existing in harmony rather than in opposition. However, an important consideration of extended role practice, by a CNS or an NP, is whether it will result in a standard of service that is at the very least comparable (ideally superior) to the one that it replaces. The RCN (1999) suggest a checklist of relevant considerations to help direct individuals and teams considering advanced nursing practice roles in breast care (see Table 16.4).

In summary, clearly all ANP roles in breast cancer care must be subject to the same scrutiny in terms of role definition, a clear route for post holders in terms of qualifications and experience, transparent documentation of competence and appreciation of accountability and litigation issues. However, it is likely that generic contentions regarding both roles will continue, and both have their strengths and weaknesses.

Of course, another argument for not regarding CNS and NP roles as being in opposition to one another is that both may begin to be increasingly superseded by the recent introduction of Nurse Consultant posts. This new advanced nursing practice role was introduced because of ongoing perceived

Table 16.4: Checklist for extended roles in breast cancer care

- Is this new skill/role consistent with nursing practice?
- Is it consistent with my current job description?
- Does it fit current priorities – nursing and organizational?
- What changes will it entail?
- Will I need to stop some parts of my current role/care?
- Do I need accreditation?
- How will I get it?
- Do I need additional skills/training?
- How will I get them?
- How will I document them?
- Do I need a training period before I take on new responsibility?
- Do I have a mentor for this change?
- How will I evaluate my performance in this new role?
- Have I got clinical supervision?
- How will it improve patient care?

Source: Adapted from RCN (1999)

limitations with the existing clinical career structure in nursing, which had resulted in expert nurses leaving because of the lack of practice-based promotional posts and to improve their earnings. Sub-roles of Nurse Consultants are expert practice; professional leadership and consultancy; education, training and development; and practice and service development. They will possess skills and competences similar to those of CNSs but with greater breadth and complexity (NHS Executive, 1999). Contentions have arisen as to whether such posts should be less specific in their focus (existing, for example, in general oncology), or whether they may be suited to site-specific cancers such as breast cancer. At the time of writing only four Nurse Consultant posts in breast care specifically have been approved and only three of these appointed. Thus the success, impact and proliferation of such posts remain to be appraised in the future.

Concluding Thoughts

For me, the concerns with regard to ANP roles in breast care relate not to who exists (NPs, CNSs or Nurse Consultants), but to why and how. The why, of course, should have patient care at its core. Indeed, opportunities for improving patient care and developing the professional value of nursing should always remain a priority over politics and power struggles. Complementing rather than competing with existing medical or nursing models can only serve to enhance both patient care and all professional groups. Indeed, complementing is essential if we are to avoid the temptation of becoming all things to all people. The necessity to demonstrate explicitly the value of ANP roles to patients with breast cancer continues, and research into the impact of such roles on patient outcomes is critical but remains problematic and somewhat elusive. Extended roles integrating medical tasks are welcomed if they do not compromise nursing care. Finlay (2000) reminds us to open horizons rather than merely add to the burden of nursing.

The how relates to appropriate selection, training and implementation of ANP roles. CNS and NP roles (both separately and blended) are valuable and necessary in our increasingly complex healthcare systems (Hamric et al., 1996). There needs to be teamwork between individual professionals in the context of not just service delivery but also institutional cooperation and negotiation (regarding, for example, workforce planning, recruitment, training and quality assurance) (Read et al., 1999). Of course NP or extended CNS roles are not for everyone and any role changes must be voluntary and not coerced. No ANP roles should ever be implemented without lengthy consideration of the prerequisite issues common to all (see Table 16.5).

Table 16.5: Prerequisite issues common to all ANP roles in breast cancer care

- Time (to adequately conduct role)
- Training (formal and informal, by whom and level)
- Qualifications (and background)
- Litigation – an appreciation of the legal implications of extended roles. Inexperience is not considered a defence and ANPs are expected to conform to higher standards than a junior nurse (Eliott Pennells, 1998)
- Accountability – approval and sanction of employer
- Documentation (explicit and meaningful)
- Resources
- Evaluation (rigorous outcome measures)
- Sound motivation

It may be supposed that an essential difference between CNSs and NPs is the prolonged patient contact enjoyed by CNSs throughout the whole disease process. They may therefore offer improved continuity, the absence of which is a noticeable criticism aimed at the medical model of rotating junior doctors (Pennery and Mallett, 2000). An intriguing dilemma for me is to what extent NPs need a background in breast cancer care prior to undertaking the role. Some existing post holders fulfil the NP role with backgrounds such as practice nursing and theatre nursing and receive what is often comprehensive training in the extended role tasks. However, my experience from the nurse-led follow-up clinic is that patients may ask numerous questions about all aspects of their disease and management other than those relevant to that consultation or task. It is my extensive knowledge of breast cancer that allows me to address rather than defer such concerns. I am unable to say how my effectiveness would have been appraised without this knowledge. Perhaps this further supports the notion of a working model that blends the two roles, rather than pitting them against one another.

Of course, unresolved issues pertaining to ANP roles in breast care remain, not least regarding training, pay, accountability, legislation and nurse prescribing. Insisting on consistency in role titles might go some way to resolving the first two of these. Currently ANP roles in breast cancer have a misleading variety of titles (including breast care nurse, breast care sister, clinical nurse specialist, nurse practitioner, specialist nurse practitioner and breast nurse clinician), hold different grades and are qualified to differing levels. This lack of consistency renders them somewhat meaningless with regard to expectations of colleagues, managers and patients, and is undoubtedly an obstacle to instigation of new posts that have an appropriate clinical focus and job description offered at an equitable level of pay.

I would urge post holders to contribute to professional debate and ensure posts revolve around evidence-based discovery of the differences various healthcare professionals offer and identification of the best professional to enhance patient care at that time, rather than jumping on a fashionable bandwagon. Salvage and Smith (2000) wisely advise letting go of resentments and boundary disputes and instead directing efforts towards capitalizing on the wealth of skills that all professionals can bring to bear on solving health problems and improving services for patients. Finally, I would echo the sentiments of Marsden (1995) who suggests nurses must continue to be flexible and responsive to change if they are to retain control of ANP roles, thus ensuring that they are truly nurse-led, rather than arising from pressurized, hurried or badly thought-out implementation. Breast cancer care is a dynamic and exciting area in which to work and I hope that you will share my confidence that we can look forward to seeing nurses (in various roles) very much at the forefront of this care in the future.

References

Armstrong S, Tolson D, West B (2002) Role development in acute nursing in Scotland. Nursing Standard 16(17): 33–8.

Ball C (1997) Planning for the future: advanced nursing practice in intensive care. Intensive and Critical Care Nursing 13(1): 17–26.

Ball C (1999) Revealing higher levels of nursing practice. Intensive and Critical Care Nursing 15: 65–76.

Bigbee J (1996) History and evolution of advanced nursing practice. In Hamric A, Spross J, Hanson C (eds) Advanced Nursing Practice: An Integrative Approach. Philadelphia, PA: W.B. Saunders, p. 16.

Bousfield C (1997) A phenomenological investigation into the role of the Clinical Nurse Specialist. Journal of Advanced Nursing 25(2): 245-56.

British Association of Surgical Oncology (BASO) Breast Specialty Group (1998) Guidelines for Surgeons in the Management of Symptomatic Breast Disease in the United Kingdom. London: W.B. Saunders.

Burstein H, Winer E (2000) Primary care of survivors of breast cancer. New England Journal of Medicine 343(15): 1086-94.

Cancer Research UK (2002) About Cancer: Statistics - Incidence and Mortality [http://www.cancerresearchuk.org/].

Castledine G (1996) The role and criteria of an advanced nurse practitioner. British Journal of Nursing 5(5): 288-9.

Castledine G (1997) Framework for a clinical career structure in nursing. British Journal of Nursing 6(5): 264-71.

Clarke M (1967) A clinical role for senior nurses in social psychiatry. International Journal of Nursing Studies 4: 331-40.

Department of Health (1992) The Patient's Charter. London: HMSO.

Department of Health (2000) The National Health Service Cancer Plan. London: Stationery Office.

Department of Health (2001) Your Guide to the NHS. London: Stationery Office.

Department of Health (2002) About CHI. London: Stationery Office.

Edwards K (1995) What are nurses' views on expanding practice? Nursing Standard 9(41): 38-40.

Elder R, Bullough B (1990) Nurse practitioners and clinical nurse specialists: are the roles merging? Clinical Nurse Specialist 4(2): 78-84.

Elliott Pennells (1998) Specialist nurses. Professional Nurse 13(6): 382-3.

Expert Advisory Group on Cancer (1994) A Policy Framework for Commissioning Cancer Services. London: Department of Health.

Ferrell B, Grant M, Funk B, Otis-Green S, Garcia N (1997) Quality of life in breast cancer, Part 1: Physical and social well-being. Cancer Nursing 20(6): 398-408.

Finlay T (2000) The scope of professional practice: a literature review to determine the document's impact on nurses' role. Nursing Times Research 5(2): 115-25.

Garvican l, Grimsey E, Littlejohns P, Lowndes, S, Sacks N (1998) Satisfaction with clinical nurse specialists in a breast care clinic; questionnaire survey. British Medical Journal 316: 976-7.

Hammond C, Chase J, Hogbin B (1995) A unique service? Nursing Times 91(30): 28-9.

Hamric A (1989) History and overview of the CNS role. In Hamric A, Spross J (eds) The Clinical Nurse Specialist in Theory and Practice, 2nd edn. Philadelphia, PA: W.B. Saunders.

Hamric A, Spross J, Hanson C (1996) Preface. In Hamric A, Spross J, Hanson C (eds) Advanced Nursing Practice: An Integrative Approach. Philadelphia, PA: W.B. Saunders, p. x.

Horrocks S, Anderson E, Salisbury C (2002) Systematic review of whether nurse practitioners working in primary care can provide equivalent care to doctors. British Medical Journal 324: 819-23.

Irvine D, Brown, B, Crooks, Roberts J, Browne, G (1991) Psychosocial adjustment in women with breast cancer. Cancer 67: 1097-1117.

Jary J, Franklin L (1996) The role of the specialist nurse in breast cancer. Professional Nurse 11(10): 664-5.

Lawson P, Emmerson P (1995) Nurse practitioners: agents of change. Health Visitor 68(6): 244–5.

Luker K, Beaver K, Leinster S, Glynn Owens R, Degner L, Sloan J (1995) Information needs and sources of information for women with breast cancer. Journal of Advanced Nursing 23: 1–9.

Maguire P (2000) Psychological aspects. In Dixon J (ed), ABC of Breast Diseases, 2nd edn. London: BMJ Publishing Group.

Marsden J (1995) Setting up nurse practitioner roles: issues in practice. British Journal of Nursing 4(16): 948–52 .

McArdle J, George W, McArdle C, Smith D, Moodie A, Hughson A, Murray G (1996) Psychological support for patients undergoing breast cancer surgery: a randomised study. British Medical Journal 312: 813–16.

McCreaddie M (2001) The role of the clinical nurse specialist. Nursing Standard 16(10): 33–8.

McGee P, Castledine G, Brown R (1996) A Survey of Specialist and Advanced Nursing Practice in England. British Journal of Nursing 5(11): 682–6.

NHS Executive Clinical Outcomes Group (1996) Guidance for Purchasers: Improving Outcomes in Breast Cancer – The Manual. London: Stationery Office.

NHS Executive (1999) Health Service Circular: Nurses, Midwives and Health Visitor Consultants: Establishing Posts and Making Appointments. London: Department of Health.

NHSME (1991) Junior Doctors: The New Deal. London: National Health Service Management Executive.

Pennery E, Mallett J (2000) A preliminary study of patients' perceptions of routine follow-up consultations and examinations of patients after treatment for breast cancer. European Journal of Oncology Nursing 4(3): 138–45.

Physician Insurers Association of America (PIAA) (1995) Breast Cancer Study. Washington, DC: PIAA.

Read S, Lloyd Jones M, Collins K, McDonnell A, Jones R, Doyle L, Cameron A, Masterson A, Dowling S, Vaughan B, Furlong S, Scholes J, Levenson R (1999) Exploring New Roles in Practice: Implications of Developments within the Clinical Team (ENRIP Executive Summary). Sheffield: School of Health and Related Research (ScHARR), Sheffield University.

Richards M, Baum M, Dowsett M, Maguire P, McPherson K, Morgan D, Sainsbury R, Sloan J, Wilson R, Blamey R, Leake L (1994) Provision of Breast Services in the UK: The Advantages of Specialist Breast Units, Report of a Working Party of the British Breast Group. London: Guys Hospital.

Royal College of Nursing (1975) New Horizons in Clinical Nursing. London: RCN.

Royal College of Nursing (1988) A Report of the Working Party Investigating the Development of Specialties within the Nursing Profession. London: RCN.

Royal College of Nursing (1997) Nurse Practitioners: Your Questions Answered. London: RCN.

Royal College of Nursing (1999) Developing Roles: Nurses Working in Breast Care. London: RCN.

Royal College of Nursing (2000) Clinical Governance: How Nurses Get Involved. London: RCN.

Royal College of Nursing (2002) Advanced Nursing Practice in Breast Cancer Care, London: RCN Direct.

Salvage J, Smith R (2000) Editorial: Doctors and nurses: doing it differently. British Medical Journal 320: 1019–20.

United Kingdom Central Council for Nursing, Midwifery and Health Visiting (1992) The Scope of Professional Practice. London: UKCC.

United Kingdom Central Council for Nursing, Midwifery and Health Visiting (1994) The Future of Professional Practice – The Council's Standards for Education and Practice Following Registration. Position Statement on Policy and Implementation. London: UKCC.

Weston J (1975) Whither the 'nurse' in nurse practitioner? Nursing Outlook 23: 148–52.

Index

Printed in the United Kingdom
by Lightning Source UK Ltd.
133429UK00001B/127-132/A